# Erich Schiffmann
# on the Practice of Yoga

The purpose of yoga is to facilitate the profound inner relaxation that accompanies fearlessness. The release from fear is what finally precipitates the full flowering of love. In this state you will love what you see in others, and others will love you for having been seen. This is the softened perception of the world that yoga promotes.

Therefore, the apparently simple benefits that accrue from the regular practice of yoga can change your life in very profound ways. Do not underestimate the value of being balanced, centered, and coordinated, of being strong and light, of being more flexible, without pain, experiencing the subsequent feelings of invisibility or transparency, and of being more sensitive. . . .

Yoga will make you sensitive to the stillness, the presence, the hush, the peace of God. This deep inner stillness is at the core of your being. It is the ground, the joy of your being. The radiant peace you'll experience is what happens naturally when the creative energy of God is allowed to flow through you unobstructed.

# THE
# SPIRIT
# AND PRACTICE
# OF MOVING
# INTO
# STILLNESS

◆

## Erich Schiffmann

Photos by Trish O'Rielly

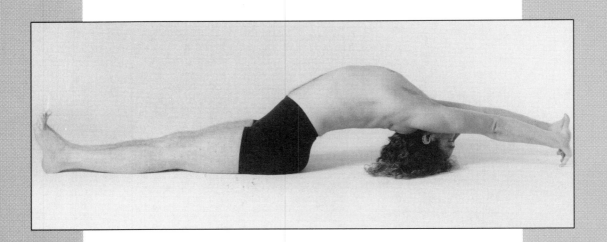

# YOGA

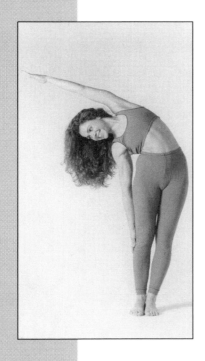

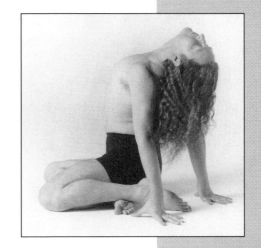

**POCKET BOOKS**

New York   London   Toronto   Sydney   Tokyo   Singapore

*To my mother*

The author of this book is not a physician and the ideas, procedures, and suggestions in this book are not intended as a substitute for the medical advice of a trained health professional. All matters regarding your health require medical supervision. Consult your physician before adopting the suggestions in this book, as well as about any condition that may require diagnosis or medical attention. The author and publisher disclaim any liability arising directly or indirectly from the use of this book.

An *Original* Publication of POCKET BOOKS

POCKET BOOKS, a division of Simon & Schuster, Inc.
1230 Avenue of the Americas, New York, NY 10020

Copyright © 1996 by Erich Schiffmann
Photos copyright © 1996 by Trish O'Rielly

Library of Congress Cataloging-in-Publication Data

Schiffmann, Erich.
  Yoga : the spirit and practice of moving into stillness / Erich
Schiffmann.
    p.   cm.
  ISBN: 0-671-53480-7 (pb)
  1. Yoga.   2. Aṣṭāṅga yoga.   I. Title.
B132.Y6S398
291.4'3—dc20                                        96-41662
                                                         CIP

First Pocket Books trade paperback printing December 1996

10   9   8   7

Cover design by Brigid Pearson
Text design by Stanley S. Drate/Folio Graphics Co. Inc.

Printed in the U.S.A.

# Acknowledgments

First, I'd like to thank Kathleen Miller for her preliminary editorial work when the book was in its formative years. I'd like to thank Tom Miller for his wonderful final editing. Love to Leslie, my wife, for her patience, encouragement, humor, insight, feedback, and support during my long hours of writing. Special thanks to Trish O'Rielly for her excellent photography and Dr. Jim Dreaver, my dharma-jousting partner.

I would also like to thank all my teachers. They've each inspired me in their own unique way. Jim Fowler at the Krishnamurti School, Brockwood Park, England (there's always something special about your first yoga teacher); Sri TKV Desikachar of Madras, India; Jean Bernard Rishi, Paris, France; Mary Stewart, London, England; Dona Holleman, Florence, Italy; Vanda Scaravelli, Fiesole, Italy; BKS Iyengar, Poona, India; Krishnamurti, India; and, most notably, Joel Kramer, Bolinas, California.

Prior to meeting Joel, even though I had been doing yoga for years, I had not yet learned how to do yoga—not really. I could perform most of the poses fairly well, but I hadn't yet discovered what it was all about. I was still looking to others to tell me what to do. Not surprisingly, and even though I loved it, I felt like I was doing someone else's yoga. It wasn't genuine yet. It wasn't mine. Joel taught me how to go within and run energy through my body. Within the first ten minutes of our first lesson, I was a changed man. From then on, yoga was mine.

I would also like to thank the many people whom I have been lucky enough to have in my experience, those that called themselves "students." I'm still learning from them. They give so much. They kept me going when times were tough.

Mostly, I want to thank my mother and father, my first gurus. They encouraged me to follow my calling, to honor my deepest feelings, and to help others as best I could. I felt loved by them, and I felt safe. That feeling of being safe and loved, though dim in my awareness a lot of the time, was always there deep within me giving me faith, hope, and courage in a world that can be very confusing. For that I thank them both with utmost, heartfelt gratitude. There is no greater gift than love. For me, they were the specific embodiment of God's Love.

I would also like to thank my older brother, Karl, for giving me my first yoga book on my tenth or twelfth birthday. "What a stupid present," I thought at the time. "Why did you waste my birthday present on that?" I found the book in one of my drawers a few years later.

Creation flows,
for life is the movement of Being.

Immerse yourself in stillness
and become consciously one with the flow.

Conscious union is yoga.

# Contents

## PART FOUR

# Introduction

People often ask me how I became interested in yoga and whether or not I was flexible when I first started. I usually say that I was reading Krishnamurti books in high school, and somewhere in one of them he said that if you really wanted to get your head together, if you wanted to achieve enlightenment, clarity, or peace of mind, otherwise known as Self-Realization, Awakening, or God-Realization—that is, if you wanted to understand what he was talking about—it helped if your body was as healthy and sensitive as possible, and he recommended yoga, meditation, and a vegetarian diet. I thought, "Well, if any of this actually helps, it's worth a try." And so I took up the practice. But it wasn't exactly like that. And, no, I was not flexible when I first started. I could not touch my toes, for example. But it came fast. I progressed quickly. I remember being able to balance on my head for a few seconds the first time I tried, but I was not able to cross my legs into the Lotus position.

My older brother, Karl, had earlier given me my first yoga book, *The Spirit and Practice of Yoga* by Michael Volin and Nancy Phelan, which I promptly put into a drawer and forgot about. I still have the book, by the way, and Karl now says he has no recollection of ever giving it to me. At some point, however—I must have been thirteen or fourteen—I remember finding the book and looking at the pictures. They had an exotic appeal. I remember liking the sheen of the man's skin, the look in his face, and thinking he appeared healthy—not in a get-fit way, especially, but in a mystical, holy, deeply healthy, appealing way. I started dabbling with the postures. I'm not sure why.

There were not very many poses in that book, maybe fifteen or twenty, but I tried them all. I especially remember attempting *Uttanasana*, the Standing Forward Fold, where you bend forward from you hips and touch your face to your legs. This wasn't possible by any means, initially, but after several weeks I bent over and was almost touching my face to my legs. I was really close. And so, I went for it. I pulled with my arms and stretched even harder, and I managed to touch my face to my knees for a brief moment. And I got such a rush! Energy sped through my whole body. It felt electric—almost scary, but not. It was actually intensely pleasurable, exhilarating. I was there just a moment, but when I stood up I was different. Something in me had changed. I realized I was tinkering with something powerful. I wasn't suddenly a zealous convert, nor did I become particularly disciplined about any of this yet, but in my mind I was beginning to think of myself as someone who was "into yoga."

About the same time I remember going into a health food store in Redondo Beach, the first time I had ever been in one (one of the few around, as I recall), and there on the counter was a book entitled *Metaphysical Meditations* by Paramahansa Yogananda. I liked his name, it had a certain roll to it, I liked the title of the book, it sounded mystical and intriguing, but I especially liked his photo on the front. He had long hair, which I liked, and like the other man, he looked holy. And though I remember being somewhat hesitant or embarrassed about buying the book, I went ahead and bought it anyway. I enjoyed the book, though I don't think I actually understood most of what it was about—maybe I did—but, mostly, I liked the way I felt when I was reading it. I joined the Self-Realization Fellowship soon after that, devoured all of Yogananda's books, especially *Autobiography of a Yogi*, and did their weekly lessons and practiced their exercises and meditations.

In my bedroom at the time I happened to have two small clothes closets, just big enough to stand up in. At Yogananda's suggestion, I put all my clothes into just one of the closets and made a meditation chamber out of the other. I put a small rug on the floor, a pillow to sit on, candles, incense, his books on a little stand, and pictures of the gurus, all five of them, on the wall. And I would go in there and meditate. I also put the guru pictures on the wall above my head near my bed. I think my father thought I was a nut. I also put Yogananda's picture on a bolo tie and wore it most of the time.

I must have been fourteen when all of this was happening because on my fifteenth birthday I took a bus to Encinitas to do a weekend silent spiritual retreat at the Self-Realization Fellowship on the cliff above the Pacific Ocean. I remember I wasn't yet old enough to drive. The resident monks gave a tour at one point. As we entered what used to be Yogananda's bedroom, one of them said, "You can still feel his vibration in here." And I could. I remember feeling pleasantly surprised. It had that magical, holy feeling. I don't remember much else about that weekend, except for the fragrance of peppermint tea and that I wasn't yet able to talk about what I was feeling with anyone.

I started reading all kinds of books about Eastern religion, yoga, spiritual biographies, and meditation. I remember reading *Siddhartha* by Hermann Hesse in English class. It was one of the few times in years that I was excited about school.

Soon after this my best friend, Bob Ackerman, gave me a book entitled *Think on These Things* by Krishnamurti, saying, "This is the best book I've ever read. You've gotta read it." And because Bob was recommending it, I gave it special attention. And I fell in love. I was totally wowed by what the man was saying. I dropped out of the Self-Realization Fellowship and read almost nothing but Krishnamurti for the next several years. All this time I was meditating, or at least trying to, reading, going for walks (that's what Krishnamurti did) and tinkering with the yoga poses, meanwhile thinking I would grow up and be a painter, an artist. Often, I'd simply climb a tree and sit in it for a long time. I actually built a tree house in a wooded area of the Palos Verdes golf course for this purpose.

I read Krishnamurti all through high school, and my intention was to attend art school in San Francisco. As it turned out, my parents either couldn't afford to send me to art school or they didn't think it was a good idea, so when I finished high school, instead of going to art school like I had hoped, I took the year off to work and save money for school tuition. During that winter I spent a month living in an apartment in downtown Los Angeles taking care of Blackie, our childhood baby-sitter who was more like my grandmother than anything else. She was a friend of my grandmother, probably a baby-sitter for my mother, too. I spent a month in downtown Los Angeles taking care of her after a cataract operation. In the evenings I would walk to the Bodhi Tree Bookstore and read, and it was there that I found a new book by Krishnamurti entitled *Brockwood Talks*. These were transcriptions of talks Krishnamurti had given at a school named Brockwood Park in England, a Krishnamurti high school, it turns out. After returning from the bookstore I would go to my room, sit in a straight-back chair, read a little more Krishnamurti, and then try to meditate.

It was during one of these meditation attempts that it dawned on me that I would really rather go to Brockwood the following year instead of art school. I figured I could attend Brockwood for a year, meet Krishnamurti, meet other people who were interested in Krishnamurti's teachings, learn yoga the way Krishnamurti did it, eat the way Krishnamurti did, learn everything about him I could, and then come back to California and go to art school. It seemed like a daring thing to do because I had never thought about going to a foreign country, I certainly couldn't afford it, and mostly, I assumed I would not be eligible because Brockwood was a high school and I had just finished high school.

I remember writing the school a very sincere letter and putting it into the mailbox with a silent prayer or desire that I be accepted at Brockwood as a student, even though I had already completed high school here in the States. I waited nervously for their reply and was ecstatic when they said yes. I told my friends I'd be going to school in England, a Krishnamurti school, but I was unable to explain why. I just knew I had to go. It was more like some primeval animal instinct or latent spiritual urge than anything else. I was on the scent of something.

That was a magical year for me. Krishnamurti was as enlightened a man as I had ever met. He epitomized everything good. He was an excellent speaker, he was serious, he was handsome, he was sensitive, courteous, mystical, shy in person, and powerful on stage. And besides being an accomplished hatha yogi (someone who practices physical yoga)—he practiced yoga three hours a day—he was also what's called a *jnani*, one who has attained Self-Realization through the so-called mental door. He affected me profoundly and permanently, and I value tremendously my time at Brockwood. I did not need to take exams that year because

I had already finished high school in California, so I was able to take classes without the pressure of examinations. What a luxury. Everyone should experience this at some point, the joy of learning without the background noise of knowing you are going to be tested on the material. My whole attitude toward school and learning changed that year. I took art, horticulture, biology, history, and yoga. Yoga classes were taught in the Krishnamacharya-Desikachar tradition, now known as Viniyoga, by a man named Jim Fowler. This meant, among other things, that all the classes were private. There was no such thing as a group yoga class. Since this was the case, I was only able to take one yoga class per week. This meant that if I wanted to do yoga, I'd have to do it on my own outside of class. So, right from the start, I attempted to establish my own daily practice. I was not successful at this, but I tried.

Jim was an excellent first teacher. He taught me the basics, and I felt inspired. He would always take your pulse before, during, and after class. The idea was your pulse should go down by the end of the practice. I kept track of my pulse like this when I practiced on my own, too. Mine rarely went down. He also drew little stick figures of what we had done together and put them in a notebook so I could practice outside of class. This is where I first learned to do yoga shorthand.

During that year I went to London on the weekends fairly frequently with others from Brockwood. Whenever possible I went to the British Museum to hang out in the Buddha statue section, staring at the Buddha statues, feeling their presence, marveling at the artists' skill, and really liking that mystical feeling. The feeling of holiness in those rooms had a special appeal to me. It felt clean, pure, without a lot of dogma or mental trickery. The Buddhas were meditating, and they were sitting in Lotus for the most part. And so that's what I wanted to do. I wanted to meditate, and I wanted to be able to meditate sitting in Lotus. I just wanted to do that. It didn't make a lot of sense.

Toward the end of the school year I asked Krishnamurti what he would do if he were me, in terms of learning yoga more seriously. He suggested I study with Desikachar in Madras, India. So I wrote Desikachar and asked him whether or not I could come to India to study with him. He said yes, and I made plans to live in Madras for a year. I went the following September and, for the most part, loved it tremendously. My first reaction when landing in Bombay, however, was repulsion. If I could have, I would have turned around and left immediately. The smells, the sounds, the noise, the people, the traffic, the smoke, the water, the pollution, every form of disease walking down the street . . . was all so strange. My first thought was, "I came *here* to learn yoga?" This place was filthy. I had always associated yoga with purity, cleanliness, Krishnamurti, the Buddha statue . . . and this is where it was born?

Desikachar had an interesting teaching style. All the classes were privates in those days, and I was seeing him three times a week. I'd come in, sit down, and we'd start talking. He'd ask me how I enjoyed living in India, how I liked the food, how was it living near the beach, and so on. He'd tell me about his kid, he'd ask me more questions . . . and in the back of my mind I was thinking, "Well, when are we going to start with the yoga? I mean, I did come halfway around the world to be here, and I'm only going to be here a limited time, and the minutes are going by, my hour is nearly up. . . ." But the conversation would continue like this until I actually asked him a yoga question and got him talking about yoga. Once I realized that this is how it worked, I came prepared—with hundreds of questions. And that's how the syllabus of our time together was organized. It was all based on my curiosity, my pulling it out of him. I liked that it was like this, though at first I thought it was strange, that he was not very giving. I was used to going to school, being crammed with information, and internally recoiling from the overwhelming onslaught of largely unwanted and seemingly irrelevant information. But this was fun. It made what I was learning absolutely relevant to me. We progressed at the rate my understanding was able to go and in the directions my interest led.

I lived in Madras for a year, at first in a small, upstairs apartment with a friend of mine from Brockwood and then on the grounds of the Theosophical Society. I had become a member of the Theosophical Society in London on someone's advice as soon as I knew I was going to India. I lived in a beautiful old bungalow near the beach for about $40 a month and did most of my own cooking. After about nine months a Canadian friend who was studying murdungam, an Indian drum, came down with hepatitis. He tried to heal himself naturopathically. It seemed to work because all his symptoms and yellow coloring disappeared. Soon thereafter, however, it came back with a vengeance. He became delirious, his speech became slurred, and he had difficulty walking as his failing liver began to poison his brain. He was in the hospital for a week or two before he finally died. I must have become infected from him. I didn't know what it was at first. I just thought I was tired (exhausted, actually) because it was so hot and humid in Madras that summer. It was one hundred and six degrees and ninety-nine percent humidity. Riding my bike to Desikachar's house became an ordeal. I barely made it across the Adyar bridge one day. The doctors thought it was malaria because I was getting high temperatures and vomiting on a weekly basis, both malaria symptoms. But they couldn't be sure, they said, unless they were able to test my blood during one of those onslaughts. When I finally turned yellow, we knew. Anyway, there I was at the hospital on my twenty-first birthday getting cortisone shots, watching my friend die, and thinking to myself, "That's me in two weeks."

The Indian government would not let me get on the airplane to leave the country because I was too sick, and I didn't write my parents about my illness until it was over because I did not want them to worry. I was ill for about two months. My bilirubin count was nearly fatal, they said. When I was well enough to travel, I boarded the plane for England. I was going to spend a week at Brockwood before returning to California. I still had art school in the back of my mind.

A friend from Brockwood picked me up at the airport. She was all excited. The current yoga teacher at Brockwood had just left. I could have a job teaching yoga at Brockwood if I wanted it! "Are you kidding?" I said. Wow. Of course. This, as it turns out, was one of those pivotal, unexplainable times when life opens a door and offers a new direction. I walked on through without hesitation. It seemed perfect. It was a better plan than I could ever have designed. "I'll do this for a year and then go to art school," I thought. I was still weak from the hepatitis so I did not start immediately. I stayed at the school, gained strength, and started teaching second semester.

I lived and taught at Brockwood for the next five years. I loved Brockwood immensely, but teaching yoga there was difficult for me some of the time because it was a high school. Teenagers, for the most part, are not yet serious about yoga, and yet there was an unspoken understanding that most, if not all, of the students should take yoga. It was assumed that anyone at Brockwood would *want* to do yoga. This was not enforced, by any means, but I'm sure Krishnamurti thought it was a good idea. So the students would sign up for yoga as one of their classes, just as I had, and they would come for yoga, for example, in between math and biology. Many of them did not take it very seriously, and I often found it frustrating. When I did finally leave Brockwood, I was thrilled to be teaching people who were coming to class of their own volition, giving it their all, and paying me besides. These five years were good for me, though. I got a lot of practice teaching. I was teaching Desikachar style, so that meant a lot of privates every week. I worked hard.

One day at the annual Krishnamurti Talks held every summer in Saanen, Switzerland, near Gstaad, an elderly woman in the Krishnamurti circle introduced me to the daughter of a friend of hers, who happened to be one of Iyengar's senior pupils and the senior Iyengar teacher in Europe. Her name was Dona Holleman, and she lived in Italy. I did yoga with her several times that week in her room at the hotel where she was staying and at a chateau in the hills above Gstaad. Dona was amazing. She opened up a whole new world and awareness for me of what it meant to do yoga. She was precise, articulate, fun. She could do the poses better than anyone, and she was an excellent teacher. She had a way of being able to explain the poses that made them seem magical. I subsequently visited her during Christmas, Easter, and summer breaks when Brockwood was on holiday. I learned a tremendous amount from her and I took lots of notes.

I was also fortunate enough to spend time with Dona's friend and mentor, Vanda Scaravelli, at her home in Fiesole, Italy, and in Rome, as well as when she visited Brockwood. Vanda was Krishnamurti's close personal friend and his hostess when he was in Switzerland. She had a uniquely beautiful teaching style that communicated the way yoga should feel on the inside. She lived yoga, it was obvious, and just to see and be with her was a joy.

My practice improved dramatically during this period, partly because Dona was such an inspiration, and partly because my attempts at establishing a daily practice were finally kicking in. I was practicing daily on my own for several hours at a time with intensity and enthusiasm, and even when I was just sitting around I found myself wanting to stretch. My body was like a new toy. I would try to put my legs behind my head while watching TV, for example. I was in Dona's circle for several years.

When Brockwood was not on holiday, and I was in England, I spent my weekends in London studying with one of Dona's students, Mary Stewart. Mary was also a godsend. I had very little money at this time, and she gave me free instruction and allowed me to assist her classes. I learned a tremendous amount about teaching this way. She even invited me to stay at her home. I ate with her family and slept in the guest room. She was very kind. I was almost too naive to appreciate just how generous she was.

During the summer of 1976, Iyengar was teaching in London, and because of my associations with Dona and Mary, I was able to attend his classes. All I remember is that the classes were packed, he had an enormous amount of energy, and that during Virabhadrasana I, the Warrior Pose, he came over and slugged me in the chin. Apparently, I was pulling my chin down too much. I never did that again when he was around. In spite of this, I was very impressed by this man. He was an extremely creative practitioner and teacher, and I wanted to study with him.

I went to Poona, India, during the summer of 1977 to study with the great Iyengar. I was apprehensive about going to India again because of my previous experience, but I vowed to be more careful this time, not to drink the water or buy any food off the streets. Someone was generous enough to pay my way. I was there with friends from England, Scotland, and Australia, and I had a blast. I'd arrive at the institute every morning at seven to watch Iyengar practice. I observed him closely and wrote down everything he did. He was extremely creative and extremely internal when he was practicing. You could tell he was thoroughly immersed in his experience. Class would begin as soon as he was finished and would last three hours. We'd then walk to town, eat, go to our room and take notes, then nap. I would then walk to the institute again to watch Iyengar do his afternoon practice, an hour of headstand and shoulderstand variations. This was followed by a pranayama (breathing) class, which was followed by the evening class. We'd then walk back to town, eat, return to the hotel, and write down everything we could remember, then sleep. It was a lovely summer.

One incident I remember most clearly from that summer occurred at the end of class one day. It had been a very intense, difficult class, and during Shavasana, the Relaxation Pose, I went particularly deep. I remember being very quiet, very centered, and yet very wide awake. Iyengar must have noticed this because he came over to me afterward and said, ''You see! It takes Krishnamurti twenty years to get your mind quiet. I can do it in one class." And he had a point. His methodology worked. It wasn't just physical, as is the common criticism of his teaching. Many people attempt to discredit him by saying his yoga is not spiritual. But here it was! Spiritual in the most practical, grounded, obvious way. And it was equally obvious from what he said to me that his intent all along was to impart the *experience* of yoga—not just put everyone through the paces, physically speaking. The whole point of all this physical, hard work—and it was very physical and very demanding—was to get into a deep meditative state. And, for me, it worked. I am extremely grateful to have learned this from him.

When I returned to Brockwood after being with Iyengar, Krishnamurti asked me to show him what I had learned. This was at a time when Iyengar was just beginning to use chairs as props for various yoga poses: backbends, forward bends, shoulderstand, etc. So I went to Krishnamurti's room and had him sit backward in the chair and do a backbend. He loved it. He had a little difficulty getting up out of the chair after the pose, which is not uncommon, and so I assisted him. He must have been in his early eighties at this time. Thereafter, every day for about a week, Krishnamurti would come up to me and enthusiastically say, "Isn't the chair a wonderful invention!" meaning he really liked using the chair for backbends and that he had been doing it daily. Soon after this he invited me up to his room again. He wanted to show me his pranayama practice. I think he said he was able to inhale for a minute or two and hold his breath for some equally incredible length of time.

The following Christmas I went home to visit my folks. One afternoon at the Bodhi Tree Bookstore I came across an article in the *Yoga Journal* entitled "Playing The Edge" by a man named Joel Kramer. I was totally wowed. Here was an article I could relate to. It was the perfect blend of Krishnamurti and yoga. I wrote Joel a letter as soon as I had returned to England asking if I could visit him the next time I was in the States. He wrote back saying, in effect, "Of course." But he also said he had a teaching engagement in England soon and that he was very interested in meeting Krishnamurti. Would it be possible, he wanted to know, for me to set up a meeting between them? "Sure," I said. "Easy. Come when K is here, and I'll introduce you." So he came to Brockwood a few months later, I introduced him to Krishnamurti at lunch, and they were able to talk.

Joel and I did yoga together in the early mornings and late afternoons. Joel was a wealth of information and experience. He taught me the fundamentals of how he did yoga, much as I am presenting them here in this book: how to breathe, how to stretch and run energy through your body in the poses, and how to "play your edge." It was a whole new way of doing yoga for me. It felt like the real thing, authentic, like the way the ancients probably practiced, and I was hooked immediately. This was a little awkward, I recall, because I was teaching yoga one way one day, and almost totally differently the next. But I had changed. I had been transformed. I was "ripe," as Joel put it.

It took me a while before I was able to describe what had happened, but as I look back, I can see that this is when yoga finally became mine. I finally "got" how to do yoga. It finally became clear. It's internal. It's a way of listening inwardly and of being guided from within. Therefore, put simply, the basic technique is to go within and listen and then do as the within is prompting you to do. I had learned from Joel how to learn from my own practice and thereby be my own best teacher, rather than always going to someone else for information, inspiration, or technique. Yoga was no longer just a discipline, no longer something I did "because it's good for me" or because it might help get my head together. It became an inspired, creative act—more meaningful and more fun!

Let me give you an example of what I am talking about. In Iyengar's classes, for example, he would say, "Move your little finger this way" or "Stretch the skin here"—and I would, and it always felt right. And then he'd say, "Move *this* skin" or "Rotate your arm in this direction"—and, again, I would, and it always felt right. But I had no idea where he was coming up with all this marvelous information, this detailed insight into how the poses worked. But when Joel taught me how to create a line of energy, suddenly all the intricacies that Iyengar had been talking about began happening by themselves. I would run energy down my arm, for example, and this skin would move this way, and that skin would move that way, and my little finger would move and my arm would rotate, just like Iyengar was saying. But instead of "me" doing it or being told what to do, it was coming from inside as a result of the energy flow. Suddenly I knew where Iyengar was coming up with all his information. He was being guided from within. I could now run energy through a line, feel what was happening, and then describe it to someone else as "Move here" or "Stretch that." But the "move here" and "stretch that" was clearly not the main event. These were the effects, the incidentals, the froth on the wave. The main event was the energy flow and going after the feeling of perfect flow. The main thing was getting in touch with the within. Once you get that, it's yours.

I left Brockwood several months after Joel's visit. This was part of going with the flow for me. Brockwood was beginning to feel stale, and I needed to move on.

Since that time I have fundamentally been my own teacher. This does not mean I do not learn from others. It means I learn from others when I am guided to do so, and that at all times I am in touch with the teacher within. What I especially enjoy, however, is the fact that every time I get down on the floor and do my yoga, it always feels new. It's not that I learned how to do yoga in the past and now I'm doing it. Each session is a learning event. It always feels as though I am in the midst of a personal yoga lesson designed especially for me. I have also been fortunate enough to have been invited to teach all over the world. For twenty years I have not needed to exert my will on my own behalf, and yet, inwardly anyway, I have lived like a king. Everything comes to me.

Most importantly, however, I've learned to relax and trust the movement of life. Life has demonstrated its trustworthiness. I've learned to willingly go with the flow and thereby enjoy life more fully. Whenever I am worried or fearful, I simply endeavor to relax and become fearless for a moment—if only long enough to take a leisurely breath or two, and either to close my eyes or gaze into the sky and temporarily forget about my problems, the way I did as a child. And then suddenly, or gradually, it doesn't matter, whatever was worrying me pales in comparison to the actual, ever-present, benevolent immensity of life that is right there, here, staring me in the face; and I come back to a more accurate perception of life, of the dynamics of the situation that was troubling me, and of what to do to resolve it. And this is yoga! Yoga is not merely touching your toes, or standing on your head, or folding yourself into a lotus pretzel. It's about how you do what you do, and how you live your daily life on a moment-to-moment basis.

My guess is that if you also will learn to meditate and do yoga and pause occasionally throughout the day to be still, to breathe, to relax, and to feel the energy or life force within you and all around you—the life force that *must* be in you for you even to exist—that you, too, will feel the palpable joy of "union with the Infinite"—*yoga*. The word *yoga* means yoke, or union. And you will feel healed, renewed, strong in mind and body, and your life will take on new meaning and new, fulfilling directions that you are not personally responsible for. It's worth the small effort required.

This book is a how-to instructional manual. It deals specifically with how to practice yoga, how to meditate, and the art of listening inwardly for guidance. It is a how-to book surrounded with philosophy that, hopefully, makes the how-to more relevant. It contains that which I have learned over the years.

I thoroughly enjoyed writing this book. It took a long time, over ten years, but I loved every single difficult, simple, frustrating, flowing moment of it. It was a tremendous learning experience for me. I thought I knew what I was going to write when I began. But the more I wrote, the more I learned. And the more I learned, the more I changed my mind, until, finally, clarity emerged. Foremost of these learnings was the realization that Knowing happens, that spontaneous intuitive revelation flows into your mind, when you pay attention inwardly, are receptive, and listen. The theme or technique of yoga, therefore, and indeed the theme of this book, is to move into stillness in order to be guided from within, and then to be brave enough, and willing, to do as the within is prompting you to do—even when you cannot explain your behavior to yourself or others. In this way you will be an inspired, inspiring, and meaningful presence. I hope you enjoy the book.

Erich Schiffmann
Pacific Palisades, California

# PART

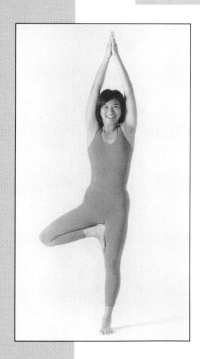

## ONE

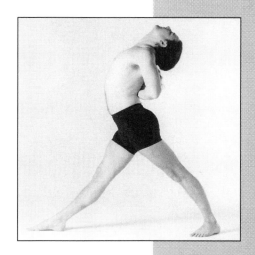

# 1

## STILLNESS

## The Peace Within You

Imagine a spinning top. Stillness is like a perfectly centered top, spinning so fast it appears motionless. It appears this way not because it isn't moving, but because it's spinning at full speed.

Stillness is not the absence or negation of energy, life, or movement. Stillness is dynamic. It is unconflicted movement, life in harmony with itself, skill in action. It can be experienced whenever there is total, uninhibited, unconflicted participation in the moment you are in—when you are wholeheartedly present with whatever you are doing.

For most of us, however, most of the time, our lives do not resemble a perfectly centered top, spinning so fast it appears motionless. Our lives are more like a top in a somewhat wild, erratic, and chaotic spin. We know we're alive because at least we're still spinning, but we are not quite perfectly centered, and we are not spinning anywhere near full speed. We don't have as much energy as we'd like, we are not experiencing as much aliveness as we might, nor are we experiencing the peace of stillness or the joy of being.

Stillness, therefore, is a higher energy state than what we're used to. This is because we are rarely wholehearted, or unconflicted, about anything. When you are not wholehearted, when you'd rather be someplace other than where you are, parts of you shut down and begin not to participate. Your energy circulation becomes constricted, and the creative life force is unable to flow through you unimpeded. Your energy flow, the amount of life force flowing through you, begins to diminish. The source of the energy does not diminish, but the amount that flows through you does. This leads to ill health, low energy, lowered vitality, lack of enthusiasm, depression, frustration, unhappiness, and suffering. None of this feels good.

When you *are* wholehearted about something, however, when you are where you want to be and are participating fully in the moment you are in—sometimes enthusiastic, sometimes mellow—you will experience a new sense of aliveness. You will experience a surge of energy, renewed vigor. This is not because there is

3

actually an increase in energy, but because you are not constricting it quite so much. There is now a better energy flow. There is less conflict, less friction, less not wanting to be where you are, and therefore—for you—there will be the *experience* of more energy.

This occurs whenever you are not attempting to spin clockwise and counter-clockwise simultaneously. Spinning in opposite directions happens when you act on opposing desires, when you are conflicted about what you are doing, not wholehearted—granted, this is most of the time. Stillness happens when you relax inside and are in harmony with yourself.

This is the point: When you experience *yourself* in stillness—that is, when you give your undivided attention to experiencing the truth about *you*—you will experience the conflict-free, calm, dynamic peace of perfectly centered abundant life energy. This exquisite peace deep within you is actually the experience of God, or the harmony of oneness felt within you as you. It's how God is experiencing Himself–Herself now and always. It is the phenomenological feeling-tone of Being, or Existence, and it is the truest thing about who you are. When you experience the peace within you, you will spontaneously undergo a fundamental transformation in the way you think about yourself and how you see the world. Nothing will seem quite the same ever again.

# Yoga

Yoga is a way of moving into stillness in order to experience the truth of who you are. It is also a way of learning to be centered in action so that you always have the clearest perspective on what's happening and are therefore able to respond most appropriately. Yoga is not the only way of doing this, of course, but it is an excellent way. It is an ancient process designed to help you uncover and discover your true nature so you can live daily life with that new awareness.

As you move into the depths of stillness, subtle and powerful changes will become apparent in your life. These will be both profound and entirely welcome. You will become familiar with the creative God Force inside you, the energy at your core. The world will look more beautiful because you're seeing it as it is, without the distorting influence of your conditioning. You will feel different, happy for no apparent reason. It will seem as though you have undergone an important change, a rebirth, as though you've become a new person, and yet you will feel more yourself than ever before.

Moving into stillness in order to experience your true nature is the primary theme of yoga simply because everything about you—every thought, feeling, and emotion, as well as every aspect of your behavior—is predicated on the way you feel about yourself. The way you feel about yourself determines how you think, what you do, and how you interact with the world. It's the basic factor that governs the quality of your life, the degree to which you are interested in living, and the way in which you interpret what's happening.

When your evaluation of self changes, when you feel differently about yourself, everything about you changes: your thoughts, feelings, emotions—every aspect of your behavior. The way you interpret and respond to the events in your life will also change. You will perceive the specific circumstances of your daily life differently because you'll have a new awareness and vantage point. You'll have less fear, fewer worries, more enthusiasm for life, and you will spontaneously become more effective in all you choose to do.

Accordingly, the way you interpret and respond to what happened in your past will also change. You'll look back and say, "Oh, so that's what was really going on!" And now, because you are seeing the situation differently, with a clearer and more mature understanding, you will find yourself able and willing to release old hurts, attitudes, and response patterns that were founded on your earlier limited understanding and that are now no longer appropriate. It feels good to let go of the past and be new in the now.

The way you anticipate and imagine your future will also change. The greater your understanding, the more grand your vision. Your imagination will no longer be distorted by the fears and imagined needs of the ego, but will be grounded in Reality. The future will look bright. You will spontaneously become optimistic about the future well-being of yourself and humanity and everything associated with the earth, sky, and universe: Creation. Therefore, everything about you and your world will change relative to your change in self-image: present, past, and future.

Here is our situation: We are ignorant of our true nature, our real identity. We don't know who we really are. This is because we have never experienced ourselves directly. We have never stayed "home" long enough to experience the truth about ourselves. We were not encouraged to do this. Instead we accepted as true what other people told us about ourselves. And, unfortunately, we were taught by people who, in all likelihood, and through no fault of their own, did not actually know.

For example, when you were a child and your mother praised you for being "good," you defined yourself as "good." You began to think of yourself as a "good" person. When your father scolded you for being "bad," you defined yourself as "bad," and you began to think of yourself as "good" and "bad" at the same time. Other people said other things about you, everyone seemed to have informed opinions, and since you didn't know—you were just a child—you believed them all. There was no reason not to. They seemed to know.

Before too long, and not surprisingly, it became very confusing because we were defining ourselves and forming our self-images based on other people's contradictory evaluations of who we are. From very early on, a fundamental conflict was introduced into our psyches revolving around this basic and most important issue: Who am I, really? And because we were not encouraged to find out for ourselves, we believed what other people told us. The result is that we feel guilty, ashamed, embarrassed, and confused about who we are. We feel judged.

If you feel guilty, ashamed, embarrassed, or confused about who you are, if you feel judged, you will invariably have difficulty giving and receiving love. It will not feel natural to you to express love easily. And when you are not giving or receiving love, when the energy of love is not circulating or passing through you easily, you gradually become bitter, you lose your natural sweetness. You unknowingly restrict your primary source of nourishment and therefore become hungry on all levels. You become unhappy or ill. You become unpleasant company. You forget how to love, and you forget how it feels to be loved. And all of this happens, to whatever extent, because guilt makes you feel that you are not worthy of love, that you do not deserve it, that you have none to give, and that in fact you are unlovable.

To some degree, this is the conclusion many of us have unconsciously taken on without further scrutiny. We take it for granted. We believe it's true. We think our guilt is justified and that punishment is our just reward. Our basic belief is, "I deserved the suffering I experienced in my past, and I deserve the suffering I am experiencing now. And the future probably holds a fair bit of suffering and hardship for me also. And then I'll die—and who knows what that's like? It's probably pretty horrible, too. I mean, life's not easy. Let's be realistic here. . . ." And yet, all of this rigamarole is due to a fundamental misperception of Reality. All the guilt, unworthiness, justified suffering, self-hate, unhappiness, and un-lovableness, as well as the subsequent inability to give or receive love easily, have come into being because of an inaccurate and incomplete perception of who we really are.

When you experience the truth of who you are, you will not feel guilty, ashamed, embarrassed, or confused. You will experience instead the tremendous relief of clarity—relief because you are not the unworthy, undeserving person you thought you were and because the internal pressure caused by these fundamental misperceptions is finally being released. When this happens, you will experience a healing sense of relief followed by a profoundly soothing inner peace, an even "at-easeness"—a stillness.

# Levels of Stillness

There are two levels of stillness. The first level involves learning to relax, become centered, and meditate. The technique involves sitting or lying down and being absolutely still—without reading a book, talking, watching the television, or listening to the radio. It involves deliberately pausing, stopping all physical movement, becoming relaxed, calm, and quiet inside, and just being—consciously being conscious. It's about being centered and still in the moment you are presently in.

For a few minutes, every form of external activity stops. Then, in that physical quietness, you turn your attention inward and focus on yourself. Focus on what it feels like to be you. Experience you. Immerse your conscious awareness in your own unique feeling-tone, the feeling-tone of the Universe expressing Itself as you. Do this deliberately in order to consciously experience the truth of who you are.

*LEVEL ONE* ◆ The first level of stillness is about being with yourself in order to know yourself. This is accomplished by being wide awake and aware as you deliberately relax into yourself. The idea is to consciously enter into a state wherein you temporarily suspend everything you think you know about who you are, including anything you have ever been taught, and simply be attentive to what's going on right there where you are. You practice being quiet, both physically and mentally, as you pay attention to the sensations in your body, the various thoughts in your mind, and your current experience of being conscious and alive. You practice simple body-mind awareness, being conscious of the moment you are now in, and thereby experience with clarity the energy of you. You consciously experience yourself as you actually are. In this way you open yourself to a new, truer, less distorted experience of you and the world.

When you are able to relax and quietly suspend all your firmly held false ideas and limiting beliefs about who and what you are, only what is true will remain. You will then experience your ever-existing truth for yourself. This is like polishing a mirror—removing the grime—and seeing yourself clearly for the very first time. And though this is not as easy as it sounds, it is also not particularly difficult.

Let me clarify something first, however. In order to let go of the false beliefs you have about who and what you are, it is not necessary to know which beliefs are true and which are false. In fact, you probably don't know, and this is the problem. If you knew, you would not be uncertain about your true identity. If you knew, you would not be experiencing conflict and inner turmoil; you would be experiencing peace. Therefore, let go of them all! Let go of everything you think you know about who you are, and see what's left.

When you let go of everything you think you know about yourself and stay with what's left, when you willingly abandon the contradictory evaluations of who you are and courageously reach deeply into yourself in order to experience yourself directly, you will come upon a new experience of who you are. You will sense the creative energy that is the life of you, and you will then define and think about yourself in a new and expanded way. And since the way you think about and define yourself is central to your perception, behavior, and experience of the world, your world will spontaneously change as your self-concept changes and comes into closer alignment with what's really true.

***LEVEL TWO*** ◈ The second level of stillness involves living your daily life with this new and growing inner certainty of who you really are: in other words, meditation in action.

This is not always easy, and it takes a little getting used to, for it means staying in touch with the deepest truth about yourself in the midst of daily life. This involves continually letting go of the judgments, evaluations, and contradictory opinions about yourself that arise in your mind throughout the day and in your relationships with other people. You do this by staying centered in your peace. You thereby learn to be suspicious of any suggestion—from yourself or others—that speaks of your guilt, your unworthiness, or your unlovableness. You learn it is appropriate to disregard any remaining inner self-criticism because in Level One you experienced yourself in a new way: as fundamentally lovable, innocent of all blame, and therefore deserving of every good thing.

Having experienced the truth about yourself in Level One, albeit momentarily, you had an insight—a glimmer of clarity, a moment of experience—about an inner truth *that you can't quite ignore.* You experienced yourself in a new way and now know your deepest truth, even though you may not yet fully believe it. Part of you knows the truth, but you're not totally convinced, and understandably so. Besides, when you are surrounded by others who are instead convinced of other things, it is doubly difficult to overcome your doubts.

This is similar to what it must have been like for Copernicus when he first suspected that the world was round. He had an insight into the way things are, yet part of him probably still believed the flat-world theory. And because he was surrounded by other flat-world theorists, and because he couldn't yet prove the world was round, it would have been difficult for him to be fully convinced or convincing to others.

The way to experience the truth of who you are (Level One) is by letting go of all your learned preconceptions about yourself and then staying present and open-minded for the experience. The way to stay in touch with your truth (Level Two), and confirm it to yourself over and over until there is absolutely no doubt, is by continuing to do what you did in Level One, but doing it now moment by moment during the day. This means, essentially, letting go of pretense and self-critical judgment and allowing self-acceptance—letting yourself *be* who you truly are. Again, you do this by staying centered in your peace, for only when you are at peace will you have the clearest perspective. By staying centered in your peace in the midst of daily life, you will validate your new perception of yourself and gradually become fully convinced. As a consequence, you will then be convincing to others.

# How to Start

Let's look at two excellent techniques for developing stillness and peace of mind. Both of these use your breathing as the primary focal point and both involve learning how to sit absolutely still. Sitting absolutely still—practicing conscious physical immobility—can teach you how to be in the conflict-free, higher-energy, "stillness" state for more of your daily life. You can learn what it feels like to have all your energy perfectly aligned and in harmony, like the spinning top. You can learn to participate fully in your experience of the now and still be relaxed. You can learn to be perfectly centered. And, of course, the more familiar you are with the feeling and experience of being centered, the easier it will be to stay that way. And since moving away from your center has been the source of all your suffering, the sooner you notice yourself going off, the better.

The importance of Level One (meditation) as an aid to the stable attainment of Level Two (meditation in action) cannot be overemphasized. The more familiar you are with the feeling-tone of your own centered being when you are "home" and alone, the more obvious it will be when you move away from it, and the easier it will be to find your way back to center in the midst of a busy life.

## Counting Backward

In this exercise you will be counting backward from fifty to zero, synchronizing the counting with your breathing. You'll count the even numbers as you exhale and the odd numbers as you inhale.

Sit with your back straight and your eyes closed. If you can sit comfortably on the floor, do so. Otherwise, use a chair. Be comfortable.

Begin by breathing in gently, fully. As you exhale, mentally say "fifty." As you breathe in again, mentally say "forty-nine," exhale "forty-eight," inhale "forty-seven," exhale "forty-six" . . . and so on.

Count backward on both the in-breath and the out-breath until you reach "twenty," then count only on exhales. Silently count "twenty" as you exhale. Then, instead of counting "nineteen" on the in-breath, do nothing, just inhale. With the next exhalation count "nineteen" . . . and so on until you reach zero.

When you reach zero, stop counting, but stay aware of the natural flow of breath in exactly the same way as when you were counting. Watch the breath as though you were going to count, but don't count. As you do this, practice sitting absolutely still. But don't *hold* yourself still. Simply be so relaxed that no movement occurs.

Be very aware of how you feel as you do this—how peaceful, energized, calm. Notice how pleasantly alert you are, how serene, fearless, at ease. Familiarize yourself with this feeling, with the feeling-tone of being centered and at peace, and rest here another two or three minutes. Absorb the stillness. Then prepare yourself, open your eyes, and return. This will take six or seven minutes.

As you do this exercise, breathe normally. Do not do deep breathing or control the breath in any way. This is important. You are learning not to be in control. You are learning to get out of the way. Therefore, rather than controlling the breath, allow it to flow freely in and out at its own natural pace. Yet, stay aware of the breath. Keep track of the numbers. As the breath comes in, count. As the breath goes out, count. And when you reach zero, stay aware of the breath nonverbally. There should be no strain in your breathing as you do this. Keep it soft and easy.

As you count backward, you may be more aware than usual of your mind darting rapidly from one object of attention to another. You may be unusually aware of sounds, physical sensations, or thoughts. You may lose count altogether. None of this matters. All of these things are evidence that the technique is working. You're becoming more aware.

The value of this technique lies in its ability to help you notice where your attention is from moment to moment, what's in your mind, and the contents of your consciousness. The counting is not only a centering device and a way of developing concentration, of training your mind to focus, it also acts as a backdrop on which your thoughts become very apparent.

For now, however, do not do anything with the various thoughts or sensations that arise. Simply be aware of them and continue counting. Gradually become more aware, more quiet within yourself, and increasingly dynamically still. As you immerse yourself in your stillness—and this is something that improves with each attempt—you will experience an unexpected and immensely satisfying sense of contentment and ease. Feel the peace.

## Mindfulness of Breathing

Sit on the floor with your back straight and eyes closed. If you are unable to sit on the floor, use a chair. Be comfortable.

Begin with a somewhat deep and gentle inhalation. Hold the air for a moment, then release it slowly in a long, thin exhalation. Do this three times. Then, focus your awareness in your body and *feel yourself breathing*.

As attentively as you can, note the changing sensations throughout your body that accompany each breath. Tune in to the subtle differences in sensation between the inhalation and exhalation. What does it feel like to inhale? What does it feel like to exhale? How do you know which is happening? And where in your body do you actually feel the breathing taking place? The most obvious sensations will be in your abdomen, chest, or nostrils, but you can feel the movement of breath elsewhere, too. In fact, there may be nowhere in your body that you cannot feel it. Experience what's happening.

Make no attempt to regulate or control your breathing as you do this. Again, practice letting go of control. Allow the breath to flow in and out on its own without your intervention. Some breaths will be deep, some will be shallow. Every breath will be different. All you need to do is be aware. You will experience the unbroken flow of breath when your mind is in an unbroken state, your attention continuous and one-pointed. That is the quality we want to cultivate, undivided attention to the instant of conscious experience you happen to be in.

Sit motionless, experience your whole body breathing, and then ride the breath into the sensation of yourself. *Feel* you. Experience the feeling-tone of the vibrating energy in your body, the overall sensation of "you." Practice becoming still and familiarize yourself with the actual feeling of stillness and peace.

If you find it difficult to concentrate on the subtle sensations that accompany breathing, say "in" to yourself as you breathe in and "out" as you breathe out. When your attention strays, notice this and then return it to the constantly changing sensations throughout your breathing body.

Be thoroughly relaxed as you practice this technique. Sit tall and be absolutely still. Give yourself your own undivided attention, ride the breath into the feeling-tone of you, and concentrate on that feeling. Immerse yourself in it. Feel you. Do this for five or ten minutes. Do it for a few moments whenever you can. Do it now, if possible. This will prepare you for the next chapter.

## Coming Back to Center

Motionless sitting is probably the easiest way of learning to be centered. Being centered, however, does not require that you be physically motionless. You learn to be centered, and you become increasingly familiar with the energetic feeling-tone of stillness through the practice of motionless sitting, and you immerse yourself in it as fully as you can when you can, but you then carry that feeling-tone with you into the motion of your life.

For as many moments of the day as you can, come back to center. Relax into where you are, breathe, and consciously be present in the now. Do this as you are driving, working, in the midst of a conversation—anything, everything—all day long.

And think of it like this: The feeling of stillness is peace, and the feeling of peace is joy. Therefore, come back to center and feel the joy. Do this frequently throughout the day. Come back to center as many moments of the day as you can, and let the joy you feel permeate everything you do.

# 2

## THE CORE OF GOODNESS

This is the most important theme in this book. It is also one of the most heartening ideas you might ever hope to be true. Because it is so important, let's go slowly.

As you sit quietly and immerse yourself in the peace and stillness of your own centered being, you will gradually begin to experience yourself in an undistorted manner. You will sink below or rise above your usual sense of self and instead come upon the undistorted, clear, conscious experience of Being—your Being. You will experience yourself as the specific conscious expression of an infinitely expressive Consciousness, Mind, Presence, or God. You will thereby intuitively know that you are more than physical and human, that your spiritual existence is guaranteed, immortal, eternal, and true, and that your Original Nature is absolutely good. You'll know that you are creative energy, Spirit, a unique expression of God's infinite Self-Expression, and that at your core is Goodness. This is what you'll experience because, in some mysterious and uncompromising way, this *is* what we are. We are all made of God Substance, Consciousness, Love.

As you sit in stillness, experiencing the energetic feeling-tone of "you" (Level One), you will invariably begin to feel exquisite inside. You will begin to feel at ease, deeply relaxed, natural, perhaps for the first time in a long time. And as you relax, and as you feel the energy you are made of, you will begin to feel loved. You'll find yourself feeling this way, inevitably, eventually, as you relax inside and allow yourself to become increasingly in touch with the loving goodness that is already in you—and it **is** already in you because that is how you were built. Love is the all-constituting substance of Being. It's what you are made of. And you did not create yourself.

When you sit quietly and let go of every false self-definition, of everything you think you know about who you are, and then **be** what's left, what remains is the untarnished presence of who you've always been and still really are. This untarnished presence manifests—shines—as pure, clear awareness and unconditional love. When you experience your essence, you will feel this natural lovingness within yourself *without having to do anything!*

13

When you feel the loving goodness inside yourself *as* yourself—as who or what you really are—you will acquire new self-appreciation. You will realize there is no basis for being self-critical or self-condemnatory, or for harboring guilt for some known or unknown transgression in the past, and that you have done this until now simply because you have accepted as true certain erroneous ideas about yourself. It's obvious to you now that when you wipe the slate clean and take a look at yourself for yourself, when you experience yourself as you actually are, you encounter a very different you from the ''you'' you thought you were. It now makes sense to disbelieve what was never true and embrace the new self-appraisal. You are You; God's specific Self-Expression.

You will then no longer think of yourself in self-deprecatory terms, and you will, as a natural consequence, loosen and release every remaining tendril of self-condemnation and self-hate. It will be reasonable to do this, though not always easy. It will no longer feel sane, however, or true or realistic, to be self-critical. And since your behavior has always been a by-product of the way you feel about yourself, you'll notice in yourself an effortless behavioral change occurring in response to this new self-evaluation. You will become more loving, more understanding, and more truly compassionate, naturally. This is a vital stage of personal maturation and is of utmost social value.

Difficulty arises, however, because we are afraid to let go of what we think we know and be what's left. We're reluctant to ease up on the tight sense of control we exercise over ourselves because life is hard enough as it is. We don't want it any harder. ''If I stop controlling myself to be one way rather than another, who knows what might happen? If I let go of every pretense and instead be genuine, things might get worse. Who knows what devil might be lurking in my depths?'' But it's also beginning to dawn on us that we have blindly believed false and inaccurate concepts about who we are, and have been ignorant of our true nature until now simply because we have been taught otherwise, and that maybe we're different from how we've thought ourselves to be, and that it's time, now, to experience what's really true—once and for all, come what may.

It requires tremendous courage willingly to release all of our firmly held beliefs and face ourselves directly. Courage is required because we don't know what we'll find. We're afraid our worst suspicions will be confirmed, or that we'll uncover aspects of ourselves we'd rather keep concealed. And we may! But underneath it all, or surrounding it all, embracing it all is the creative energy of Consciousness, Identity, or Presence that we *really* are—grounded in love and goodness.

But at first we don't know this. We don't know that goodness is at our core. We don't know that happiness is the natural state, that this is what we'll find. So we feel trepidation. We're suspicious. And we're likely to think all this talk about love and goodness is nothing but, at best, pure fantasy. But, in actuality, we're not absolutely certain this *isn't* what we'll find. We don't really know whether it's true or false. We don't really know whether goodness or evil is at our core, or if we are some blurry mixture of the two.

Therefore, we need courageously to desire to know the truth, and then we need to go within and experience ourselves directly. Therefore, *want* to know the truth, once and for all. Want to know *your* truth. Let go of everything you think you know about who you are, suspend every idea you now have about what's true and what isn't, and open your mind to what's actually so—to the living truth of you.

This is the most logical, important, life-affirming thing you can do. You'll be glad you risked experiencing yourself with clarity. But it can be frightening, unnerving, unsettling. However, if loving goodness is both at your core and is the surrounding all-pervading presence of Consciousness that you are—and this is something you will only ever know by experiencing it within yourself as your deepest truth—then the more clearly you experience yourself as you really are, free of any overlay of conditioning and in spite of your fears, the more *love* you will experience. If love is what's in there, then love is what you'll find when you go within. But you won't be convinced of this until you go within. Therefore, take the chance. It's worth the risk. And it's inevitable. You're bound to succeed. You will no longer be so afraid to know what else is true about you, which will further encourage you to relax deeper, trust more fully, and genuinely be yourself without inhibition or pretense.

You will discover and know that love, goodness, and creative consciousness are what constitute your being because you will **experience** these attributes within and as yourself. You will simultaneously realize that you did not put them there because you did not create yourself. You were created by the creative God Force. The inherent creative goodness within you is not a mental construct that you attempt to adopt, not pretense or self-deception, not something you conjure up. It's something you discover. You go in empty-handed, not knowing, and this is what you find. And when you allow yourself wholeheartedly to experience the core feeling-tone of the love that you are, you will spontaneously feel happy. You won't have to lift a finger or change yourself in any way. It's the way you were built. It's what you are. The emotional feeling-tone of love and goodness is happiness.

There will be an overwhelming sense of authenticity about this experience. You will have no doubt about its truth. You will be convinced. You will also realize that it is not egocentric to be appreciative of the creative energy that you are. Nor is it arrogant, presumptuous, or conceited to feel good inside about yourself, or to be happy for no apparent reason, or to acknowledge that you are a perfect creation of the God Force.

You understand instead that it is egotistical and arrogant to believe anything else, for you are not a self-created separate energy. It is not any more narcissistic (in the pejorative sense) to experience self-love or self-appreciation than it is to appreciate a lovely flower or a spectacular sunset. The wonder and beauty of you is not your doing, and appreciation will be the natural response of anyone who realizes this truth. What a relief! You are not who you thought you were. You are the infinite Oneness in specific Self-Expression. How wonderful to be affiliated with the great God Force.

In order to experience the natural joy of Being—in order to be happy!—we do not have to fulfill any conditions that are contrary to our original nature of loving goodness. We especially do not have to be other than the way we are. In fact, it has been the lifelong attempt to be some way other than our natural being that has made us frustrated and unhappy. And of course! You cannot be anything other than you. Therefore, let yourself be yourself—be you!—and live your truth without inhibition. Discover the truth by letting go of old concepts. Make space for the new. Release every idea you have about who you are, and then be the you that remains. Being you is not a substitute for what you can never be. It is the gracious acceptance of what you have always wanted and have never been without.

Think of it like this: The farther you are from knowing your truth and experiencing the love you are, the unhappier you will be; the closer you are, the happier. Keep it simple. It works like this because goodness *is* at your core and because happiness *is* the feeling-tone of your original nature. But, really, whether you are "close" or "far," you are always only a thought away. Your original nature is not, in fact, far away from you. It is not elusive. It is not someplace other than where you are, nor is it something you evolve or transform into or earn. It's right here, yours, already.

Become your already-existing naturally happy truth by spending quiet time alone every day to meditate. At least once a day sit down for a few minutes by yourself, stop moving, stop thinking, and just *be*. Deliberately be still. Close your eyes, relax, breathe, be aware, and consciously experience your present moment of conscious awareness. Immerse yourself in your own unique feeling-tone. Feel you. Bask in the exquisite experience of being alive, of conflict-free high-energy peace, and become thoroughly familiar with the core tone of who you are.

This is like dipping cloth into dye. Each dip of the cloth strengthens the cast of the dye and enhances the color. Here, however, you are dipping yourself into you. You are experiencing you. Each time you do so, you become more you; that is, your sense of the authentic you is enriched. Each dip into the silent experience of you washes away more false ideas, which enables the real you to shine forth more clearly to yourself and others.

As you do this, something new and very interesting will gradually begin to happen. You'll find yourself becoming more intuitive. Your mind will seem to expand, and your inner voice will start talking to you more clearly, guiding you, telling you what to say, what to think, where to go, what to do with your life. As you will discover, this is the source of right action. I will say more about this later.

Therefore, as you directly experience the living truth of who you are, two wonderful aspects of being become apparent. First, you come upon the core of goodness. This will promote a new, expanded, and truer sense of self. It will give your life new meaning, and you'll find yourself feeling happy for no apparent reason. Of course, there is a reason. Happiness and love is the stuff of which you are made. You can obscure your awareness of it, but you cannot get away from it. You cannot actually change it.

Second, the inner feeling—or inner voice—starts speaking to you with more clarity. Or rather, it's not that the inner voice now speaks with more clarity, but you'll start hearing it more clearly. It will become more obvious to you, and harder to ignore. This internal communication from the deeper regions of Being can become, if you are willing, your new guide to appropriate action in daily life. You will feel good inside about who you are and be increasingly effective in all your actions.

Let's move now into a practice mode with regard to all that has been said so far. We'll continue with three more exercises. These have been specifically designed to help you experience the loving goodness truth inside you.

One of the first things you may notice as you sit in stillness is that your body vibrates or hums. The center of this hum is in the area of your heart and throughout the length of your spine, your core. This is where love vibrates most obviously. The purpose of the next two breathing exercises, then, is to direct your conscious feeling-awareness into the area of your heart and core and thereby increase your sensitivity to the vibratory hum. You'll feel the love vibration inside yourself that will cause you to feel profoundly loved and profoundly safe, and you will thereby spontaneously become more loving—more of a pleasure to be around. This is good for you, and it's good for others! These exercises are worth a few minutes of your undivided attention. Enjoy them.

## Heart Breathing

Lie on your back with your eyes closed and palms flat on your chest. Begin by gently breathing in and out, aiming the breath into the chest so that you feel the wishbone at the base of your sternum expanding with each breath. Do this for a minute or two.

Then allow your breathing to flow in and out naturally, effortlessly, without any intervention on your part, and simply station your awareness in the center of your chest at the base of the sternum—where your hands are—and feel what you feel. Feel yourself breathing. As attentively as you can, note the changing sensations in the area of your heart that accompany each breath as it flows in and out.

Breathe in and out of your heart, lie absolutely still, be relaxed, and allow your breathing to flow freely and easily. Make no attempt to regulate your breathing or control it in any way. Some breaths will be deep, others shallow. Every breath will be different. All you do is remain aware of the ever-changing sensations that accompany breathing in the area of your heart.

As you practice this technique, let each breath remind you to stay centered and present in the now. When your attention strays, notice it has done so and then bring it back to the feeling-awareness of the ever-changing sensations in your chest. Do not think about the breath, nor about the meaning of love. Simply experience what's actually there to be experienced. Stay with what's happening. Shift from thinking mode to feeling mode, and experience your unique feeling-tone emanating from your heart center. Be especially on the look out for pleasurable sensations of warmth, expansion, or spaciousness, and notice how the movement of breath seems to fan and increase these sensations. Willingly give your undivided attention to this exercise for ten minutes.

## Expanded Heart Breathing

Sit on the floor with your spine straight and eyes closed. If you are unable to sit on the floor, use a chair. Be comfortable. Take a moment to become quiet and prepare yourself.

When you are ready, begin with ten or twenty fairly deep, gentle, continuous breaths, endeavoring to achieve full expansion of your chest and rib cage. Allow the sternum to rise and swell forward as you breathe. Go ahead and exaggerate it, but be very, very gentle.

Then inhale fully, again lifting upward with the sternum and expanding your chest. Hold the breath for a comfortable length of time, somewhere between five and twenty seconds, and as you hold your chest gently open at full expansion, *feel* the sensations in the area of your heart.

Feel the obvious sensations—the physical sensations of stretch and fullness accompanying chest expansion, the feeling of satisfaction, of air-hunger being satiated, and of air-hunger arising again as the seconds go by, your heart beating, your desire to exhale—but feel the deeper, subtler energy as well. Feel the energy of love in the area of your heart as you hold your chest open. Then exhale quietly, releasing the breath at a comfortable pace and relaxing deeply. Do this twelve times.

With this technique you are increasing your sensitivity to the vibratory feeling-tone in the area of your heart. Think of this as a vortex of energy in the vicinity of your physical heart but not your actual physical heart. You will be able to feel this vortex of energy with increasing clarity with practice. Do not attempt to hold the breath as long as you can. Hold the breath only as long as is comfortable. You should still be able to exhale smoothly, quietly, without panic. There should be no strain whatsoever. Exhale when you receive the inner cue to do so and keep the breath soft, strain-free, and peaceful. This is not a contest. It does not matter how long you hold the breath. Use the technique to increase your sensitivity to the inner feeling.

When you have completed the twelve breaths, sit absolutely still for another minute or two and simply be aware of how you feel. Station your awareness in the area of your heart and core and feel what you feel. Stay aware of the changing sensations that accompany breathing in the area of your heart, the sensations throughout your core and body, the space around your body, and especially the overall energetic feeling-tone of you. Willingly let go of everything you think you know about who you are, and allow yourself to experience you with clarity.

## Who Am I?

Sit with your spine straight or lie flat on the floor on your back. Close your eyes and take a few moments to become quiet and still. Relax your body and allow yourself to become intimately aware of your breathing. Observe the natural flow of breath in and out of your body.

Then put aside everything you think you know about who you are and ask yourself the question, "Who am I?" Ask the question but *do not answer it*. Instead, *feel* the answer. Feel who you are. Feel the energy of you. Answer not in words but in the direct experience of the energy that you are.

When your attention wanders from this very personal self-experiencing and you notice yourself thinking other thoughts, ask yourself, "Who is thinking this? Who is having this thought?" The answer will always be "I am." Then ask yourself again, "But who am I?" Then again immerse yourself in the feeling-tone truth of you.

When you notice yourself suddenly aware of a particular sound or sensation, your attention pulled away from the feeling, ask yourself "Who is hearing this sound? Who is experiencing this sensation?" The answer will always be, "I am." Then again ask, "But who am I?" And again blend with the feeling-tone truth of you. Find out who you are through direct experience. Keep bringing your conscious awareness back into the conscious experience of you in the now.

There is no adequate mental answer to the question. The vibrant silence is the answer. And so, be still and know.

# 3

## WHY YOGA?

The first time I saw someone practicing yoga I had mixed feelings. On the one hand I was highly attracted, there being something profoundly "right" about what I was seeing; on the other hand there was a mysterious, exotic, and ancient air about it that made me nervous. I had never seen anything like it before. It seemed powerful, almost bizarre. The man I was watching obviously knew what he was doing, and he seemed to have access to a hidden reservoir of energy.

Questions like "Why in the world?" and "What for?" raced through my mind. Reactions like "So what," "crazy," and "fanatic" filtered through, and yet I was deeply impressed. I wanted to know how twisting and bending your body could have anything remotely to do with God, life, meaning, or happiness. What was yoga all about? What relationship could it possibly have with anything? With my life, my perceived problems, global issues, despair, hopelessness, the alleviation of suffering, making a difference, enlightenment . . . ? And like many things in life, we can never know in advance the full impact something is going to have on us. Reasons for our initial involvement may pale and lose importance as we move deeper. We change and learn, often in unexpected ways.

The simple perspective I have come up with, through all the years and thousands of hours of practicing yoga and meditation since that first exposure, is that yoga makes you feel good. It's relaxing. It's energizing. It's strengthening. You feel better at the end of a session than before you began, and life runs more smoothly when you maintain a consistent discipline than when you don't. Yoga enhances your experience of life. It changes your perspective. You thereby find yourself spontaneously embracing a larger, more accurate conception of who you are, how life works, and what God is. You start seeing things differently, with less distortion—which results in more peace of mind, better health, more enthusiasm for life, and an ever-growing authentic sense of inner well-being.

As you practice yoga and meditation regularly, this subtle sense of feeling good gradually becomes so pervasive, so natural and genuine, so much a part of you that it carries over into the whole of your life. And in doing so it helps clarify your deepest longings, motivations, and aspirations, thereby restoring optimism, hope, meaning, and purpose to life.

This transition will be smooth and easy much of the time (even unnoticed) because it's so natural, but some of the time it may not be smooth or easy. It may be damn hard and painful. But this is only because growth hurts when you resist change, and most of us have an inclination to resist change in an attempt to remain comfortable by staying the same. But life is change. Change happens, especially when you're involved in a powerful transformative process such as yoga. You grow. You can't not change. That's just the way it is. It's how things work. Therefore, in order to stay comfortable as you grow, you must flow with the changes and not attempt to remain the same—just as you buy a new pair of shoes for your son or daughter when their feet have outgrown the pair they've been wearing. It's not reasonable for them to continue wearing their favorite shoes when they no longer fit. You get rid of the old ones and buy a new pair. But the reason you need new ones is that their feet have grown. Growth has occurred. Their foot grew, the shoe became too small, their foot hurt. Pain is not an inherent part of being a foot. Nor is it an inherent part of growth.

Your feet cannot be comfortable in a pair of shoes that has become too small. Nor can an emerging flower be comfortable by staying inside its protective husk that has gradually become too tight. Nor a growing chick inside its shell. Nor can you be comfortable in old belief structures and limited self-concepts. You must slough off the husk and allow yourself to open and bloom. You must willingly let go of any belief structure that limits your awareness and causes your experience of growth to be painful. You must let go of that which until now has been a protective coating or shield—and bloom. With the blooming will come a new sense of self and new appreciation for life.

The confidence necessary to do this will accrue naturally from the practice. You learn to open up by relaxing, being fearless, and becoming increasingly defenseless. Defensiveness, or shielding, is what creates the discomfort associated with growth. Changes start happening, changes that may not always be initially welcome, and rather than flow with the change and grow, many of us choose to stop the process and stave off the change in an attempt to remain the same a little longer. We contract in order to protect ourselves. We stop the practice the moment it starts working, usually when we start changing in ways we had not anticipated. This is because that which is good for us is not always recognized as such right off the bat. It's not uncommon to become fearful, defensive, and self-protective, to mistrust the process and revert to old ways of being. The problem with doing this, however, you discover, is that it hurts *more* not to change. Increasingly, then, you embrace change. You realize it's the movement of fulfillment. And when you are no longer resisting growth it will be experienced by you as less traumatic and more joyful. It feels good to go with the flow and grow.

We all like feeling good. We all want peace of mind. We all enjoy being joyful, peaceful, energized, and relaxed. Surely, there's no confusion about this. Yet most of us would readily admit that we are not feeling as good as we might. We may, in fact, believe that anything more than a transient, spurious happiness is not actually attainable. But we would also like to feel better and actually be happy. We want the truth, come what may, but we'd also like the joy and fulfillment of a meaningful life if at all possible.

We all have different visions of happiness and fulfillment, and different strategies with which to pursue them as we attempt to ascertain what's true. Yet, regardless of our differences, all of us are doing those things that we think will make us happy—or at least less miserable, less susceptible to future suffering. The way we do this is based on our current personal understanding of how life works. We pursue different courses of action because our understanding, inclinations, and circumstances vary. The essential motivation is the same, however. We want the truth—and we want to be happy.

You may want something other than just "feeling good," however, something more than a vague, nonspecific happiness. You may want a new car, a washing machine, a master's degree, or a better relationship. You may want spiritual enlightenment. But would you still want the new car, the washer, the degree, the relationship, or the enlightenment if in having it it did not also make you feel good? Would you want these things if they made you feel bad?

It's difficult to want something, even if it's good for you, if you think you'll feel worse as a result of having it. Therefore, we must be very alert for self-deception. How much of your pursuit of truth is tainted or twisted by what you want that truth to be? If Truth causes you to suffer more than you already do, would you still want it? This is an important question, one that leads many people not to want to know the truth, and one that you are answering one way or the other as evidenced in the way you live your life.

The various things we desire and pursue, therefore, and the many ways we attempt to grow and change are what we perceive to be the means to happiness. We think, "If only I were ten pounds lighter," "If only I weren't so shy and fearful," "If only I could do that pose better," "If only I had some money," "If only someone loved me, if only things were somehow different, if only I were different from how I am . . . then I'd be happy." We think that having this or that, or being this or that way, will do the trick.

The problem, though, is that we don't actually know what will make us happy. We've received many of our desires, things we thought would make us happy, changed ourselves in every conceivable way, and still feel largely unsatisfied. The fulfillment of desire is generally not very satisfying in the larger sense. We realize that what we thought we wanted wasn't it after all. It didn't give us lasting happiness. A new desire always arises. Besides, there are many things in this world that can temporarily make us feel good, but that are not very good for us and that eventually make us feel bad.

The thrust of yoga, in contrast to the pursuit of your desire as a means to happiness, is aimed at the monumental, life-changing discovery of who and what you truly are. This is how yoga works, how it makes you feel good. It helps you experience the truth, your truth—which, you discover, is goodness. Your basic nature is happiness.

You don't know this at first, however. You don't know this is what you'll find. But when you do experience your truth, free of every idea you now believe about yourself and free of every hope you have about what that truth is, you will spontaneously feel exquisite inside and be happy. And this is no small thing. This is big, huge. And when you are in touch with that basic goodness, with the pure Consciousness that you are, all that you desire will be in alignment with your deepest truth and will therefore come to you easily as a manifestation—or proof—of your congruence with Truth. The fulfillment of desire will then be fulfilling because you are in accord with Truth, in harmony with the Oneness.

The ramifications of knowing your truth will be enormous. You will begin to live with a security, a confidence, and an inner psychological peace born of an unshakable conviction in your own personal worth. You will experience self-love and appreciation and will thereby begin to feel full enough to reach out and love others. You will also feel increasingly grateful to the creative God Force for the privilege of citizenship and the joy of participation in the endless creativity of the event called life.

Now, let's start with a brief overview of the what and why of yoga. What are the benefits of practicing yoga? And why would this be of interest to someone who has never been involved with yoga before?

Let me say first that yoga, like brushing your teeth, is an acquired preference. When I was young I didn't like to brush my teeth. It required my parents' daily reminding to get me to do it. Now I brush my teeth not only as a prevention against tooth decay, but because I prefer the way my mouth feels when it's clean.

The same has been true with my yoga practice. At first it took conscious discipline and deliberate effort to establish a daily practice. Now I practice not only because it's good for me, but because I prefer the way I feel when I do. I feel clean and new, much like the way brushing my teeth makes my mouth feel. The entire motivation has changed. Yoga helps keep my energy-tone at a level I like. This can easily become your most compelling reason for doing yoga. Then, just as you gladly brush your teeth every day, so will you gladly practice yoga. Brushing once a week is not the same as spending a few minutes daily.

Please understand that what I am attempting to describe and put into words is an activity that is essentially nonverbal. Words, by their very nature, will never quite convey the meaning. The description can never fully communicate the described. The explanation is pallid and anemic in comparison to the richness of the actual experience, and it's the actual experience of yoga that concerns us.

Words, however, can prepare you for the experience. They can foster motivation, which inevitably leads to success and understanding. The word *water*, for example, will not quench your thirst. But it may encourage you to continue looking for water until you find a well or drinking fountain. The words and analogies I have chosen, therefore, though not entirely precise, are accurate enough to give you a foretaste of my meaning. Be playful with the analogies, as I have been in using them, and listen for the meaning that lies beyond the word.

# Balance, Strength, and Flexibility

One of the most obvious things about having a body is that it tends to stiffen and tighten the older you get, much like a plant that is tender and supple when young and becomes hard, dry, and woody with age. When you were young, you were probably very flexible; most children are. As you have grown older, your range and ease of movement have probably diminished. Perhaps you're not as spry as you once were, you move more slowly, and you may be experiencing more aches and subtle pains. You may also have noticed that you're less energetic, less resilient to change, more prone to injury, and that injuries take longer to heal. You may not feel quite as alive as you used to feel.

Given the way most of us live and think, this is neither surprising nor mysterious. Nor is it something that happens suddenly. It creeps up slowly, and you notice it gradually. Your awareness of this gradual decay and loss of vitality, however, can spark a very real commitment to the discipline of yoga.

As your body tightens, not only is it less comfortable to be in, like a shirt that has shrunk and is now too small, it actually becomes less efficient and more prone to disease and degeneration. As your body tightens, it literally begins to choke itself. This internal constriction inhibits the circulatory system, not only of your blood and other fluids, but of the essential life force. And when the circulatory system (which irrigates, oxygenates, and feeds the cells) is inhibited, the cells' food supply is diminished. This gradual undernourishment contributes to the overall aging, drying, and hardening of the body. Nerves, glands, and muscles, as well as the different energy networks in the spine, all become subject to a slow death precipitated by the lack of nourishment inherent in this internal strangulation.

With yoga you can dramatically retard, even reverse, the tendency to stiffen as you age. You can actually bring the suppleness of youth back into your life and be more flexible, durable, and stronger than you were as a child. You can learn to focus your physical and mental energy more effectively and thereby be more vital, creative, and efficient in all your activities.

There are many physical benefits that accrue from regular hatha (physical) yoga practice. The three most obvious are the immediate increase in your balance, strength, and flexibility.

**BALANCE** ◆ Improved balance refers not only to the heightened physical coordination you will acquire, but to the balance of power between the left and right, front and back, and high and low aspects of your body.

Most of us are not balanced and therefore do much of what we do asymmetrically. We may be stronger on our right side, for example, and weaker on our left. We can turn our head or twist our spine farther in one direction than we can the other. We can cross our legs with the left leg on top, but not the right. We can bend forward with ease but not backward.

None of this would matter much except for the fact that being asymmetrical and unbalanced creates a certain inevitable level of stress and strain throughout your body. Parts of you work overtime, other parts are neglected. This can lead to injury, pain, or just plain discomfort. Working toward a balance within yourself will bring a welcome harmony to the overall feeling-tone of who you are.

Yoga creates symmetry throughout your whole body, making you strong and flexible in a balanced way. It also teaches you to balance the mental impulse to push, control, and be assertive with the complimentary impulse to yield, surrender, and be passive. This balanced attitudinal equilibrium, rather than hampering the energy of either impulse, heightens the effectiveness of both.

**STRENGTH** ◆ When you feel tired and weak, you also feel heavy. You literally feel heavy, a burden to yourself, as though you had to drag yourself around. When you feel energetic and strong, however, you feel light, and life doesn't seem so difficult. The weaker you are, the heavier you will feel. The stronger you are, the lighter you will feel. A consistent yoga practice will make you strong and light.

This may not sound like much. But if, for example, you were twice as strong as you are right now, you would feel twice as light. It would seem as though you were half your current body weight. Imagine weighing half your present weight. You would feel very light and buoyant, and your everyday experience of who you are would be dramatically different.

The whole tone of your body will change as your strength increases. You will have an easier time handling your own body weight. You will feel sturdier and more sure of yourself. You will have a lighter step, your experience in the world will become a pleasure, and life will seem and be easier. If this interests you, then work to increase your strength. Do this by exercising it, using it. Be happy when a pose challenges you in this way.

**FLEXIBILITY** ◆ As you free your body and become more flexible, you not only restore lost movement, you actually erase all the tensions and internal conflicts that would otherwise accumulate and eventually erupt as pain. The more flexible you are, the harder it is for pain to lodge in your body. Pain and tension are forms of blocked, stuck, misplaced, and misused energy. Being more flexible opens these energy blockages and frees your energy circulation. Your entire body will feel clean and new as the stuck parts are freed and released.

Pain often comes from neglect (a form of misuse) and is always a signal to take care. Toothaches, backaches, and headaches are all symptoms of such neglect or abuse. They are forms of asking for help and should be listened to, not ignored. Healthy teeth do not hurt, and healthy backs do not ache. Toothaches hold you in "tooth-consciousness," backaches in "back-consciousness." If you have ever had either, you know what I mean.

The healthier your teeth are, however, the less "tooth-consciousness" you will experience. The healthier your back, the less "back-consciousness." And the healthier your whole body is, the less "body-consciousness" you will experience. This will produce a state wherein you feel transparent, clear, clean, almost invisible. And because your body is operating perfectly, it will not demand your attention in uncomfortable ways. Your awareness and life experience will again feel pure and untainted. This is probably the way you felt when you were young.

Easing the grip of body-consciousness will spark the growing awareness that "you" are much more than mortal. The healthier you are, the less concerned you will be with your body. This frees your mind to discover itself. It is interesting how it comes full circle. At first, yoga makes you more sensitive and more conscious of your body; otherwise, due to neglect, misuse, or abuse, pain will be calling you. But now, because of the care you have taken with yourself, your awareness and self-definition are free to expand beyond your body to new levels of experience and learning.

The gratifying result of being supremely healthy is that your body becomes barely noticeable, much like having your car in perfect running order. When your car is perfectly tuned, your driving experience is of the ride, the scenery, and the people you are with. You are not worried about whether the car is about to break down or not. The way to alleviate worry and transcend "car-consciousness" is by taking care of your car, not by ignoring it and leaving its well-being to the whims of chance. The way to transcend worrisome body-consciousness is by taking care of your body. The idea is not to become obsessed with your physical form. Simply give it enough care and attention so that it functions as the perfect instrument and comfortable embodiment it was meant to be.

# Sensitivity and Self-Trust

These three things—balance, strength, and flexibility—will enhance your overall sensitivity. This is essentially what the discipline of yoga is all about. It is an awareness process wherein you attend to very subtle shifts in sensation and feeling as you do the poses, or *asanas*. You immerse yourself in the various sensations of stretch and listen for the intelligence of your body to advise you about what to do—like whether you should be stretching more or less, for example. You practice using your intuition in this very specific arena of yoga asanas. In so doing you simultaneously exercise your body as you refine your sensitivity to inner guidance.

The beauty of being more sensitive lies in the discovery that beneficial things naturally start feeling good, better than before, and therefore become attractive to you. Things that are bad for you no longer hold the attraction they once may have had. Your diet, for example, may undergo an effortless change. Certain foods you previously enjoyed may no longer be so appealing, and previously uninteresting foods may now entice you. Lifestyle habits may also change without conscious determination.

An ever-increasing sensitivity, therefore, will initiate an easy self-corrective process that reinforces self-trust. Self-trust means we have the confidence necessary to follow through and pursue things that feel right. This is very important. It means that we can now openly trust ourselves to pursue what is attractive to us and avoid what isn't. Until now, this is exactly what has gotten us into so much trouble. We've pursued things and situations we found attractive and have ended up paying for it, in one way or another. And we have thereby learned *not* to trust ourselves. It makes sense not to trust if it keeps getting us into trouble, and pretty soon this mistrust feels normal.

With the cultivation of sensitivity, however, your likes and dislikes will change. You'll discover that what now attracts you *is* in your best interest. You can therefore safely allow yourself to pursue what attracts you, what you like. You can trust yourself to trust yourself. It's no longer dangerous, but safe—smart. And it's fulfilling. It *will* make you happy.

Of course, what you are really learning is that self-trust is the most intimate way of expressing your trust in God and the universe. You are not a separate creation, remember, and you did not create yourself. Trusting yourself, therefore, is actually trusting in the intelligence of the Creator who made you. It is your personal demonstration of your trust in the universe and Infinite Mind, and your confidence will be well reinforced because of your ever-increasing sensitivity. This basic self-trust is the foundation of all yoga and the prevailing quality of those who have learned to be their own best teachers.

# Love

All this becomes especially interesting as you notice how thoroughly your life is shaped by your thoughts and the way you interpret what's going on. Every thought, feeling, and emotion manifests in one form or another in your body and in your life. As you become more sensitive to the inner feeling of who you are, you will notice this with surprising clarity. You will also learn a very simple truth: Loving thoughts feel good, and unloving thoughts feel bad. Unloving thoughts are like self-inflicted poison darts, whereas loving thoughts are the natural response to reality when it is clearly perceived.

This simple understanding will initiate a natural change of mind that will culminate in the primary and most important theme of yoga: learning to love and be loved. You will gladly allow the energy of love to circulate freely through you once you start feeling it. You'll no longer be so afraid of love, at war with love, because it will feel so much better to be loving than not. In this way you will gradually become the conduit for love to shine through unobstructed, undiluted—pure and perfect.

But what is love? What do we really know about it? How much of our beliefs about love are true, and how much is merely our imagination?

Love is the most practical thing in the world. It's what's needed most. And this is what it is: Love is the willingness to see that which is Real in each and every thing. It's the willingness to let go of what you think something is in order to see it clearly—as it really is. Love, therefore, is the supreme healing power because it looks beyond what appears to be true to what *is* true.

As you begin to see all things in this new way, you'll find that you and the world are different than you thought they were—and magnificently better. You'll sense that there is, indeed, authentic cause for hope and joy and an optimistic outlook. The more realistic you are, you discover, the more optimistic you become. We are not victims doomed to death and suffering and short-lived transient joys, but beings alive in a creative universe, uniquely specific expressions of a creative, eternal, universal Consciousness, Mind, or Infinite Presence, God.

You welcome love—that is, you become able to see that which is Real in each and every thing—by clearing your mind of prejudice and beliefs and then being with things as they are. Only when your mind is clean of preconceptions, even if you're right, can you see and relate to what is actually true. With regard to other people, for example, love is the willingness to let go of your ego reactions to the way people are presenting themselves in order to see them as they really are. To love another is more a matter of letting go of everything you think you know about that person, so you can be with him or her in the now with a clear and uncluttered mind, than it is to have ideas in advance about what it means to be loving and then attempting to behave "lovingly." When you do this, people will feel as though you are extending love to them, that you are being loving, when in actual fact you will have merely withdrawn your preconceptions in order to be clean with them in the now.

You learn to love by learning to forgive. Forgiveness is the deliberate withdrawal of judgment. It's the deliberate letting-go of criticism, condemnation, and *conditions-needing-to-be-met-before-I-see-you-anew* with regard to yourself, others, and everything else, in favor of seeing the deepest truth. It's about removing the filter in order to see clearly. Not judging yourself or others puts you in the position of perceiving accurately. Each one of us is the specific expression of Infinite Consciousness, whether we know it or not and whether we are acting like it or not. Everyone is some aspect of the same infinite thing that you are. Your willingness to see yourself and others in this way is transformative. It encourages everyone to relax, be fearless, and therefore be less defensively aggressive.

This is something you will want to learn simply because the perspective and love that come from forgiveness feel infinitely better than anything coming from blame or judgment. Love feels better than non-love. Is this a surprise? The conscious realization of this fact, however, will propel you into a perception of yourself and the world that will work to enhance and preserve this secure sense of overwhelming love.

# Self-Realization

***FIRST DIMENSION*** ◈ Yoga can be seen as having three interwoven themes or dimensions. The first involves getting down on the floor and actually doing the exercises. The exercises purify and heal your body by making you balanced, strong, flexible, sensitive, energized, and relaxed. They promote radiant health. They also increase your mental stamina by training your mind to concentrate and sustain a focused attention. In combination, these culminate in the experience of stillness and peace. This is why I refer to the practice of yoga as a way of moving into stillness.

This first theme is exceedingly important because when you experience yourself in stillness and feel the peace within you, you will come upon a new awareness of who you are. This new awareness will convince you that "you" are part of a greater whole, that you are not a separate energy nor a separate consciousness. You are an individuated and specific expression of one energy, one Consciousness, one Infinite Mind—much like a single wave on the ocean is a specific expression of that ocean. Waves are not separate energies. They are individuated and unique, one of a kind, but they do not exist apart from the ocean.

Similarly, we are not separate entities somehow disconnected from the One and Only, the All. We are individually specific and unique, yet inseparable from the whole. We are individuated conscious expressions of Infinite Conscious Being, Infinite Mind, God, the Father-Mother, the one I Am, the Self. There is no "you" or "me" apart from It. We are It in specific manifestation. We are Consciousness being specifically conscious.

Ego is when the wave—you or me—mistakenly believes that it stands alone and that, somehow, it is essentially separate and different from the ocean and from other waves. The ego sense is not real, not accurate. It is not an actual energy or presence. It is imagination, misunderstanding, a false sense of Self—the result of an incomplete perception of who we are. It is a misidentification, a limited understanding of the facts based on our conditioning and the data we receive from our five physical senses only. It is thinking we are one thing when we are really something else. It's how we define ourselves prior to knowing what's really true.

It is not surprising that misidentification occurs, because from the wave's vantage point on the surface of the ocean, it does look separate. It looks out, sees other waves, and defines itself as one among many. The underlying sameness is not obvious at first glance.

This is how we feel, mostly. We feel separate and distinct from one another, alone in a vast universe, with our underlying sameness not readily apparent. We look out and see "others." Separateness is what's obvious. But when the underlying oneness begins to be obvious, it will steadily become *more* obvious, and pretty soon there will be a complete transformation both in the way you think about yourself and the way you see your world. Your existence will then be different, more in harmony with life, because you'll be seeing yourself and the world in a new way.

We are both the wave, individual and unique, *and* the ocean. Both. At the same time. We are Consciousness, Infinite Mind, God, in specific expression.

Because we *are* Consciousness in specific expression, we are each our own best contact point with that Consciousness. Your mind is your personal best entry point into the awareness of Infinite Mind, your own closest touch point with the creative God Force, which is the life of you and everything else—just as a wave's closest contact point with the ocean is itself. When you realize this, and then take the time to immerse yourself in stillness, you will experience this Godness-Goodness within you as you. As you do this, you awaken to the spiritual meaning of yoga and the spiritual essence that is the real you.

**SECOND DIMENSION** ◆ The second dimension of yoga deals with meditation and communion. This involves an enhanced way of using your mind based on your newly emerging perspective of yourself as a mind in Mind, and it is the direct result of having experienced yourself in stillness. This "new" way of using your mind is the basis for expanded thinking, for experiencing personal power, for obtaining inner guidance and insight, for intelligent decision making, and for the sure conviction of the inherent goodness of life. It involves voluntarily giving up your own limited knowledge in glad exchange for the wisdom of the whole. This is the wave asking the ocean, your mind asking Mind.

When you experience yourself in stillness—that is, when your mind is at its most focused, energetic, present, alive, relaxed, and wholehearted—you will "hear" the voice of God whispering in the depths of your being. You will recognize this "voice"—sometimes called the inner voice or little voice—as the voice of your Soul, the voice that speaks your deepest and most genuine desires.

You will then intuitively understand that the Will of God, or the intent of the universe, and the desires of your heart are one and the same. They are not at odds with one another. They do not conflict. In fact, and this is the point, they are not two. This realization, by the way, is tremendously reassuring. It quells fear and restores faith. You will then *know* that your mind is part of the one Infinite Mind, the Mind of God, that there is no difference, and that there really is an inner voice happy to guide and direct you throughout your life. You will also know that it is in your best interest to listen most attentively to that voice, that it is none other than your own deepest wisdom.

***THIRD DIMENSION*** ◆ The third dimension is the natural consequence of having clearly experienced your truth: The more familiar you are with the creative God Force in you, the more you will see It and recognize It in others.

This is a monumental theme, and this idea has the power to transform both your individual world and the world at large. No longer will you see an evil, hostile world filled with alien and antagonistic forces. And no longer will it seem reasonable to complain, criticize, and condemn everything you see for being so blatantly imperfect. Instead, you will smile inside as you begin to see the very same creative energy with which you have become familiar within yourself as the energy and life of all things and people. All the world will take on a friendly and nonthreatening glow as you see ''your'' energy everywhere.

When you see *your* energy in someone else, you will have a sudden moment of recognition. At first you may be confused, not knowing why you recognize them or who they are. Then it will dawn on you. You are seeing yourself. You are seeing the thing in you that you call ''you,'' but you are seeing it in them! It's exactly like seeing your reflection in the store window as you walk by, or looking into a mirror and clearly seeing yourself.

When you see yourself in someone else, you are seeing the Self. The term Self-Realization is actually a very accurate description of what happens when you understand the deeper meaning of yoga. Realize means ''to make real.'' When the Self becomes real to you—and it will when you experience it within and then see it without—then the notion of a shared Self and common Source will become a conscious reality for you. You will realize that both you and ''others'' are simply different faces of one infinite Person, one Infinite Consciousness, one Infinite Mind or Being, God. The spiritual overtone of life will become supremely evident. You will see no difference between yourself and others.

Fear will then fade away and disappear because you are experiencing the oneness of yourself and the world. You will no longer be sensing anything in anyone else that is worthy of your fear. In fact, just the opposite is occurring. Everything you sense now confirms your new trust, your new perception, and strengthens your new impulse to relax and be fearless instead of defensive and aggressive.

Fear will fade because the deepest truth about all things and all people is that *everything* is made of the same energy as you. Every specific thing is Infinite Conscious Being in specific form. What is there to fear when this is what you are relating to? And love, remember, is the willingness to see this. Love, therefore, conquers fear. It makes you fearless. It exposes fear for what it is—a misperception of the facts.

The purpose of yoga is to facilitate the profound inner relaxation that accompanies fearlessness. Fearlessness is the natural attitude of anyone who understands that there is nothing to fear. Scary things seem to exist only in your imagination. Every perceived enemy and imagined threat is a misperception of the facts and therefore an illusion. When you see the true nature of things, you will see their God Essence and know there is nothing to fear. And you'll relax. It's simple. And because you are no longer fighting to save your own life, and because others are not forced to defend themselves against your defensive aggression, everyone can relax and become more pleasant.

The release from fear is what finally precipitates the full flowering of love. In this state you will love what you see in others, and others will love you for having been seen. This is the softened perception of the world that yoga promotes.

Therefore, the apparently simple benefits that accrue from the regular practice of yoga can change your life in very profound ways. Do not underestimate the value of being balanced, centered, and coordinated, of being strong and light, of being more flexible, without pain, experiencing the subsequent feelings of invisibility or transparency, and of being more sensitive. You will not only loosen all the negative connotations associated with body-consciousness, you will gain the positive experience of your own inner stillness.

Yoga will make you sensitive to the stillness, the presence, the hush, the peace of God. This deep inner stillness is at the core of your being. It is the ground, the joy of your being. The radiant peace you'll experience is what happens naturally when the creative energy of God is allowed to flow through you unobstructed. And it's the conscious awareness of this ever-present feeling-tone, the feeling-tone of the creative God Force, Consciousness, that will guide you intuitively through life and help you make your most important decisions.

Let's conclude this section with several exercises designed to help actualize all of this. Their primary purpose is to facilitate a new self-awareness coupled with the conscious experience of fearlessness and love.

## Mirror Gazing

With a mirror, practice gazing into your eyes. First, look into the center of the pupil of your left eye, for about a minute. Make eye contact with yourself in that one specific eye. Both of your eyes will be gazing into the one reflected eye, but it will feel as though your "energy" is predominantly coming out of your left eye. Gaze softly. Then switch eyes. Gaze into your right eye for about a minute, and feel the energy coming out of your right eye.

Then stare at your third eye, the point between your eyes at the bridge of your nose. Stare softly and let your vision expand peripherally until you are able to see into each eye simultaneously. Practice being on the same visual light beam with yourself. There will be a wonderful clarity about what you're seeing when you "get in there." Look yourself in the eyes and see yourself seeing yourself. This is a very interesting exercise.

## Gazing with a Friend

Practice gazing into the eyes of a friend. Sit a comfortable distance apart and then gaze into the friend's left eye as he or she gazes into your left eye. Do this for about a minute. Then gaze into the right eye as he or she gazes into your right eye. Do this for about a minute. Then gaze into the left eye as he or she gazes into your right eye—you're now visually connecting with one another—and then switch and gaze into the friend's right eye as he or she gazes into your left eye.

Now gaze into one another's third eye, the point between the eyes at the bridge of the nose, and allow your vision to expand peripherally until you are able to see into each eye simultaneously. There will be a sense of clarity and connection when this happens. You will be in the same world together, the same moment together, and you'll see each other seeing one another. When you lose the connection, again stare at the point between his or her eyes and again allow your vision to expand peripherally until you've reconnected. Attempt to sustain the connection.

## Eye Contact During the Day

During the day practice looking in the eyes of others. Don't be obnoxious with it, but do be interested in "going in there" and *seeing* them. Practice connecting with your eyes. You'll notice they are probably coming out of one eye more than the other. If they are not in the eye you are looking at, move your attention to the other eye and see if they are there. Go back and forth until you find them and then beam in on them. Connect visually. Let them see you seeing them.

You're not just connecting with your eyes when you connect in this way. You are connecting mentally. You are becoming one with that "other" one. You're being in the same world together, acknowledging one another's existence. You're looking beyond the surface identification to the real person inside, and you're learning to see the thing in you that you call "you" in the other person. This is called "seeing the Self," seeing your Self. Practice seeing the Self in others. Practice seeing the ocean in every specific wave.

## Ah

Sit with your back straight and eyes closed. If you are unable to sit on the floor, use a chair. Be comfortable. If you prefer, lie flat on your back.

Begin with a smooth, deep inhalation. Hold the air for a moment, then open your mouth about an inch and release the breath in a l-o-n-g, s-l-o-w exhalation. Silently whisper "ahhhh . . ." for about ten or twenty seconds. Then close your mouth, breathe in deeply again, and again let the breath out in a long, slow fashion through your open mouth. Do not attempt to exhale as deeply as possible. Just soften without strain.

Do this twelve times and then be still and experience the energy you are made of. Feel what it feels like to be you. Experience yourself as the Infinite Mind that you are.

This technique uses soft, long exhalations to facilitate an unusually profound inner release. The idea is consciously to let go of all muscular holding as you expel the breath and thereby relax as deeply as you can without effort, especially in the area of your throat and core. As you relax you will feel safe, cradled. And because you are feeling safe, it will make sense and be easy to relax even further. Therefore, keep letting go, deeper and deeper, level after level. Put down your emotional shield, release all unnecessary physical tension, saturate yourself with the peace-filled feeling-tone of fearlessness and safety, and experience the soothing nature of lovingness that is the energy you are.

As you sit motionless, be aware of the sensations in the area of your heart as well as your overall feeling-tone. Also be aware of the space around your body and sense how far you extend. Do you really feel a limit? There should not be the slightest hint of strain.

It is essential for your own peace of mind that you become familiar with the conscious release from fear, if only in moments. The ensuing knowingness of an all-pervading security issues forth from this deep inner release. As you consciously immerse yourself in the energetic peace of fearlessness and safety, you will experience a renewal of optimism that will clarify your priorities and aspirations. Your life will acquire new meaning as you establish the inner conviction that you live in a friendly, nonthreatening, purposeful universe.

Apply this technique whenever you sense fear. Exhale and relax, then breathe in the creative life force. You will feel stronger immediately.

## Sensitivity

Sensitivity grows through use, and the way to become more sensitive is by exercising your senses. Therefore, go for a walk in nature and be as sensitive as possible. Hear your footsteps on the ground, feel your feet as you walk, listen to the various and ever-changing sounds in your environment, be aware of what you are seeing, look at everything, breathe, and savor the fragrance of the air. Be sensitive and aware every way you can. Then carry that sensitivity with you during the day. Practice shifting from thinking mode to feeling-sensing mode.

## Practicing the Presence

Sit quietly with your eyes open or closed and become intimately aware of your breathing. Allow the breath to flow freely in and out at its own natural pace. Make no attempt to regulate or control it. Some breaths will be deep, others shallow. Every breath will be different. All you do is remain aware. There should be no strain.

Ride the breath into the conscious feeling-sensation of "you," immerse yourself in stillness, and then mentally say, "God is Love and therefore so am I. God is all there is of me. God I am." Repeat these sentences slowly, over and over. Say them in your mind and concentrate on the feeling-sensation of you. You are the specific location of Goodness, Consciousness, I Am-ness. Be thoroughly relaxed and experience yourself deeply. Be like the wave relaxing into the ocean. Feel your truth. Experience the fact of your existence. Let go of any desire to be one way rather than another, and instead, *feel* what's actually so. What does it feel like to be you right now? What does it feel like to be Consciousness being specifically conscious?

Gradually let go of the sentences and enter into the silent experience of you. The more you immerse yourself, the more pleasurable it will be. If you lose your focus, repeat the sentences until you again feel centered, then release them. Dissolve the apparent separation between you and your Self, your mind and universal Mind. Practice being wide open like space and see what happens. Be involved. Experience the Awareness-Presence that you are and enjoy yourself. Do this in a relaxed and attentive manner for five or ten minutes.

# 4

# WHAT DOES IT FEEL LIKE?

Have you ever been on a long airplane flight or train ride? Or worked at your desk for hours without stopping? Or done anything where you've been stationary for extended time spans? Most of us have. You're in the seat of the airplane or car, for example, cramped and unable to move much; your back, neck, and legs ache; your shoulders stiffen and become increasingly tense; and the very inactivity makes you uncomfortable, antsy, and tired. Surely, this is familiar.

At the end of the trip when you finally climb out of your seat, what do you do? Just naturally, without even thinking about it, you move and stretch. Haven't you done this? You can observe people at airports doing this all the time. You stretch, wriggle, writhe, arch your back, shrug, and circle your shoulders, turn your head, stretch your neck . . . and this makes you feel better. It helps get the kinks out.

A similar thing happens first thing in the morning when you wake up. Actually, most people do not stretch on waking, though you have probably done it occasionally, and you've certainly seen animals do it, especially cats and dogs. If you try it tomorrow morning, though, if when you awaken you stretch, wriggle, and writhe for a few moments—squeezing and stretching your muscles, exhilarating yourself with the feeling of stretch and energy flow, and allowing yourself to assume various spontaneous contortions—you may be surprised at how nice it feels and how quickly you wake up. Yoga is something like this.

Yoga is a sophisticated system for achieving radiant physical health, superb mental clarity and therefore peace of mind, as well as spiritual insight, knowledge, and understanding. It is a complete system for total psychosomatic-spiritual health. It's a way of learning to live in happy harmony with life. And, as with a cat stretching as it awakens, yoga wakes you up—gently—and makes you feel wonderful. The more yoga you do, the more awake you will become, both literally and figuratively, and it feels wonderful while you are doing it.

In yoga you stretch as though it were first thing in the morning, much like a yawn. Do it now. Yawn. Open your mouth and initiate a yawn. Observe how the yawn comes from deep inside you and reverberates outward. Feel the energy of the yawn radiating outward into the atmosphere. Notice how pleasant it feels.

Do it again. This is the action and feeling to become familiar with . . . that of expanding and stretching yourself open from the inside out.

Now do several slow neck rolls. Sitting erect, lower your chin toward the breastbone and allow your head to hang limply. Look downward or close your eyes, and simply relax in this position for ten or twenty seconds. Breathe softly. Allow the stretch to penetrate. Feel what's happening. Then raise your head, tip it to the right, and allow your head to relax toward the right shoulder. Experience the sensations of stretch along the left side of your neck as you allow the stretch to penetrate and deepen. Relax, so the stretched part elongates. Be here ten or twenty seconds. Then tip your head to the left and be here for the same length of time, relaxing. Again, allow the stretch to penetrate, experience the sensations of stretch, and savor how it actually feels. Then come back to center.

Now tip your head to the right and slowly roll your face downward toward your chest, rolling your head to the left so your left ear comes near the left shoulder. Then do the reverse: Roll your face downward toward the chest again and tip your head to the right. Go one direction then the other, slowly, gently, ten or twelve times. Notice that doing this with your eyes closed enables you to experience the various sensations with more clarity. Then come back to center.

Now do several head circles or neck rolls. Move your head in small then large circles, first one direction then the other, slowly. Writhe gently into the area of your neck, letting your head move around as though it had a life of its own. Feel what you're doing as you do this. Intuitively "follow" the various sensations of stretch. Press gently into tight areas. Pay close attention to every subtle sensation. Make it sensual, full of feeling. Be spontaneous. Creatively explore this area of yourself. Don't mindlessly swing your head from side to side or attempt to make the biggest possible arc. Be mindful. Go slowly and concentrate on experiencing the changing sensations of stretch. Be attentive to where it's painful, where it's pleasurable, and where there isn't much feeling. Experience the various sensations as attentively as you can, whatever they are, and be curious about what's in there. Do this for the perfect length of time. Stop when you feel you've done enough. Bring your head back to center, be still, and then be aware of how you feel.

Now stand erect with your feet apart, your arms outstretched in the air, and gently stretch and slowly writhe as though it were first thing in the morning, you've just woken up, and you feel like stretching! Do a whole body neck roll. Writhe with your whole body. Stretch everywhere, energize everywhere. Flood all parts of you. Wake yourself up—gently, slowly, sensually. Make it feel good. And immerse yourself fully in what you're doing *as you are doing it*. Stretch your whole body open from the inside out. Press into the various tight spots you find. Release the contracted areas, pent-up energy. Do this for a minute or so. Be attentive to where it's pleasurable, where it's painful, and where there isn't much sensation. Feel deeply. Concentrate on experiencing the ever-changing sensations of stretch. Experience every part of yourself. Immerse yourself so fully that you're momentarily not thinking about anything else. Then stop the gentle writhing, stand still for a few moments, and be aware of how you feel after having done this.

These are excellent examples of what it *feels* like to do yoga. They also convey the friendly attitude and total involvement you should bring to your yoga practice. The main difference between these examples and the actual practice is that yoga is more deliberate. You will be moving in perfect coordination with your breathing and assuming very specific positions.

The various asanas are actually very precise tools. Each yoga posture, or asana—pronounced AAH-suh-nuh—is a specific shape or template in which the stretching occurs. The idea is to use these tools or shapes to help create more space in your body. Your body is the visible and tangible portion of your energy field, and each pose is like a map into a specific area of that field. You create more space by undoing the tight spots, releasing tensions. Therefore, a large part of the practice is about deliberately roving through your body looking for the contracted, painful areas. Using the various poses as maps into yourself, or places to look, you then endeavor to stretch, open, and release the contracted areas. This is extremely pleasurable once you get a feeling for it.

Think, for example, of massage. When someone asks you to rub their neck or shoulders, usually it's because they are experiencing some degree of pain or discomfort in that area. Your job is to look for the tight, sore, and tender areas and then rub, deliberately pressing into and flirting with the knots of tension that cause the pain. These knots are the areas you are attempting to undo, ease away, and erase. As you do this, however, it is not effective or intelligent to go directly into the sore area and press as hard as you can. The tight area will contract further and become even less willing to release its excessive grip and open. Therefore, you proceed slowly. You approach the contracted areas with care and come at them from various angles—circling the area, pressing with varying intensities, gradually working your way into the center of the tightness and dissolving it altogether.

In yoga you do much the same thing, but differently. Using the pose both as a map and tool, you deliberately explore yourself, looking for tight, sore, or painful areas within yourself. You look for them so you can erase them. You then gently stretch them, press and squeeze them, breathe into them, relax and release them, and thereby ease away the tension and open the contracted area. This allows new energy to flush through you, nourishing undernourished areas, soothing chronic pain, and improving energy flow throughout the whole of you—revitalizing you. You can actually increase your vitality and improve your experience of you. This is done slowly, carefully, with sensitivity and feeling— enjoying what you are doing. You creatively and intuitively make subtle internal adjustments in the poses as you deliberately search for even the smallest knots of tension. This is not an attack against yourself, remember, and it should not feel like one. It's a loving gesture.

This is like going through your garden and pulling out the weeds. If you do this daily, eventually you'll have only baby weeds, and your work will be considerably easier. When you are really weed-free, the poses will feel clean, and there will be the experience of free-flowing, unobstructed energy.

Like the yawn, the early morning stretch, the neck roll and massage, yoga feels wonderful. And why not? You're releasing tension, relieving pain, and improving energy flow. It's liberating, energizing, healing. It's exhilarating. As you move inward and take care of every part of yourself, as you sweep through your energy field and ease away the pain—pulling out the weeds, creating more space and comfort, flooding yourself with new life—you'll not only realize you are taking superb care of yourself, that you are undergoing a deep cleansing and healing, and that you are truly making yourself more radiant, but your outlook on life is changing. You'll find yourself being different, and as a consequence, you'll understand the world and everyone in it differently, too.

More importantly, though, you'll realize you are not becoming different . . . you're becoming who you've always been. You're consciously "becoming" the genuine, authentic You—the You that is the Son or Daughter of God, the Father-Mother. This is radical! It's not just "feeling good"—and it's not just physical.

This is only an approximation, remember. It's as close as I can get to describing what yoga feels like to me. Actually, yoga is more studied than simple stretching. It's slower, more deliberate and conscious. It does not have the same random exuberance as an early morning yawn and stretch, for the most part. Yet it feels better! Sometimes you will press firmly as you stretch, other times you'll stretch with less intensity and be soft. Your intent will change and flow according to the need. Sometimes you will stay on one specific spot, remaining motionless, letting the stretch penetrate; other times you will work the area more generally. Yoga has many moods. One is not better than another.

The idea is to be increasingly sensitive, appropriate in the moment, so that each moment of practice feels perfect, alluring, desirable—and then to be as wholehearted as possible. The more yoga you do, the easier this will be, and the better you'll get at doing it. Getting "better" at yoga is not only a matter of becoming stronger and more flexible, of becoming more proficient in the poses, but of getting better at finding the specific alignment in each pose—moment by moment by moment—that feels perfect to you, *and* of wholeheartedly immersing yourself in the experience. The ability to immerse yourself in your conscious experience of the poses and meditations, to be more and more fully present in the Now, is what will cause this awareness to infiltrate naturally into the rest of your life. This, of course, is what it's all about.

Your breathing is the key. Breathing brings the poses to life. It's what animates the stretches and gives yoga its fluidity and flow. As you immerse yourself in the flowing rise-and-fall rhythm of your breathing, you'll begin to sense that really there is only one breath; even an hour of yoga is just one long continuous stream of breath flowing in and out. The idea, the training, is to make your awareness as continuous as the breath. You do this by staying with the breath continuously, breathing consciously. Therefore, pay attention to your breathing; listen to it, feel it, taste it, savor and enjoy it. This flowing awareness of unbroken continuity will bring an integrated and increasingly meaningful sense to your practice.

What makes asana practice especially interesting, however, is the fact that you are working with an energy field–*your* energy field. You are not just stretching and squeezing muscles, bones, skin, and tissues—simply being therapeutic. You are changing your energy pattern, the way your energy flows. The pattern is expressed in your muscles and tissues, and this is where you'll feel the changes taking place, but what you're changing is the underlying pattern. Consistent asana and meditation practice will improve the way your energy flows, and this will change the way you experience yourself—transforming the way you perceive and relate to the world.

The various asanas and meditations have proven themselves to be especially effective at relaxing tense, painful areas of your body and in strengthening weak areas. They have powerful therapeutic value in dealing with physical and psychological problems. They improve circulation and glandular function. They retard aging. They increase the strength, stamina, and flexibility you need for other activities. They increase your sensitivity. They enhance your looks, your posture, your skin and muscle tone. You'll find it easier to sit comfortably in meditation and remain attuned to the creative life force energy within you. The practice of yoga will help bring a welcome, renewed vitality to your life. You will feel more alive as you allow the creative life force to flow through you unobstructed. This feels good.

Learning yoga will often feel as though you are learning something you already know how to do. This is not surprising since we are all familiar with the wonderful feeling of stretching and yawning after a restful sleep and of spontaneously taking a deep breath in clean mountain air. Yoga is a way of consciously bringing these natural surges into daily life. The joy and refreshment of a deep, full breath in combination with the exhilaration of a deep, strong stretch is rejuvenating. To deepen your breath is literally to inspire yourself, and to stretch, expand, and allow greater openness in your energy field is to experience, acknowledge, and embrace a bigger sense of who you are. As you embrace the fullness of yourself without inhibition or apology, you will be able more fully to participate in the world in a constructive and meaningful way.

Be happy you know how to practice. The practice will make you happy.

# PART

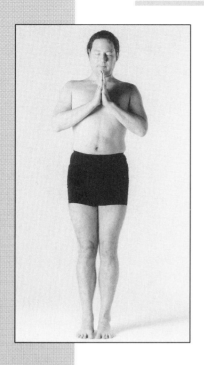

# TWO

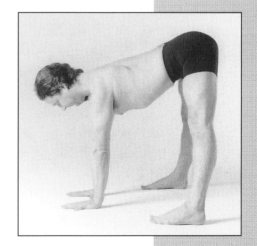

# 5

## ASANA FUNDAMENTALS

There are three fundamental themes of asana practice. They are: 1) ujjayi breathing, 2) lines of energy, and 3) playing the edge. I will explain each of these separately in the following chapters and then illustrate their application as we go through the poses.

First, let's look at the fundamental building blocks that comprise the basic poses. The building blocks are made up of the seven primary types of movements your body can make. Every yoga posture is simply one possible combination of these basic movements. Advanced postures are deeper extensions and different combinations that, being more intricate and efficient, enable you to exercise several areas of your body simultaneously.

## Asana Building Blocks

The seven primary types of movement are:

- ◆ *flexion* (decreasing the angle at the joint—such as chin to chest)
- ◆ *extension* (increasing the angle at the joint or a return from flexion—such as the head returning to erect alignment)
- ◆ *hyperextension* (a continuation of extension beyond the starting position or beyond the vertical plane line at the ear—such as dunking your head backward)
- ◆ *abduction* (sideward movement away from the midline—arms or legs moving out to the sides)
- ◆ *adduction* (return from abduction—bringing the arms back to the sides)
- ◆ *rotation* (left, right, inward, and outward)
- ◆ *circumduction* (when a movement describes a cone—such as arm circling).

In addition there is *hyperflexion* (a term used when the upper arm is flexed beyond vertical), *lateral flexion* (lateral bending of the head or trunk), *supination* (outward rotation of the forearm), *pronation* (inward rotation of the forearm), *inversion* (turning the sole inward, weight on the outer edge of foot), *eversion* (turning the sole outward, weight on the inner edge of foot), *dorsal flexion* (movement of the top of the foot toward the shin bone), and *plantar flexion* (movement of the sole of the foot toward the floor).

The movements of your foot at the ankle are dorsiflexion and plantar flexion, as well as inversion and eversion. These movements can be found in poses such as Dog Pose (dorsiflexion), Hero Pose (plantar flexion), and Lotus Pose (inversion). Your knees are capable of flexion and extension. These movements can be found in poses such as Hero Pose (flexion) and Mountain Pose (extension). Your hips are capable of flexion, extension, hyperextension, abduction, adduction, and internal and external rotation: Reclining Leg Stretch (flexion), Locust Pose (hyperextension), Spread Leg Forward Fold (abduction), Hero Pose (inward rotation), Lotus (outward rotation). Your shoulders are capable of flexion, extension, abduction, adduction, internal and external rotation, upward rotation of scapula, elevation and depression of scapula, and hyperextension. These movements are found in poses such as the Standing Forward Fold, Dog Pose, and the Shoulder Openers. Your neck is capable of flexion, hyperextension, lateral flexion and rotation: Bridge Pose (flexion), Locust Pose (hyperextension), Standing Side Stretch (lateral flexion), Sage Twist (rotation). And your spine is capable of flexion, hyperextension, lateral flexion, and rotation: Standing Forward Fold (body flexion), Locust Pose (hyperextension), Standing Side Stretch (lateral flexion), and Sage Twist (rotation).

The above selection can be contained in ten poses: Standing Forward Fold, Standing Side Stretch, Dog Pose, Spread Leg Forward Fold, Bridge Pose, Reclining Leg Stretch, Locust Pose, Sage Twist, Hero Pose, Shoulder Openers, and the Lotus. These are the core poses. It's important to learn these well. A skillful practice grounded in these basic postures will enable you to progress safely to more advanced postures and variations.

Using these ten as the core of my selection, I have chosen forty-five of my favorite poses to illustrate the basic principles of yoga. These forty-five poses form an excellent summary of what most people can aim for and eventually accomplish with ease.

We will go over these poses thoroughly, finding ways to make them easier or more difficult to suit your needs. Some poses will probably be easier for you than others. You may also have a natural proclivity toward either forward bending or backward bending, and toward twisting in a particular direction more than the other. If you are stiff or tight in a particular pose, it can always be traced back to one or several of the basic building blocks. Being aware of your areas of tightness and the postures and variations that are relevant to them allows you to tailor your daily practice to your own needs.

Seen in this light, being an inflexible beginner is in many ways an advantage. Because your range of movement is limited, you have no choice but to learn the basics thoroughly—proceeding gradually, step by step, with plenty of time to master the early stages before adding more difficult steps. Even if you happen to be in exceptionally good shape, avoid the natural tendency to rush deeply into the postures before learning the initial steps properly. Have patience and learn these poses well.

Before we begin, please understand that the various postures are designed to open and release the various tight areas of your body gradually. It may take you a while before you can do them all with ease. Be patient. Take your time. Enjoy the process. Keep in mind that the poses are not destinations, nor are they strange contortions to force yourself into for some esoteric purpose. They are part of an ongoing process of self-exploration and self-healing. Each individual pose is a map into a specific area of yourself, and where you are in the pose *is* the pose for you. Immersing yourself in the process is the important thing. That's what's interesting, not the achievement of elaborate postures. Involvement in the process will yield the results you desire.

Yoga done properly is not a competition, even with yourself. It's a matter of doing what you can at any given moment, of being aware of what you're doing, of building strength and endurance, and of gently working out the tight spots. But whether you're more flexible than you were yesterday is not the point. Where you are in the pose will vary each time you practice. The idea is to start calmly wherever you are and progressively work toward deeper movements by practicing the intermediary steps that lead you to the final pose. If, for example, you are unable to cross your legs in Lotus, then you need to practice the in-between steps that you are able to do now. If you do these regularly, you will eventually sit comfortably in Lotus.

Your daily practice should include all the core poses mentioned earlier, plus Headstand and Shoulderstand once you have correctly mastered them. Once your practice has been established, you can spend extra time deepening either your forward bending, backward bending, or twists, or concentrate on problem areas that need more attention. You can spend extra time on your backbends in general, for example, or your Upward Bow in particular. Or you can focus on poses that will deepen your forward bending, prepare you for Splits, or enable you eventually to bring your legs behind your head (the ultimate forward fold!). If you are unable to balance on your head, spend time with that.

Your progress will be steady and natural as you practice these basic poses regularly. For now, be happy doing them in their easy form. They are the help you need to establish your firm foundation in yoga. Always perform the poses slowly and with care. Never fight yourself. Mastery of these easy poses will make the more difficult poses easy. Most of all, learn to enjoy your practice.

The significance of everything I have put down will become apparent only as you spend private time with your own practice. The secrets of yoga lie in the doing of it, and only as your personal practice matures will your yoga become truly your own. Be sure you understand this, for it is the case with so many things. The advances you make and the depths you plumb are fundamentally up to you. My major interest is to share with you a way of doing yoga that you can apply to any posture you ever do, whatever your level of proficiency, and to assure you that the fruits of practice will carry over into all aspects of your life.

With that in mind, the best way to prepare yourself mentally for the proper practice of yoga is to think of it as a time of communion and renewal. Think of your body as the temple or home of individualized God, Consciousness in specific expression, and of each asana as a prayer. Learn to do each pose as though it were the center of all life and of all other poses. Each pose you perform will automatically suggest the whole universe of which it is a part. Nothing exists in isolation. The old masters knew this well. This is the secret of yoga.

# 6

## THE WIND THROUGH THE INSTRUMENT

Think of your body as a musical instrument, a wind instrument. Your breath, accordingly, is the wind through the instrument. As such, it is the single most important aspect of yoga technique. Traditionally considered the primary carrier of *prana*—life force—your breathing originates deep inside you, radiates outward and then inward, providing a gentle and steady rhythm for movement, stretch and release. Sometimes you will breathe softly, other times with vigor, but the breathing itself will always be a central and governing focus. Proper breathing brings the poses to life, inspires every subtle shift and movement in every yoga posture, and can help center your awareness in your conscious experience of the now.

## Ujjayi Breathing

The main type of breathing we do in yoga is called *ujjayi* (ooh-JAI-yee). Ujjayi breathing, known as the "victory breath," is characterized by an audibly hollow, deep, soft sound coming from your throat.

*The main idea is to coordinate your movements with your breathing*. This brings a graceful and sensuous quality to your practice and turns each yoga session into a fluid and creative meditation. As you become skillful at this, the breath and movement will no longer feel distinct. You will experience them as one action, inseparably entwined. You will instinctively breathe as you move or stretch, and move or stretch as you breathe.

Certain movements are always done on inhale, others on exhale. The type of breath (inhale or exhale) depends on what works most naturally on your body. Each specific movement should start with the initiation of the appropriate breath. Opening movements such as backbends and lifting arms are done on inhale. Folding or closing movements such as forward bends and lowering arms are done on exhale. For example, you raise your arms overhead on inhale, and lower them

47

on exhale. The movement, though, is initiated or inspired by the breath and is surrounded by breath.

This pattern makes sense, for it's what happens naturally. When you expand or open there's more room, so that air naturally enters; and when you fold or close, air is squeezed out. If you run short of breath before a particular movement is completed, stop moving, finish the breathing cycle you are now on (exhale if you have just inhaled, inhale if you have just exhaled), and continue moving with the next appropriate phase of breath. In this way an inhaling movement such as arm raising is always done on inhale, even if it requires some exhales in between. Always move with the breath, and only move when you are breathing. One inhale plus one exhale equals a single breath.

# Push and Yield

Every yoga posture involves a "push" and a "yield." Pushing is an active force that moves the body further and deeper into the posture, gently exploring areas of tightness. Yielding is a passive force with which you wait and listen to the moment-to-moment feedback from your body; it's a letting go of resistance that allows the active force to be successful without being aggressive. The pushing and yielding elements occur simultaneously, as in a dance. Done properly, therefore, yoga is a matter of pushing and yielding, of "doing" and "not-doing," at the same time.

The breath plays a key role in this simultaneous push-yield activity because of its ability to function both automatically and under conscious control. It's the perfect bridge between push and yield, control and surrender, doing and not-doing, and it represents a unique link between these two forces.

Skill in yoga involves orchestrating these two forces with the breath. This means that sometimes you will push with the breath into your tight areas, or challenge your endurance, or deliberately increase your sense of "fire" and energy by consciously breathing with more vigor and intensity. At other times you will ride the breath and stay soft, mellow, and be in a pose with minimal effort. With your breathing you can creatively orchestrate the tone of your practice.

# Guided from Within

Normally we think of the conscious mind as the controller of movement. But consider what it would be like steering a car, typing, running, walking, hitting a tennis ball, dribbling a basketball, anything, if you had to think consciously about what you were doing. Actually, as a beginner in yoga or anything else, you must begin by thinking. In fact, learning an activity even involves a different part of the brain than is used to perform it once you know it. This part of the brain works more slowly and uses more energy than the other, so during this initial learning phase you'll need to move gently, slowly—with heightened awareness. You'll need to think carefully about the pose, the breath, the lines of energy, and you will need to learn all the fundamentals of technique. Only when you have graduated from that halting stage, however, will you attain grace and efficiency. This is because the conscious mind is too slow. There is always a space or gap between what the mind says it wants to be doing and what the body actually does. In this gap between intention and execution, between the "ought" and the "is," there is always a loss of energy.

In yoga this separation comes to an end when you allow the breath to replace the thinking mind as the guiding impulse behind movement and stretch. This involves merging so thoroughly with the breath that you are not thinking about anything else. This moment, this breath, this now, is all-important. You immerse yourself so totally that the usual separation between you and the pose dissolves.

This makes it easier to listen to your body. Instead of pushing your body around with only your muscles or your mind, you learn to be guided from within—only moving when your body says it's ready. You learn to push when that is appropriate, and you learn to wait, hold back, or retreat when that is appropriate. Appropriateness is something you cannot anticipate in advance. Knowing when to push or when to yield is fundamentally only knowable in the living instant of each new moment. Being sensitive in this way is the result of having merged and "become one" with the pose.

As you merge the pose with the breathing, you will feel the breath gently nudging, coaxing, opening, stretching, and relaxing your muscles and various tight areas. These areas are contracted energy, contracted parts of you. Releasing them, therefore, will not only give you more energy, but it will make you more comfortable in your body as well.

Merging the pose with the breath will also increase your sensitivity. You'll feel what's happening with more clarity. You'll notice how holding the breath dulls your feeling-sensitivity, and how letting the breath flow freely and deeply increases it. You'll notice how your breathing actually fans the feeling, increasing and clarifying it, heightening your ability to sense yourself. Learning to feel, and feel deeply, is one of the more important learnings in yoga. Proper breathing will directly enhance your feeling-sensitivity.

The idea is to increase your sensitivity to the inner feeling of your body and let it guide you into the appropriate action for that particular moment. That's the secret—the primary thing to learn. The trick is gently to concentrate your attention on the steady flow of breath and ride it into the feeling-tone of the pose. The feeling-tone of the pose will then talk to you. It will instruct you about what to do, what subtle adjustments to make, whether or not to press deeper into the stretch, whether to breathe with more vigor or more gentleness, and how long to stay in the pose.

In this way you exercise your sensitivity and develop self-trust. Your yoga will become increasingly internal. It will become your own. You will no longer feel as though you are doing someone else's yoga. You will have learned how to learn from yourself, and you'll find this most important trait carrying over into all aspects of your life. You will then understand that you have truly learned how to do yoga only when you've become your own best teacher, which means being guided from within.

However, you will only hear the inner feeling talking to you if you are listening. If your mind is elsewhere while your body is doing the pose, you are not actually doing yoga. You are not "in union" with what's happening. You're close, of course. There is a semblance of yoga occurring, and doing it at all is better than not doing it, but the practice here is that of merging and becoming one with what you're doing. You're practicing yoga, yoking or "joining with." You're learning to merge, to yoke your conscious awareness with your now-experience—and you're practicing in this relatively simple and specific context where there are fewer variables to contend with. You're training yourself to keep your attention immersed in what's happening. Specifically, you're learning to stay with the flow of breath in order to stay with the feeling of the pose. The inner feeling will then guide you and tell you what to do. You will have learned how to do yoga when you've become willing to be guided from within.

In the broader context of what it means to live a yogic life, the idea is to continue this awareness all day long—not just in the poses. The poses, besides being good for you for so many reasons, are simply a specific context in which to practice being guided from within. During the day, practice this same kind of listening for inner guidance by paying attention to how you feel and then allow yourself to do and be as you are prompted. There's more to say about this later. For now, suffice it to say that asana and meditation practice make it easier to hear and follow your inner voice during the rest of your life, to let "Thy Will be done" be your basic instinct. They strengthen your ability to meditate constantly, always to be listening inwardly for guidance from Infinite Mind, and they develop the confidence required to trust yourself and go with the flow. When you are willing to be guided by the inner feeling, you will have learned the secret.

# Balance

The proper use of breath also brings a balance in the way your body opens to the stretch. When the force normally used to push the body into greater opening is balanced by the relaxation that comes from proper breathing, a new kind of energized relaxation emerges. We normally think of relaxation as a letting-go that is flaccid, a diminution or lessening of energy. Proper breathing, however, adds a vital and dynamic aspect to relaxation.

In order for yoga to feel right, a proper balance is necessary between push and yield. Too much push has a driven quality that betrays a harshness and severity toward oneself that is probably displayed in other areas of life as well. Your practice will be permeated with an emphasis on energy that is untamed, scattered, and often violent in nature. Injury, as well as an agitated, off-center state of mind is likely to result.

The other extreme occurs when ''fire'' is lacking, when there is no exploratory thrust, when it is predominantly yield. Yoga performed in this manner is dull and lethargic, all effort, energy, and intensity being avoided. There is a relaxed and sometimes sensuous quality to this, but yoga done in too yielding a fashion never develops the openings or strength that provide the energized relaxation that is so appealing and revitalizing.

Depending on your personality, you may find yourself tending toward one or the other of these extremes. If so, understand that there is an appropriate balance of these forces. If you tend toward being aggressive and overly goal-oriented, try allowing more surrender and yield into your practice. This will not slow down or interfere with your progress. In fact, learning to yield, be patient, and deliberately enter more slowly into the poses will actually increase the depth of your poses. It will help you achieve more easily what you are now attempting through excessive force. Your practice will mature in ways you had not anticipated, revealing an unexpected richness and depth.

If your tendency is to yield and not be assertive, try being more adventuresome, energetic, and exploratory. This can work to your advantage and be very pleasing, without being difficult or stressful. The analogy of an early morning yawn and stretch again comes to mind. If you were to wake up and simply hold your arms out limply to your sides, it just wouldn't feel as satisfying as it does to stretch with enthusiasm. It feels better to invest a little energy—to stretch with some intensity. It's not difficult to do this. It's exhilarating, invigorating.

An effective way of bringing a balance here, regardless of which extreme you tend toward, involves using your breathing and the line of energy technique (which I will describe later) to generate energy, but at relatively easy places in the pose. This will satisfy the hunger to push for those who like to push, and respect the tendency to yield for others. It will also teach those who like to push how to yield, and those who like to yield how to push. Done this way, your strength, endurance, and flexibility will all increase at a pace your body can assimilate and retain. You will become stronger, lighter, more relaxed, sensuous, and comfortable in your body than you will by just pushing or by just yielding.

Yoga that has a proper balance between the active and passive feels wonderful. It is not overly aggressive or torpid, but a harmonious and complimentary blend of push and yield. It is at once both vigorous and quiet, like a perfectly centered top spinning so fast it appears motionless.

Be sure you understand, however, it involves push *and* yield—both. Sometimes it is appropriate to push, and at those times it feels best to generate energy and push; other times it will be more appropriate to yield and it will feel better to surrender, let go, and be passive. And yet, even in a given moment when you are primarily pushing, there is much more than this going on. You are also waiting for your body to let you in. You are not only pushing. And if, at a given particular moment you are primarily yielding, you are also simultaneously exercising control to some degree in order mentally to direct the energy flow and continue staying in the pose. You are not just yielding. It is always push and yield.

The important idea to keep in mind is to be guided always by the inner feeling. This is one of the primary teachings of yoga. Here, in the physical practice, you listen to your body. You start easy. You do the groundwork. You listen inwardly to the subtle impulses to action that arise while you are in a posture. You then follow the impulses of the moment—stretching here, stretching there, breathing deeper or softer, making subtle internal adjustments, increasing or decreasing the intensity of the pose, whatever meets the need. The need is to do whatever is necessary to make this moment feel perfect, to do what feels best. You *learn* to do this. But you also allow yourself to do this. Your feelings, by the way, are a trustworthy guide to action because only what is best can feel best. You can therefore trust yourself to trust yourself. You have your own best interests at heart.

Therefore, by listening to the impulses of the moment and following your own inner guidance in the postures, you are actually exercising your sensitivity and developing self-trust. Self-trust, remember, is more than merely trusting yourself. It's that quality of being that arises when you realize you did not create yourself, that you are an expression of the creative God Force, and that there is an underlying spiritual orderliness to all things you are a part of. In trusting yourself, therefore, you are not trusting "you," you are trusting that deeper essence that is the source of you. Trusting yourself then becomes the most intimate way of trusting the universe and the most obvious demonstration of that greater trust.

Proper use of the breath will enhance your ability to feel, to listen inwardly, to be guided from within, and thereby to learn from yourself. It will also teach you to sustain a sharp, focused attention for longer periods of time. In combination, these strengthen your mental stamina and help you be wholehearted.

The ujjayi breathing technique in particular is a very effective centering device. As you hold your attention on the sound of the breath, the quality of your participation will improve dramatically. This new quality of undivided attention and full participation will facilitate your personal experience of yoga. A sense of oneness will then guide you and tell you what to do, and you will notice yourself becoming more creative and intuitive, not only in your yoga but in your life.

# Interest, Attention, and Enjoyment

It is difficult to pay attention to something if you are not interested in that thing. But it is also difficult to be interested if you are not paying attention. For example, you may be watching the best film in the world. But if you are thinking of something else and are not paying attention, you will miss the subtle nuances that make the film so good, and you won't appreciate or enjoy it as much as you might. Interest, attention, and enjoyment are obviously interrelated. Of course, if you are not interested in doing yoga at the moment, you should really be doing something else. Or you may be interested but unable to maintain a focused attention for an extended period of time. Ujjayi breathing can create that focus.

Each breath you take can remind you to be here now, to treat this moment as important, and repeatedly to affirm the fact that right now you are exactly where you want to be, doing exactly what you want to be doing. You will probably be amazed at how much energy is suddenly at your disposal the moment you realize this. When you are no longer wishing you were somewhere else, doing something different, you will discover that energy is the given and that energy is abundant. What would you expect but the fullest enthusiasm and response when your body, mind, heart, attention, and interest are all in one place? When your attention is no longer splintered and dissipated through conflict, indecisiveness, or half-heartedness, you will experience an increase in energy and feel more alive.

This is especially interesting because, unless you are an absolute beginner, you'll find your mind tiring long before your body. When your mind begins to tire, only then does your body start getting tired. As your interest begins to flicker and wane, you become less attentive. You start thinking of other things, wishing you were elsewhere. Your energy goes elsewhere. You treat your body and your yoga with less care, less respect; and automatically but not surprisingly, your body—following the dictates of your mind—loses its energy and also gets tired. But as you stay clear within yourself that this is what you want to be doing right now, you will be able to sustain interest and attention for longer periods of time. As your capacity for attention increases, so does your energy, your actual physical energy.

Your mental attitude, therefore, is the real source of energy and enthusiasm, and you will learn this very quickly in yoga. Interest is the key. Be interested in the quality of your participation, in discovering where your interest actually lies. Notice what attracts your attention and what motivates you. And attend to the change of tide—when do you start being less interested, and why? What brings it to life again? Notice how your interest fluctuates, how at some moments you are more interested than at other moments. This is not only the heart of yoga, it is the heart of life.

And understand, if the quality of your participation is half-hearted, fragmented, and conflicted, then that will be your experience, and it will not be as satisfying or fulfilling as it might. It's not that you *should* be wholehearted and fully attentive. It's that more and more you will want to be that way simply because being wholehearted and attentive to your present moment of conscious experience is where the greatest enjoyment lies. In this way it is possible to make every specific moment of your yoga practice enjoyable and meaningful.

It's worth the small effort required to discipline yourself mentally to be attentive and present with whatever is happening each new moment. The way to stay most interested is by keeping your attention on what's actually happening. Train yourself to stay in the now. Specifically, stay with the breath and stay with the feeling of the pose. You will only hear the pose talking to you if you are listening and paying attention. Sometimes you will practice with vigor, sometimes you will practice with softness, and most of the time it will be somewhere in between. Yoga is not mechanical. The key is interest, and the trick is to be attentive in the moment to that which elicits your fullest enthusiasm and response.

The quality of your yoga, and of your life, depends solely on how interested you are in the doing of it. Interest unleashes the energy of passion, and passion expresses itself as quality.

Therefore, especially toward the end of a session when both your body and your attention are beginning to tire, deliberately continue breathing with the ujjayi breath. It is not hard to do this, and to do so strengthens your capacity for attention. Strengthening your capacity for attention is the real key to yoga, and your breathing is the key to this capacity. This is more important than being able to touch your toes, or stand on your head, or turn yourself inside out.

# How to Do It

Ujjayi breathing is not difficult to learn. It involves narrowing the aperture in your throat by gently tightening the epiglottis, which is done like this:

Softly whisper the syllable "ha" with your mouth open. Haaaaaaaaaaaa. Stretch it out. Feel the air vibrating softly in the back of your throat. Listen to the clean, hollow sound; it's similar to the sound of the ocean you can hear in a shell. Produce this sound as you are inhaling and exhaling. Try it. Take a number of breaths this way.

Now close your mouth and continue making the same soft, smooth, deep, and hollow sound. This is easiest as you exhale, but it is also possible as you inhale. You are now breathing through your nostrils with your mouth closed, and yet the suction is coming from the back of your throat. The nostrils are relaxed and passive, and you will therefore feel the air in your nostrils only very lightly. You are not sniffing the air in. You are gently drawing the air in from the back of your throat. Breathe like this in all the postures.

Many people can do the ujjayi breath immediately. Others take longer. If you have trouble, I can only encourage you to keep trying. It is well worth learning and will have an immediate impact on your yoga. Once you get it, use as little effort as possible. Eliminate every trace of strain. Make a clean, even sound without any lumps or surges in it. Breathe as though you were drinking the air through a long, slim straw. Do not gulp the air. Draw in long, sure, thin breaths. At first it will be erratic, especially if you are new to a posture. Eventually you are looking for a smooth, deep breath.

There are several advantages to breathing in this fashion. First, narrowing the valve in the throat enables you to develop a very fine control over the amount of air flow. This will lengthen and deepen your breath considerably.

Secondly, the lungs and diaphragm are strengthened since they have to pull harder against the resistance in the throat. With the added push and pull, the lungs work more as a bellows, creating additional energy that can be focused and channeled into different parts of your body. You will not tire as easily. Once you get a feeling for the ujjayi breath, you will not want to breathe any other way during yoga. As you establish a smooth rhythm with the ujjayi breath, it will feel as though you have harnessed a strong, gentle power.

Finally, a sound in the throat naturally draws your attention to the breath. This strengthens your concentration and makes it more difficult for your mind to wander, or at least more obvious when it does. The sound lets you know whether the breath is flowing smoothly and evenly, or not. And being aware of the breath helps you be aware of your whole body, for the breath is a direct reflection of your state of comfort or discomfort, ease or strain. When your body is comfortable and free of undue strain, you will be able to breathe smoothly and deeply with a pleasant sound coming from your throat. Breathing smoothly, in return, promotes a sense of ease in the poses. When you are unable to produce an even and pleasant ujjayi sound, it means you are straining, that the pose is perhaps too difficult for you, and that you should really be careful not to overstep your present level of skill or physical conditioning. Breathing with the ujjayi throat sound is a built-in safety mechanism.

The proper use of breath acts as a very fine tool for creating and sustaining an energized relaxation, as well as for centering your awareness in the present moment.

# Preparation for Breathing

**1** Sit or stand with one hand on your abdomen and the other on your heart on a level with the base of the breastbone. Using your hands this way will help you sense what you are doing more accurately. Exhale by pulling the abdomen inward, backward toward the spine. To inhale, simply release the inward abdominal pull and allow your belly to swell gently forward into your hand. A natural suction will occur, and air will come in automatically. Do not press your belly forward, keep it strain-free, and for the moment do not allow the top hand to move. Move only the abdomen. Breathe like this for about a minute.

**2** Place your palms on the sides of your chest, level with the bottom of the breastbone; have your fingertips barely touching. Exhale deeply first. Then breathe in deeply and expand your chest, attempting to move the fingertips horizontally away from the midline. Make your chest round. Notice how the chest can be expanded in all directions—sideways, forward and backward, and upward—simply by moving the sternum (breastbone) upward. As you exhale, gently squeeze the rib cage inward with your hands; this will help create greater elasticity throughout the rib cage. Breathe like this for about a minute.

Think of "how" to breathe as a combination of the above two preparations. The inhalation starts with the gentle swelling forward of the abdomen and then moves upward to expand the rib cage fully. The breastbone rises and swells forward as the shoulder blades slide down your back. These actions increase the distance between the top of the thighs and the bottom of the ribs—the area of your waist—and it is this increased space that gives the diaphragm freedom to move. As you exhale, allow the ribs to relax and come back to center without losing the spinal length you achieved with the inhalation, and then gently pull the abdomen inward. Breathe like this in all the poses throughout the practice.

**1** Exhale fully first. This will flatten the abdomen, empty the lungs, and create room for a deep inhalation.

**2** To inhale, simply relax the abdominal contraction and allow your belly to gently swell forward a little. This part of the inhalation is passive. You do not have to do anything. Do not press your belly outward in an attempt to get more air. Simply release the inward pull of your abdomen. Air will come in effortlessly.

**3** Aim the breath upward into the sternum to expand your chest and slide the shoulder blades down your back. Actively lift the ribs upward as you emphasize the sideways movement of your lower ribs, the backward expansion and widening of your back, and the forward and upward expansion into the sternum. This will insure the full excursion of the diaphragm, pull the air deep into your lungs, and flatten the abdomen somewhat. Do not shrug your shoulders upward as you do this; keep them down and relaxed. Savor the air.

**4** Finally, pull the air all the way up into the clavicles and top of the chest. This will widen the chest across the top, smooth out the collarbones, and help move the shoulders gently back and down.

**5** To exhale, allow the ribs to relax, release the air slowly, and gently pull the abdomen in. Maintain the length you achieved in the area of your waist and keep the sternum raised and chest open. Allow the crown of your head to continue floating upward.

Breathing in this fashion fills the lungs fully. Every inhalation will actually increase the distance between your hips and lower ribs, the area of your waist, and elongate the spine and torso. This is an important movement in many of the poses and is the reason to aim the breath upward into your chest. By straightening the spine and lifting the ribs, you will gain greater freedom of movement in your waist, spine, and shoulders. The upper half of your body will have more freedom, and your legs will move more freely within the hip sockets. There will be more ''space'' inside your body, more comfort and ease.

As you breathe in this fashion, attempt to make the transitions from your belly to your chest to the clavicles fluid and smooth on both the inhalation and exhalation. You should feel a wavelike rhythm to it, as if the breath were rippling through your body.

# Breathing in Postures

There are a few very simple guidelines for breathing in postures. Imagine your lungs as a pair of balloons. They fill as you breathe in and empty as you breathe out. As they fill they rise and float, becoming taller and rounder. They expand in all directions—upward, downward, sideways, forward, and back. You can feel the air going backward into your back, forward into your chest, sideways from just below the armpits, and up, elongating your spine. Any movement that enlarges your chest or lengthens your spine, expanding the balloons, is enhanced by an inhalation. Any movement that compresses the balloons, reducing lung volume, naturally squeezes the air out and should be an exhalation.

♦ *Any time the body is folding and becoming more compact, the movement is done on the* **exhalation**.

◆ *Any time there is an unfolding, a straightening of the body or an opening of the chest, the movement is done on the* **inhalation**.

For example, in the Seated Forward Fold, you would exhale as you fold forward and inhale as you come up.

Moving into postures that curve your spine backward and open the chest, such as Cobra Pose, are done with the inhalation.

◆ *Twisting motions are done on* **exhalation**.

In advanced twisting poses, however, it becomes more complex. When the twist takes place in the lower spine, you would activate the twisting action with the exhalation. When it takes place in the upper spine, you would use the inhalation.

◆ *When the weight of your body is doing the stretching for you, release deeper into the stretch as you* **exhale**.

These guidelines are not rigid, and occasionally in more advanced postures there may be exceptions. But they work pretty well. As you learn more about yoga and develop a feeling for it, however, *feeling* becomes the most important criterion. Once you have a feeling for what you are doing, whatever feels best generally is the best. Meanwhile, these guidelines will help develop an inner feeling for breathing in postures.

Once you are in a posture, the same phase of breath that got you there is used whenever you deepen in the same direction. In other words, unless you are very warmed up, you will not get as deep as possible in just one breath. Each successive breath will take you a little deeper. In the Seated Forward Fold, for example, you would fold deeper with each successive exhalation; doing the Cobra, each successive inhalation would increase your depth.

Many postures have several opposing stretches, giving you the opportunity to use both the inhalation and the exhalation to deepen. For example, a major component of any foward fold is the deliberate elongation of the spine prior to folding foward. The folding forward is with the exhalation, but the elongation of spine is done as you inhale. Therefore, both the inhalation and the exhalation are used to increase your depth in the pose. You'd inhale to lengthen your spine and exhale to deepen the fold. If you were doing a twisting posture, you would inhale to elongate the spine, and then turn, twist, and rotate with the exhalation, over and over.

At first, it is important to segment the moves like this, to pay deliberate attention to the ujjayi breath, and to isolate and choreograph what you are doing. It will flow and be more fluid as you become more skillful.

Deepening occurs not only in the stretch but in the breath as well. Without forcing or making yourself uncomfortable, work toward a deeper, slower, and more flowing breath as you hold and deepen your postures. You will notice that if you are at all frightened, tense, or uncomfortable, parts of you will resist, your breathing will be strained and erratic, and it will feel as though you are working against yourself. Deepening the breath, however, will expand you from inside. It will also increase your intake volume of air and lengthen the time span of each breath. More air will give you more energy, and lengthening the time span of each breath will encourage a sense of calm. Being energetic and calm, your body will open with minimal resistance.

You have probably noticed how shallow and constricted your breathing becomes when you are anxious, fearful, uncomfortable, or off-center. Emotions affect breathing. Just the opposite can happen in yoga, especially in postures that work the diaphragm through deeper twisting, backward bending, or tight forward folds. Your breathing will become shallow and rapid, and at first this can make you anxious, claustrophobic, or uncomfortable. But by learning to sustain your extensions with a slower, deeper, and more regular breath, you can maintain a relaxed attitude of mind. This will encourage your body to open at its optimum pace.

In any case, do not be bound by these suggestions. They are guidelines, not rules. Understand them, acquire a feeling for them, and then use them to your advantage. Feel yourself expanding and drawing in life energy as you inhale, relaxing inside as you exhale. And become familiar with the inner sense of how your body wants to move and breathe. It will always tell you what to do. Experiment with the suggestions, discover what feels natural, and then let yourself be creative and intuitive, always guided from within.

# How to Combine Breath and Movement

The ability to coordinate skillfully your movements and stretches with your breathing so they function as one is a fundamental theme in hatha yoga. It is more than merely coordinating them, however. It is understanding they are the same. Breath and movement are one. The breath creates and fuels the movement—just as the movement shapes and changes the breath.

To combine the breath and movement, follow this three-step approach:

**1** Learn the basic movement without concentrating on the breathing; breathe normally, without restriction.

**2** Coordinate the movement with the appropriate phase of breath: Inhale on expanding movements, exhale on compressing movements.

**3** Let the breath take over. Feel the breath inspiring the movement. Then, by allowing the breath to initiate the action, create a sense of oneness between the breath and the movement. Let this be more than merely coordinating them skillfully or technically. Remember, you are a wind instrument. Let the breath move through you. Bring the pose to life with the breath. Be inspired.

Acquire a feeling for this with the following very simple arm movement. Stand with your feet together and your arms by your sides. Then:

**1** Breathe normally as you slowly raise the arms from your sides until the thumbs touch above your head, then slowly bring the arms back down. Raise and lower your arms slowly and leisurely at an even speed. Do this a few times.

**2** Now coordinate this movement with your breathing. Inhale as you raise the arms, and exhale as you lower them. Notice how the movement seems to come alive.

Do this over and over until it feels natural to breathe in as you raise the arms and natural to breathe out as they come down. Breathe slowly and deeply. Match the speed of the movement with the length of the breath. Breathe slowly so your movement is slow and smooth. The inhalation should begin just prior to the arm-raising movement and finish just after the movement finishes—so the movement is surrounded by air, cushioned. The exhalation would initiate the arm-lowering movement and come to an end after the movement is complete. Pause momentarily after inhaling and exhaling. Keep the entire movement full of air.

**3** Now do more than merely coordinate the movement with the breath. Make them the same. Make them one. Become so familiar with the breath and the movement, and immerse yourself so completely in what you are doing, that they literally feel like the same action—different aspects, perhaps, but the same—as though you could not imagine moving without the breath or breathing without the movement. Let it be fluid and graceful. Repeat this again and again. Find the newness in each repetition.

The entire movement should be infused with air. As your arms go up, it should feel as though the inhalation itself were causing your arms to move; it should also feel as though the arm movement were causing you to draw in more air. As your arms come down, it should feel as though the exhalation were causing your arms to lower *and* that the arm-lowering movement itself helps squeeze the air out of your lungs. There should be a subtle feeling of resistance, as with an accordion or bellows. You cannot squeeze air out of an accordion faster than it wants to go, for example. There is a sense of pressure, of squeeze, of resistance, because you are actually squeezing the air out. Create a similar feeling here. Do not just raise and lower your arms, as though they were empty. Slowly draw the air in and stretch outward in the direction your arms are pointing as your arms go up, and squeeze the air out and stretch outward in the direction your arms are pointing as your arms come down. It should have a pneumatic feeling to it.

This is a very simple movement. All you are doing is raising and lowering your arms. There is nothing difficult about it. But if you understand this important concept as it displays itself in this simple movement, your yoga session will turn into an absorbing, insightful, and very powerful meditation.

# Orchestrating the Tone

With your breathing you can orchestrate the tone of your yoga. The tone you desire can depend on many things. But in any case, it is always your choice. The idea is to breathe in such a manner as to make this moment, now, feel perfect. You may breathe in a soft, deeply sensuous, slow manner, or you may breathe in a vigorous, or shallow, or intense manner, or any other permutation. The form it takes at any given moment does not matter. The form will change to meet the need. Essence matters. Your job is to breathe in the way that feels most appropriate to you now, and in every given moment there will be a way of breathing that feels right.

If you want to orchestrate softness in the poses, breathe softly. If you want more fire and energy, deliberately increase the intensity of your breathing. Again, it's like playing a wind instrument. There are many ways of playing middle C. You can blow with force, you can blow softly, or you can blow in staccato. The note is still middle C, but its quality is dependent on the type of breath. In orchestrating the tone of your yoga with your breathing, you vary your breathing to create the perfect feeling-tone, the tone that lures your fullest participation. This is your yoga. You are in charge.

There are three distinguishing characteristics to skillful breathing. The first characteristic is that it is smooth, free of strain, not erratic. Smooth breathing will smooth out your poses. It is difficult to be relaxed or comfortable in a pose if there is any strain in the breath, if you are holding the breath, breathing erratically, or panting. Breathing smoothly generates an overall sense of well-being and promotes softness and relaxation in the poses.

The second characteristic of intuitive breathing is its depth. You learn to breathe consciously either more or less deeply in order to meet the needs of the moment. This can be a little or a lot—not too deep, not too shallow—always the perfect amount, and should always be smooth, steady, and strain-free.

You may be getting tired in the middle of a strenuous pose, for example, and need more energy—so you breathe with more vigor; you generate energy by breathing deeply. Or you may be at a deep edge in a pose, on the edge of pain but not pain, wherein you need to be very alert and careful so as not to injure yourself—so you breathe more delicately. You keep the heat on, so to speak; you stay right there at your edge, not letting up, but you play it with great sensitivity, orchestrating the perfect stretch with your breathing. Deepening the breath is especially good if you are experiencing resistance, feeling sluggish, or having difficulty motivating yourself. This intentional exhilaration can often (not always) initiate new energy. You will naturally breathe more deeply if you are feeling energetic or doing a strenuous pose. With soft, quiet breathing you can reach hard-to-access areas of yourself.

The third characteristic of conscious breathing is its pulse, how it brings the pose to life. This means that some of the time you will push as you inhale, for example, and yield as you exhale—or vice versa. Inhalations tend to be active and assertive, and exhalations tend to be passive and restful. Most of the time, therefore, you will push or fuel a line of energy with the inhalation, and relax, release, and clarify the line with the exhalation. Sometimes, though, it's just the reverse. You will be passive with the inhalation and push or energize with the exhalation. And sometimes you will want to push or energize with both, and sometimes you will want to be soft and clarify with both. Really, there are no rules. Your innate intelligence and growing sensitivity will be your guide.

Sometimes you will find it interesting to generate intensity in a pose or be in a deep stretch while keeping the breath soft. Other times it will be more interesting to relax in a pose but breathe strongly, deeply. Become familiar with all three characteristics of skillful breathing, experiment with all your options, and learn how each affects you. You will then know how to apply them. If you are in a soft mood, consciously breathe softly. When your mood changes, change your breathing accordingly. If you want to increase your fire and energy, increase the intensity of breath; if you want to relax in a tight situation, breathe more softly. Whatever it is you want, however it is you feel, create and match that mood with the breath. And if you want to change the mood, deliberately change the breath. You are in charge; you are master of your breath.

Be aware of how you can use the breath to orchestrate the perfect feeling-tone, but be aware also that what feels perfect is not up to you. You are not deciding where perfect is. You are not dictating where it should be, or forcing or coercing the issue. You are looking for it, finding it, and breathing into it. The main thing is always to listen inwardly and allow yourself to be guided by how your body wants to breathe. This is what determines what feels perfect at any given moment. Pay attention inwardly and do as you are prompted to do.

Monitor your mood as you orchestrate the tone of your yoga with your breathing, and be aware of whether you are becoming more or less interested in what you are doing. Monitor your interest level and the quality of your participation. Generate the depth and quality of breath that elicits your fullest participation and makes this now-moment feel perfect. Breathe consciously.

The breath brings the poses to life, and with your breathing you establish the tone of your practice. As you do this with sensitivity and skill, your yoga will become a truer, more authentic, unique expression of you.

Always remember, yoga is a living art. It is a very personal expression of the moment. The subtleties of this art involve using your breathing to elicit the feeling-tone that feels perfect to you now. The idea is to improve and enhance the quality of your participation, to immerse yourself fully in this now-moment, and thereby be guided from within with more accuracy. In this way you will not only be more effective, you'll enjoy yourself more fully.

Yoga is not mechanical, and proper breathing will bring an increasingly creative sense to your practice. It should always feel as though you are learning something new. Be glad you have the time and inclination to practice. Be thankful you have discovered yoga. Be grateful. Celebrate your realization that the energy, enthusiasm, and attention you bring to yoga now will benefit all other moments of your life as well. Practice with passionate calm.

# 7

# LINES OF ENERGY

Look at the palm of your hand and pretend for a moment that your hand is an asana, a yoga posture. The center of your palm is the center of the posture, and radiating outward from the center—like rays of light from the center of the sun—are five lines of energy, your fingers. Now gently, slowly, almost imperceptibly, spread your fingers as much as you comfortably can *and* stretch outward through them in the various directions they are pointing. Experience your hand as a mini-sun and feel the energy in your hand radiating outward from the center of the palm. Keep your hand **as relaxed as possible** as you do this, sustain the action, and feel your whole hand remolding itself to this new shape—this new energy configuration—by allowing the stretch to penetrate.

Give yourself a few playful moments to experience this exercise with your hand. Release the stretch, then do it again several times. Give this your undivided attention, and understand experientially what it means to stretch and relax with intensity. Experience what it means to stretch deliberately and still be as effortless as possible.

This is what you will be doing in the various yoga postures, the only difference being that in the poses your whole body will be involved, not just the hand. You'll extend your energy outward from your center in a relaxed manner, in various directions simultaneously depending on the shape of the posture. You'll sustain the action for the duration of the posture and thereby energize and reconfigure your entire energy field.

Now, as a living being, you are an expression, a channel, a particular configuration or pattern of energy, of creative life force. You are a unique expression of the Creator, and life force flows through you. Life force, or Mind, or Consciousness, is what you are. It is the reason for your being, the how and what of your being. Energy flows through you, enlivens you, and makes you *you*. And if the flow of energy becomes obstructed or lessened for any reason, much like diminished blood flow due to arterial constriction, then your health will suffer and problems will arise. If the flow remains unimpeded, however, if the channels can remain open, health is natural and easy.

Your body's ability to function as a clean and efficient channel is limited by stiffness, lack of strength, and lack of endurance. Your mind's ability is limited by the way it thinks about itself, by the way you think about you. The process of yoga is one of undoing the obstructions and limitations in your body and mind that inhibit the free flow of creative life force.

Each yoga posture is a specific template for this energy flow, just as your hand was a specific template in the example above. These templates have evolved over thousands of years and are extremely good at opening tight and blocked areas. As you assume each individual posture and deliberately funnel your energy and breath through the pose, you are in effect cleaning the tubes and airing out the pathways that distribute the life force. Stiff and tight areas of your body inhibit the free circulation of energy and thereby strangle your internal supply of nourishment. These are the areas where you experience pain or discomfort to one degree or another. They are undernourished—crying for help. When clenched tightly this way, they remain separate, constricted, unrelated to the whole. As they open, they begin to receive nourishment once again. Physical discomfort and pain will disappear as healing occurs. When you restore lost movement to these tight areas of yourself, you rejuvenate them, bringing life to more of yourself.

As you loosen and dissolve the physical and psychological knots that bind your body and mind, you are literally enlarging your capacity to channel the energy of life. Creative life energy will flow through you more easily, with greater volume and power; and as it does, you will experience more ease and less disease, feeling and becoming more alive. With yoga, you nourish yourself at very deep levels, which causes you to glow with radiant health. You will become increasingly peaceful inside, less conflicted, and you will experience yourself more clearly as a uniquely beautiful expression of the creative God Force.

This is important because the fulfillment of your highest potential is directly proportional to your ability to function as a clean and efficient channel. It will occur more rapidly as you recognize yourself as the unobstructed, undiminished, and undenied specific presence of God.

Yoga done properly is a matter of creating, directing, and channeling "energy" through these various templates. This involves knowing how to create a "line of energy" with specific "current."

# Your Center

Let's go back to the spread hand example for a moment. The center of your palm is the center of the posture, and the lines of energy, your fingers, radiate outward from there. In your body, your physiological center is in the area of your belly that has traditionally been called **hara**, two inches below the navel. This can best be thought of as the whole pelvic basin, or pelvic bowl, that lies below the navel and above the genitals.

This area, your center, will always be in, or moving toward, one of two positions. It will either be in **cat tilt** or **dog tilt**. In cat tilt, as with a cat arching its back, the pelvis is rotated backward around the hip joints by drawing the navel backward toward the spine, tucking the coccyx down and under and contracting the buttocks. In dog tilt, as with a dog stretching as it wakes, the pelvis rotates forward around the hip joints. The alignment of your center is a function of your pelvic positioning, therefore, and since every line of energy originates at your center, these two movements should be the first you learn.

Start by getting down on your hands and knees to practice them a few times. Tuck your hips under, press the middle of your back up toward the ceiling in cat tilt, and gaze at the floor between your knees. Then turn your hips into dog tilt, gently arch your spine downward, and gaze forward. Go back and forth several times.

Most forward-bending postures, such as Dog Pose and the Seated Forward Fold, are done with dog tilt. Most backbends, such as the Locust Pose and the Upward Bow Pose are done with cat tilt.

The first thing you think as you do any yoga posture is "Should my pelvis be in cat tilt or dog tilt?" It will always be one or the other, or moving *toward* one or the other. You take a moment to establish the alignment of your center before establishing your lines of energy.

Every yoga posture is a combination of at least two lines of energy, each line radiating outward from your center; and depending on the shape of the posture, you will have two, three, four, five, or more lines. The Tall Mountain Pose, for example, is a two-way stretch with one line of energy moving up the arms and one line of energy moving down the legs, with your pelvis in cat tilt. These two lines move in opposite directions from one another, and each line has its root at your center.

Stick Pose also has two energy lines. Here, however, your pelvis will be in dog tilt; it's rotating forward around the hip joints. From dog tilt, one line moves upward through the spine, and one line moves outward through the legs.

Tree Pose has three lines of energy. One line reaches up the arms, one line moves down the supporting leg, and one line stretches outward through the bent knee. Your center will be in cat tilt.

Triangle Pose has five lines of energy. One line reaches outward through each arm, one line travels down each leg, and one line extends outward through the spine in the direction it is pointing.

These energy lines radiate outward from your center and move your body in opposing directions *at the same time*. It is the movement and intensification of these various energy lines that help undo the tight areas and open the posture for you. It's this that gives you more flexibility. When you hold both arms outstretched and horizontal, for example, you have one line of energy moving outward through each arm in opposite directions. The outward stretch through each arm is what spreads, broadens, and opens your chest. In Triangle Pose, you not only open the chest, but elongate the spine, stretch the legs, and flatten the pelvis.

The most important line of energy in every posture, always, is your spine. Your spine is rooted in your center and grows upward, much like a tree growing upward from the earth. Other lines, your arm lines, for example, are also rooted in your center. Your arm lines do not start at the shoulders. They start at the root of your spine, travel up the spine first, and then extend outward through the arms, like branches of a tree. They are not separate appendages somehow disconnected from their source. Every line of energy is an affirmation of its source. The source is your center.

# Single Arm Line of Energy

**PART ONE** ◈ Sit comfortably erect and raise one arm to the side, parallel to the floor and straight. Keep your arm as relaxed as possible without allowing it to fall limply to your side. Experience your arm, how heavy it feels, how long it feels, how much energy is required to keep it there. Note, for example, that although your arm is not totally relaxed, it is as relaxed as possible.

Now gently squeeze the elbow straight, spread your fingers fully, and stretch outward through the arm in the direction it is pointing. From your shoulder, stretch toward the elbow; from your elbow, stretch toward the wrist; and from the wrist, stretch through your hand to the tips of your outstretched fingers and beyond. Feel a dynamic tautness in the muscles of your upper arm and hand.

This is a ''line of energy,'' a flowing stream of intention, extending from the shoulder to the fingertips. The muscles of the arm and hand should be taut enough to be on the verge of a slight tremor. Push softly and then harder. Note the change in feeling. Relax the fingers for a moment and observe how this interrupts the flow through your line of energy. Make the hand taut, fingers spread, and once again feel the energy moving through the arm in a single direction, always in the direction the arm is already pointing. Lower your arm and rest.

This is what I call ''channeling'' or ''creating'' a line of energy. This is a fundamental technique in yoga. Here you are directing energy to flow along a specific line in your body. This particular line of energy extends outward from your shoulder and remains a ''line'' whether you stretch strongly or softly.

Remember, the arm line does not originate at the shoulder. It originates at your belly. Do the experiment again and notice the difference between energizing just the arm, as though it originated at the shoulder, and then energizing it by first lifting upward into your chest—from your belly—and then stretching outward through the arm. There is a qualitative difference between the two. When it is the arm only, the arm feels separate, disconnected, and less powerful. When the arm line comes from your belly, however, it becomes the natural outward extension of a whole body event, and therefore has a sense of integrity and strength to it. Lower your arm and rest.

**PART TWO** ◆ Extend the same arm out to the side again, but instead of holding it parallel to the floor, hold it at a forty-five degree angle sloping toward the floor.

Create a downward-sloping line of energy here. First lift upward from your belly into your chest, then stretch from the shoulder downward into the elbow, from the elbow into the wrist, and from the wrist into the fingertips. Spread your fingers and stretch the skin on your palm. Push strongly for the duration of this part of the experiment.

You can create a line of energy here, but because of the slope it feels different. It may even feel as if the arm is "asking" to raise itself. Listen inwardly and feel if this is so. Keep stretching outward through the arm, and then *slowly* raise it to horizontal again. Do not rush this part. Continue stretching outward through the arm in the direction it is pointing, and see if you can sense an increase in energy as the arm comes up, an increase in intensity and feeling, almost as though you actually were putting more power into the line.

The outward stretch urges the arm to rise. You are not just lifting your arm. Your arm comes up as you stretch outward, and your fingertips circumscribe as large a circle as possible. Slowly raise your arm, continue stretching outward, and focus on the sensations of intensity and energy flow. Do you feel how it changes? Can you sense the intensity in your arm increasing as it rises? Try this a few times until you acquire a feeling for it, and then relax.

The horizontal line is more powerful than the sloping line. This is because when your arm is horizontal, it channels the flow of energy more efficiently. The difference in feeling between the two is often dramatic, though at first it may seem subtle. As you become internally more sensitive in your practice, you will sense these various subtleties more clearly. Subtle shifts in sensation and feeling will be more obvious.

The second part of this experiment is an example of *following* a line of energy and illustrates the self-corrective nature of this technique. In the last example, raising the arm intensified feeling. Lowering the arm would lessen feeling. At any time during a posture, then, if you would like more or less energy in any given line, simply search creatively for the positioning that will provide it. As you reach for an increase or decrease in energy, or for a feeling of stretch or energy flow that feels more right to you, automatically the posture will internally self-correct, realign, and adjust according to your subjective perception of what feels right.

In Triangle Pose, for example, the classical or traditional alignment of the posture is with the upper arm vertical. As you increase the amount of energy up the arm and clarify the arm line, though, and as the pose opens and becomes easier for you, you'll find that the top arm wants to be doing more than merely stretching straight up. You'll want more of a challenge. You'll want a deeper opening. If you experiment a little with the top arm, turning it in, turning it out, bringing it toward you or away, or a little forward or back, you'll find that the line can hold more energy and be a more powerful line, a more efficient line, if you reach backward with it and then fold it down behind your back to catch the thigh with the hand. That's how Stage Two of Triangle Pose came into being. The top shoulder then gets a powerful stretch, the trunk and rib cage rotate to their maximum, the chest opens more fully, and the pelvis flattens better.

The idea is to be creative and sensitive in the poses, to follow the lines into your tight areas so they can release and open, and to search for the alignment that feels perfect. Your job is to find the precise alignment of each line of energy so that the pose as a whole feels custom-made for you.

If your arm wants to roll in slightly while in a posture, be willing to let it do so. If your arm wants to roll out or come more forward or back, try it out and see what happens. Is there an improvement or not? Notice how the quality of the line changes. Note also how other parts of the posture are affected and be aware of your body as a whole. If some part of your body is asking for a change, be willing to accommodate it, trust the guidance you are receiving, and see the result. Allow your inner intelligence to dictate the alignment. You don't have to think about it, nor know in advance what you are supposed to do. Simply follow the line of perfect flow.

This is especially interesting because, as it turns out, what feels ''right'' is what will be technically correct. As you follow the line of perfect flow, you necessarily move in harmony with sound body mechanics.

This is an important theme. Listening inwardly allows you to hear and be guided by the intelligence that created you. This happens by paying attention to what feels right and what doesn't, and adjusting accordingly. As you practice, trust your inner sense of what feels right. Exercise that ability. That's the point.

Within the context of each specific yoga posture, you first establish an energy flow through that template. You then listen inwardly for guidance, trusting and adjusting, and continue listening as you continue moving energy through the shape. The more conscientiously you do this, the better you'll get at following the dictates of your inner intelligence, the intelligence of the universe as it expresses itself as you.

# Current

Current is voltage—the amount of power, intensity, or feeling you generate in each line of energy. There are three distinguishing characteristics of a good line of energy, which the following examples should clarify.

> Sit comfortably erect with one arm out to the side, horizontal and parallel to the floor, as before, and create a line of energy outward through the arm.

**CHARACTERISTIC ONE: "RELAXED AS POSSIBLE"** ◆ The first characteristic of a good line of energy is that it is as relaxed as possible. You do not want to use more energy than you need. You put the energy in, but you practice being as effortless as possible.

> Here, for example, it is possible to create a subtle current of intention outward through the arm and for your arm to remain almost totally relaxed. Do it now. Make a line of energy outward through the arm and have it be as relaxed as possible. The hand is not limp, the fingers are not drooping, and though extremely minimal, this is a valid line of energy.

Every line of energy and, therefore, every yoga posture can be done softly like this. This is more difficult in complex and intricate postures. The significant point, however, is to be as relaxed as possible—to "do" and "not-do" at the same time. This requires a certain minimum expenditure of energy. The idea is not to use more.

**CHARACTERISTIC TWO: "DESIRED INTENSITY"** ◆ The second characteristic of a good line of energy is that you generate the intensity of current that feels best.

> Gradually increase the current in your arm. Do this by squeezing the elbow straight, spreading your fingers, and stretching *outward* with more vigor through the arm in the direction it is pointing. Deliberately generate more intensity in the arm, more voltage, and thereby create a more powerful line of energy. The increase in current will define and clarify the line. You have total control over how much current you gen-

erate. Do not strain. By increasing the current slowly, you can gauge and discriminate among different subtleties with an accurate sensitivity that is crucial in advanced and intricate postures.

Stretch softly at first, then increase the current gradually. Increase it to thirty percent, forty percent, fifty, seventy-five, and for just a moment create a very strong line of energy, stretching outward through the arm as strongly as you comfortably can. Still, though, keep it as relaxed as possible as you do this.

The idea is to create the amount of current that feels best to you at the moment—sometimes strong, sometimes soft—and then maintain that level, hold it steady, acclimatize, as you release every unnecessary effort and every sense of strain. You want to be as relaxed as possible without losing the increased energy flow. This "desired intensity" will vary according to your mood, strength, and flexibility, as well as which pose you happen to be doing.

### CHARACTERISTIC THREE: "ALTERNATING CURRENT"  ◆  The third characteristic of a good line of energy is that it pulses with the breath. The breath brings it to life and pulses through it.

With the arm vertical this time, establish an upward-flowing line of energy. From your belly lift upward into the chest, from the shoulder stretch upward into the elbow, and from the elbow stretch upward through the fingertips. As you inhale, stretch upward through the arm. Use the inhalation to create and enhance the line, so that the breath and the upward stretch work as one. As you exhale, retain the upward energy flow and release every sense of effort or strain; even get the sense of increasing the line, making it longer, by *releasing* upward. Inhale again and *increase* the upward stretch through your arm, increase the current, and as you exhale, maintain the increase but release the effort required to increase the energy flow. Feel the stretch emanating from your center and moving continuously up the torso, through the arm and out the hand.

The basic pattern is to increase the current as you inhale and release any sense of strain and all unnecessary effort as you exhale. As you do this, feel how the arm pulses, the current alternately increasing and then purifying within the rise and fall of a single breath. Lower your arm and relax.

The idea is to enliven the lines with your breathing. Sometimes, as in this example, you will increase the current with the inhalation and purify the line with the exhalation, and sometimes you will do just the reverse. This is a valuable skill to perfect because it allows you to sustain a line of energy for longer periods of time without tiring and without strain. Endurance, strength, and stamina will improve quickly this way, enabling you to spend more time in the postures, thereby opening yourself to an even greater degree.

Skill in yoga involves creating the intensity of current that makes the stretch feel perfect. Being able to do this with each line of energy is a matter of inner listening and skillful tuning. If you were tuning a violin string, for example, you would turn the key just the right amount—not too much, not too little—in order to adjust the string tension and create the perfect sound. How much you'll turn the key cannot be known in advance. It all depends on the sound. This is exactly what you do with your musculature, your lines, the current, the breath, and the alignment of the pose. You can then skillfully open specific muscular and energetic blockages with just the right amount of pressure.

As your body becomes stronger and more flexible, you will desire and enjoy a stronger current more often, much like a fine horse enjoys running fast because it feels good. You will feel more alive as you are able to process more energy.

The important point, though, is to create the intensity of current that *feels* best—not too much and not too little. More isn't always better. If you create too much intensity you may not enjoy your practice as much as you might, you may get injured, and you'll eventually lose enthusiasm. It may feel as though you are attacking yourself, which becomes tiring. On the other hand, without enough intensity, if your practice is too soft or slack, it won't yield the benefits that now motivate you. The main thing is to create a balance. And loving your practice, enjoying what you're doing as you are doing it, should be your sole criterion regarding how much current to create, which poses to do, and how long to practice. It should feel good as you are doing it.

# Your Whole Body

When you read the words "Spread your fingers and stretch your whole hand," you instinctively know what to do. There is no need for me to say, "Stretch the thumb, index finger, middle finger, ring finger, pinkie." You understand that the whole hand is involved.

In the same way, your whole body should be involved when you do the poses. Now, however, the words "Stretch your whole body in Triangle Pose" might mean that one hand is limp or drooping, your legs bent, or your spine hunched over. The overall action throughout your whole body may not resemble the overall action in your hand—that quality of total involvement. You may be reaching very attentively with one arm, for example, but forget the other completely. Part of the skill in yoga is learning to involve all of yourself, just as when you spread your hand, so that all of you is activated and filled with energy. One way to remember this is to keep your hands open and fingers spread whenever possible, as well as your feet and toes. This takes a small degree of attentiveness and can act as a reminder for the rest of your body.

Keeping the image of an early morning stretch in mind as you do the poses can also be helpful in understanding the dynamic and appealing nature of this line of energy technique. When you stretch first thing in the morning, you invest energy and do it with enthusiasm, partly because it feels so good. You press outward, squeeze your muscles, and you stretch! And without even thinking about it very much, you adjust and readjust from the inside out—stretching here, stretching there, intuitively, almost uncontrollably. Adjusting intuitively is analogous to "following the stretch," and "current" is the amount of intensity, oomph, or vigor you put into the stretch.

Learning the line of energy technique teaches one part of you at a time to stretch, like separate fingers. Eventually, you are able to add them all up and hold these "separate" lines together in one continuous awareness. In Triangle Pose, then, at first there are five separate lines of energy emanating from your center, and it may feel like five different things going on. As you become more experienced at yoga and more proficient in the poses, more skillful at what you're doing, it will instead feel like one glorious happening—your whole body, mind, heart, awareness, and passion doing yoga . . . breathing, stretching, moving, listening, trusting, adjusting, all simultaneously, all of you.

Instead of having a mental image of a completed posture as your primary goal and then trying to "put" your body into that position through force or effort—so that you are fundamentally always working externally—these lines of energy are the key to an inner yoga. As you learn how the postures work and how these lines of energy move, and as you learn to follow the lines into your tight areas and open them, the completed postures will come from inside, not outside, like a blooming flower that is gently expanding outward from its center. The delicate intensification of your energy lines and your ever-improving ability to stay with the energy flow—following the lines into and through tight areas of your energy field, erasing and releasing them—is what gradually reveals the completed posture.

This will all become clear as we go through the postures together. For now, understand the basic techniques. I am going over each concept slowly and in specific detail, step by step, in order to clarify the techniques and save you time. The descriptions are accurate and stated exactly as intended. Take your time in reading and understanding these comments. The time you take now to absorb and understand these simple concepts will save you many hours, months, and years of trial and error in your practice.

Your yoga practice has already begun. If these comments are not yet clear, do not worry. You will only ever "know" or understand these techniques as you use them on a regular basis. The secrets are in the experience itself, in the doing, in the practice, and these techniques are the distillation of many years of practice.

# 8

## PLAYING THE EDGE

A large part of the art and skill in yoga lies in sensing just how far to move into a stretch. If you don't go far enough, there is no challenge to the muscles, no intensity, no stretch, and little possibility for opening. Going too far, however, is an obvious violation of the body, increasing the possibility of both physical pain and injury. Somewhere between these two points is a degree of stretch that is in balance: intensity without pain, use without abuse, strenuousness without strain. You can experience this balance in every posture you do.

This place in the stretch is called your "edge." The body's edge in yoga is the place just *before* pain, but not pain itself. Pain tells you where the limits of your physical conditioning lie. Edges are marked by pain and define your limits. How far you can fold forward, for example, is limited by your flexibility edge; to go any further hurts and is actually counterproductive. The length of your stay in a pose is determined by your endurance edge. Your interest in a pose is a function of your attention edge.

In daily life, we tend to remain within a familiar but limited comfort zone by staying away from both our physical and mental edges. This would be fine except that as aging occurs these limits close in considerably. Our bodies tighten, our range of movement decreases, and our strength and stamina diminish. By consciously bringing the body to its various limits or edges and holding it there, gently nudging it toward more openness with awareness, the long, slow process of closing in begins to reverse itself. The range expands as the edges change.

Sensing where your edges are and learning to hold the body there with awareness, moving with its often subtle shifts, can be called "playing the edge." This is a large part of what you'll be doing in your practice. Your skill in yoga has little to do with your degree of flexibility or where your edges happen to be. Rather, it is a function of how sensitively you play your edges, no matter where they are.

This is a very freeing idea. Normally, we have an idea of how the posture "should" be. We have ideas about how deep we should be able to go into a pose, what we should look like while we are there, and how long we should be able to stay. We are often more aware of where we aren't than of where we are.

This idea of the "completed" or "ideal" posture as a specific destination somewhere in the future is often a lurking presence in the back of our minds as we do the poses. Because of this, there will necessarily be a gap between where you are in the posture and where you think you should be. This gap, more often than not, contains a subtle frustration, a conflict, a feeling that where you are is insufficient—or worse, who you are is insufficient—and that if you were truly doing yoga properly and were a "good" or "evolved" person, you would be somewhere other than where you are. If this is the case, your practice will be permeated with the effort of going somewhere else. It will be future-oriented, the present moment being significant only as a stepping stone to the future. And you will miss being present.

Envisioning the postures in advance can yield dramatic results, however. And watching someone else do an advanced and difficult posture that you would like to achieve can be especially helpful, both because you see it is possible and can be performed with ease, and because your nervous system—simply by watching— receives a tremendous amount of nonverbal information about how to perform the pose correctly. Having that information in your nervous system and the back of your mind as you practice can make that pose easier for you, as long as you use it as a general guideline that you understand will be expressed differently in your body. The way to realize these changes is by focusing your attention on the process of what you are doing. This involves flirting with the tight spots, your edges, with sensitivity and attention.

The main thing to understand is that there is no such thing as a "completed" or "ideal" posture. Each posture is an ever-evolving, constantly moving energy phenomenon that is different from day to day, moment to moment, and person to person. The process of sensitively flirting with your edges and achieving perfect energy flow is not merely the means to achieve the pose—it *is* the pose.

This is what the physical aspect of yoga is fundamentally all about. Your body is limited in movement not only through its genetic makeup, but through the conditionings that have accrued over the years. As you age, this becomes more and more apparent. Yoga is a way of exploring these limits. It's not a matter of "How can I attain this or that final posture?" It's a matter of gently pressing into the various edges you encounter within the template structure of each particular posture. And your edges and limits will change as a by-product of this exploration; *you* will change.

# Intensity and Pain

You should *never* be in pain as you practice yoga. Your practice should not be a painful ordeal, but rather an expression of joy. Pain is most easily defined as any sensation you do not like, and it always invokes a natural withdrawal mechanism. When you put your hand on a hot stove, for example, instantly you take it off. Before you're even aware that your hand is on the stove, it's off. This is a built-in self-protective device.

The same withdrawal mechanism is activated whenever a yoga stretch begins to hurt. Muscles clamp down and contract in order to protect themselves from overstretching. They are suddenly less willing, fearful, and they resist the stretch—naturally. And they do this, to whatever small or large degree, before you are even aware it's happening. This is blatantly at odds with your initial intention to stretch, open, and expand your physical boundaries. Therefore, by pushing into pain you are actually working against yourself. One foot is on the accelerator, and one foot is on the brake.

Pushing and working hard are frequently appropriate and can be thoroughly enjoyable at the right moments, but they should never result in pain. You may want to approach pain and get near it, but not actually be in it. You want to be in the place where it "hurts good," where you know you are dealing with what needs to be dealt with—the contracted parts of your energy field—but where it's not so intense that you resist, tighten up to protect yourself, or prevent yourself from going too far.

The ideal state for practice is to be as willing and relaxed as possible, as nonresisting as possible, so that one part of you is not in opposition to another. You can then comfortably press your edges open. The practice becomes one of being relaxed and willing at your deeper edges; and this isn't necessarily easy. It's difficult to stay relaxed in the midst of a high-intensity stretch.

You want to stay within your comfort zone where you are safe and, at the same time, press into the various tight areas. By pressing, stretching, and breathing into your tight areas, you can ease them open, thereby expanding the boundaries of your comfort zone. It's like being inside a bubble and gently pressing outward from inside to expand its shape, so that you experience more space and comfort within the bubble.

Pain lurks just beyond your deepest edges as a reminder that you have gone too far. It's important for anyone who spends time nudging edges open with yoga to have a healthy understanding of pain—and to have a feeling for the distinction between pain and intensity.

The word *pain* actually stands for a variety of different possible sensations ranging anywhere from sharp and intense to subtle and dull. Physical pain may arise from a variety of causes; a pulled muscle, for example, or from a stretch that is too intense. Psychological pain often involves the feeling that you are in a place you don't like, doing something you would rather not be doing.

Herein lies one of the reasons for the frequent confusion between intensity and pain. A powerful stretch, whether or not you have gone too far, will generate an intense sensation. Someone who is not used to intensity or is excessively worried about getting hurt may be afraid of the intense sensation and resist it. *Re-*

*sisted intensity becomes pain*. Therefore, even relatively mild levels of intensity can be experienced as pain if you go beyond your psychological edge.

If fear prevents you from going deeper or staying longer in a posture, it is wise to avoid overriding the fear by being brave or courageous, since this makes injury more likely. Instead of pushing past psychological limits, open more slowly by finding a less intense level of stretch just before fear enters. Hold the position there as you deepen the breath, relax, and acclimatize to the stretch. By playing the edge of fear like this, you never have to experience psychological discomfort.

This can have a very profound influence on all aspects of your life. One of the things you learn in yoga is to enjoy working with intensity. Intensity is simply more "energy" at any given moment, more feeling. Happiness and sadness, for example, can both be experienced with more or less intensity. If you are unable or unwilling to deal with an increase in intensity, however, not only in your yoga but in your daily life as well, your range of life experience will necessarily remain limited and narrow. Yoga can teach you to enjoy and learn from a broader range of experience. It will encourage you to seek out and process more intensity. The more you do this within the safe arena of yoga practice, the more it will influence all of your life. This is not as intense as it may sound. More intensity isn't even noticeable as you become strong and open.

This has two distinct advantages. First, you will be able to allow more pleasure into your life. More good will come to you because you are open and receptive, no longer pushing it away. You will experience more joy and find yourself able to handle the heightened intensity of happiness. Haven't you noticed that even in the midst of joy, something you thought you wanted, there is often a part of you that wants to turn it off? Or at least turn it down a bit? It's difficult to handle intensity of any kind, even if you like it. Yoga can change this for you forever. As you are able to generate more energy and process more intensity in the poses with enjoyment and full willingness, you will correspondingly be able to receive and process more goodness in your life.

Secondly, yoga teaches you to experience the so-called "negative" emotions and intensities without being overly disturbed by them, without having to run away from them. They will feel less intense than they previously would have. You will then be able to learn from the "bad" and painful experiences in life without being bowled over by them. And therefore, because your full range of life experience is being broadened and enlarged in all directions, you are now able to learn from both the "good" and "bad," making your life that much richer.

It is important to learn how to generate voluntary intensity deliberately and willingly, by deepening the breath, increasing the current, strengthening your lines, and flirting with the various edges that arise in each pose. This is best learned in postures that are easy for you. In these postures any intensity you experience is largely self-generated. Learn to create voluntary intensity in these easy poses and in the early stages of any pose you do, and then delicately press into your tight areas in order to nudge them gently to greater openness. This will prepare you for the intensely pleasurable sensations that come with the territory of advanced yoga. Intensity is pleasurable when you are prepared for it, when you are able to let go into it; it becomes unpleasant when you resist it or generate too much. Skill in yoga involves creating the perfect amount of intensity—not too much, not too little.

# Minimum and Maximum Edges

Every pose has a "minimum edge" and a "maximum edge," as well as a series of intermediary edges between these. Most of us are aware of the maximum edge; it is the easiest to detect. This is the point where the stretch begins to hurt. It is the furthest point of tightness beyond which you should not go. If you were to force yourself beyond this point, you would definitely be in pain and might easily hurt yourself or pull a muscle.

The minimum edge is where you sense the very first sensation of stretch, the very first hint of resistance coming from your muscles. For example, bending over and touching your toes may tax you to the maximum, but about halfway down (or less) you can sense the first edge. This is where you initially become aware of a stretch.

It is important to be aware of your very first edge, your minimum edge. Taking your time to open that edge is like preparing to go through a series of gates. You must go through the first gate before you can go through the second, and the second before the third. The real key to depth in postures is going slowly, making sure you have thoroughly opened your early edges.

As you come into a pose, look for your very first edge. Do not rush past it. When you feel that edge, stop. Stop moving, deepen the breath, clarify your energy lines, and wait for it to open. You will know the first edge has opened when the sensations of stretch begin to diminish. At that point you will naturally want to go deeper into the posture. Rather than having to push your way in, you will feel drawn into the pose. As you are drawn deeper, a new edge will soon appear, and the sensations of stretch will come back. Wait for the sensations at this new edge to diminish before going deeper.

Do this over and over. Wait for the sensations of stretch to diminish somewhat and then go deeper. It will feel as though you are sneaking into the pose, not barging your way in. Proceed slowly, edge by edge and gate by gate. Apply pressure and wait for the musculature to open. Then you can move deeper into the pose, apply more pressure, all the while orchestrating the tone of the pose with the breath and current, again waiting for the musculature to open and the sensations of stretch to diminish. Continue working like this until the musculature will no longer release. Then stay where you are and be motionless. Retain the sense of energy and stretch, and release every hint of strain. Be as relaxed as you can be; do and don't-do. When you sense that it is nearly time to come out of the pose, delicately accelerate your energy for a moment. Finally, release the stretch altogether and come out of the pose.

While you are at each new subsequent edge, deepen the breath, define and clarify your lines, and pay close attention to the actual feeling of the stretch. Keep tabs on whether you are enjoying yourself or not. If not, why not? Find a way of doing the pose that is enjoyable. And then be interested: Are the sensations of stretch increasing? If so, it's a sign that you are too deep in the posture and should back off a bit. Are the sensations staying the same? If so, stay where you are, deepen the breath, and wait for the sensations of stretch to diminish. And when the sensations of stretch have diminished somewhat and you are able to relax with intensity, you will instinctively know it is time to go deeper.

Proceed step by step, edge by edge, paying close attention to what you are doing, being sensitive to the changing sensations of stretch. Remember, yoga is essentially an awareness process wherein you attend to these subtle shifts in sensation and feeling. The attention you give to these changing sensations of stretch is what exercises and develops your sensitivity. You will become sensitive to subtler and subtler sensations.

When the sensations of intensity no longer diminish at the new edge, it means your muscles are not yet ready for a stronger or deeper stretch. You can flirt with these tight areas by pressing into them gently, by changing the strength and character of your breathing, by increasing and decreasing the current in your lines, by staying in the posture longer, or by doing several repetitions of the pose—but do not force your way through them. Respect your tight edges. Work with them sensitively. Lure them to greater openness.

The more you do this, the better you'll get at it. Instead of telling your body when to move or what to do, you're learning to wait until it's ready. You wait for the inner feeling to tell you when to move. You listen for the inner cue to action, and this becomes easier and easier to detect. When you feel the energy flowing freely and the sensations of intensity beginning to wane, that's the sign. If you go too fast, however, the sensations will increase instead of diminish. There will be pain—a roadblock to the free flow of energy. This is feedback that you have gone too deep, too fast, too soon. Be interested in the feedback you're receiving from your body while you are in the pose.

Let's take an imaginary pose and rate it from one to ten. ''One'' is the beginning of the pose. ''Ten'' is as far as you can go before reaching pain. There is no pain in the one-to-ten range, though the sensations of stretch will become increasingly intense as you approach ten. Anything beyond ten we will not consider.

As you proceed from one to ten, the intensity will gradually increase. At one you will not feel much, but somewhere around two or three you will feel your first edge. Most of the time we rush past these early edges, looking for the real stretch deeper in the pose. It's important, however, to find your first edge and acclimatize yourself there before deepening. It is the opening of this early edge that allows the later, deeper openings to occur. If your early edges are not fully open, your body will not be ready for the intensity of the deeper extensions. Somewhere around eight or nine and inching into ten is what I would call your maximum edge, the deepest extension or degree of intensity you are now capable of sustaining without pain or discomfort. Remember, never push yourself into pain.

If your limits in a posture are marked by pain, and if the intensity of the stretch continues to increase as you come closer and closer to your maximum edge, how do you tell the difference between pain and intensity? Easy! The answer is obvious. If you do not like the sensation and you do not want to be there, it's pain. It's totally up to you. This is your yoga. You are not here to punish yourself or do something you don't want to do. You are learning to generate an intensity that is attractive, pleasurable, that you like and want. It's something you are actually looking for. At your maximum edge, just before pain—but not in pain— is an intensity that is extremely pleasurable. Therefore, go slowly. Take your time. Don't miss that perfect point. Increase the intensity of the pose gradually and deepen the pose with care. This will teach you to enjoy and assimilate greater amounts of energy and intensity.

The feeling-tone of a perfectly orchestrated strong stretch at a deep edge has a seductive quality to it. It's intense, pleasurable, exhilarating, and invigorating. Your body will like it. This should not be surprising, however, because by stretching your body to full openness, you are freeing yourself from the constraints of tightness, contraction, and pain. You are increasing your internal energy flow, flushing new life through your system, opening and nourishing yourself at very deep levels; and all of this is good for you and therefore feels good. But if you unawarely press too deeply, too quickly, into a posture, then the pleasurable and attractive sensations of intensity will become painful and unattractive. If you happen to go too far into a stretch—"too far" meaning you do not like it—then ease out of the pose until you do. Center yourself in your breathing, regain composure, and then slowly go in again, being more careful this time.

Be clear about this: If you start not liking the stretch *for any reason*, then move out of the pose until you find a place you do like. Reasons for not liking where you are can be physical or psychological. You may be stretching the muscle too much, or you may not be in the mood. Either reason is valid. Never be in a place you don't want to be. If you do not like it, change it. Adjust. Find the degree of stretch you can totally immerse yourself in.

Sometimes you will want to flirt more seriously with your various resistances and with the common reluctance to stay with an intense, and perhaps uncomfortable, sensation for an extended period of time. But doing this when you want to do this is different from doing it when you do not want to. If you avoid feedback and spend a lot of time being uncomfortable or in pain, you are not going to enjoy doing yoga. You will not look forward to your practice. You will not be working with the principles of opening. And by encountering unnecessary tension and resistance, you will not be doing your body any good, either.

# Edges, Breathing, and Wholeness

Since your movements and stretches will be coordinated with your breathing ("Move when you breathe, and breathe when you move") the most subtle and sensitive way to play your edges and fine-tune the feel of your stretches is with your breathing. Without the sensitive use of your breathing, your stretches cannot be precise. The muscles and lines are not sensitive enough in themselves, nor sufficiently delicate, to fine-tune a stretch accurately.

The overall feeling in your muscles and body is the *sound* of yoga. The sound is a feeling, a tone, a feeling-tone; it's very much like singing a note. And if a particular line of energy is not tuned just right, it will either feel "flat" or "sharp." Continual readjustment is necessary to stay perfectly tuned. I usually create a line of energy that is slightly flat, just below perfect tension and with low current. I then deepen the breath as I increase the current to fine-tune the line. This enables me to press delicately into an edge from the inside out without invoking the stretch-reflex withdrawal mechanism; and if I happen to go too far, I soften my breathing, back off the edge somewhat, decrease the current in my lines, then try again. In this way it is possible to create a strong current of energy in any given line, or flirt with a maximum edge, or perform a difficult and advanced posture without forcibly pushing beyond physical and psychological edges. The moment you do that, remember, your intention will fragment, and your attention will wander. You will begin to resist what you are doing, part of you wanting to continue and part of you wanting to stop.

The hallmark of practicing yoga properly, however, is wholeness, wholeheartedness, not being in conflict. The idea is to generate wholeheartedly the optimum intensity of energy by consciously creating an increase or decrease in current. You then use this energy to extend your boundaries and limits, to expand your comfort zone, basically—both physically and psychologically speaking. Yoga is not about "pushing through the pain," "overcoming the pain," "no pain, no gain," or about being excessively willful. If you are having to be brave and courageous in order stoically to withstand excessive intensity, you are pushing too hard. You are forcing the issue, fighting. *Never fight yourself.* Yoga is not about fighting. There is no advantage to this and there are many disadvantages. Ease up when necessary. Intensify when appropriate. Practice skillfully.

The optimum degree of intensity is the amount that elicits your fullest attention; sometimes this will be a lot, and sometimes this will be a little. The correct amount is the amount that helps you be one-pointed and whole. It is the amount that feels perfect to you now. Too much is a strain, and too little is not sufficiently interesting. Your mind will wander in either case. Getting "better" at yoga means getting better at generating the perfect degree of current, intensity, breath, and feeling so that, in that moment, you are consciously one with what you're doing—whole, not conflicted, and exactly where you want to be.

Therefore, learn to be more interested in the feeling-tone of your body than in how deep you are in the posture. Learn to create an energy flow that is attractive to you. Do this by pressing into your edges with the perfect degree of current and the perfect pitch of breath. Realize this is not a function of how flexible you are. A stiff body can do this just as beautifully as a flexible one. The beautiful inner music—the inner feeling—is the yoga, not the achievement of elaborate postures. And be assured, your body will grow more beautiful and become strong and flexible by being played beautifully.

This is where the concept of push and yield most meaningfully displays itself. The art of yoga lies in how well you play your edges, how delicately you flirt with your limitations, how well you lure yourself deeper into the postures, how sensitively you balance the desire to achieve results with the relaxation of nondesire and surrender, and how thoroughly you immerse yourself in the process and enjoy what you are doing. And again, the primary tool you use is your breathing. Your breathing orchestrates the feeling-tone of the poses as it brings them to life.

Keep in mind that the various poses are like maps into your body. Having a map, however, does not infer a specific goal or a predetermined destination of where you should be in the pose. The idea is to use the map to explore—to look deliberately for tight, blocked areas within yourself—open them, and thereby create lines of clean energy flow. This requires that you be delicate, deliberate, and exact, not in the sense of "blueprint," but in the sense of being increasingly inwardly sensitive for the specific alignment and intensity of stretch that feels most right. This entails pressing for greater depth in the poses, greater openness, yet also remaining passive and yielding. You knock on the door, breathe, wait, then go deeper when the musculature lets you in.

Use your breathing and energy lines to nudge into your edges, being watchful and patient. Do not barge in, but also don't just remain passive. Apply pressure in specific areas, increase the intensity gradually, breathe, and wait for them to release. Lovingly persuade the tight areas to open, breath by breath by breath. Communicate nonverbally to the various tight areas that it is in their best interest to relax and open. Do this by finding easy places in the poses where you can establish an energy flow, then bring this flow into the contracted area.

Again, never push yourself into positions that cause you to resist the stretch physically or emotionally. Always start from comfort and safety, and only increase the stretch after you're comfortable where you already are. Then feel free to go after your deeper extensions and stronger stretches. Use as much ambition and desire as you want. Push as much as you want. Let go as much as you can. But learn to do all of this with sensitivity. Deepen the breath and increase the force in your lines at relatively easy stages, then wait and be patient. Your body will open and let you in when it's ready. By staying at easy stages of the pose longer, you will increase your strength and endurance. You will need these in order to hold the increased flexibility that will accrue through time and practice.

Skill in yoga is a matter of harmonizing your breathing with your energy lines as you flirt with your edges. It's a matter of getting all three just right, of changing them when necessary, and of adjusting and readjusting in order to create the feeling-tone that is the most attractive to you in that moment. It's a matter of adjusting the tension and stretch of your muscles, and the pitch of your breathing, to produce the perfect feeling-tone. You can make it exquisite. The more perfect it is, the more one-pointed and focused your mind will be.

# PART

## THREE

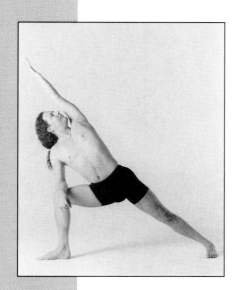

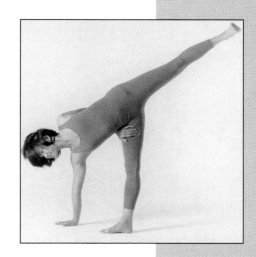

# 9

---

# THE ASANAS

## THE OPENING

# 1 Sit Quietly First

Always start your yoga session sitting quietly. These few minutes provide an interval in which to let go of your usual daily concerns, gather your energy, become centered, and affirm your motivation to practice with one-pointed enthusiasm. During this quiet time, be aware of any specific poses you feel like doing. These will come to mind spontaneously, much like the way specific foods come to mind when you think about what to eat. Pay attention to these subtle requests, for they will clarify the content of your practice.

Start your session in this fashion:

**1** **Sitting Down.** Begin by sitting erect on the floor in any comfortable position. Take a moment to survey your surroundings. Feel the energy in the room, observe the colors and shapes, and be aware of how you feel. Then close your eyes and breathe in deeply, gently. Savor the air for a moment as you hold the breath, then release it slowly. Do this three times, reminding yourself that you are an integral part of the universe. Pay attention to your posture, the feeling-tone of you, and be relaxed and motionless. Then say a short prayer or invocation, such as ''I am grateful for this time of communion and renewal in which I may meditate and practice yoga.''

**2** **Centering Through Breath Awareness.** Then turn your attention inward, sit absolutely still, and become intimately aware of your breathing; practice the Counting Backward exercise or the Mindfulness of Breathing exercise given in

Chapter One if you found them helpful. At this point, do not control or regulate your breathing. Allow it to flow freely in and out according to its own natural rhythm. Note the changing sensations throughout your body that accompany each breath, stay aware of your "now" feeling-tone, and let each breath enhance this awareness. When your attention strays, notice it has done so and bring it back to the feeling-tone of your breathing body. Do this for a minute or two.

**3** **Deepening the Breath.** Now deepen the breath with the ujjayi throat sound, placing your emphasis on a long, smooth exhalation. Breathe deeply for about a minute and then begin your asana session. Carry the centeredness you attain here into the poses, always staying focused on the breath. All of this can take as little as three to five minutes.

At the end of your asana session when you are resting in either Shavasana or Padmasana, again say a small prayer of thankfulness and immerse yourself in the feeling-tone of you.

# Benefits: The Opening

The Opening portion of every workout is a time of warming up, setting the tone, coming into the now, and pointing yourself in the correct direction for practice. There are many possible openings. They are like chess openings that get you into the game. They center your attention on the breath and loosen the limbs, torso, and spine for the various poses that follow.

# Benefits: Sit Quietly First

Centering. Establishes flow of breath. Inner attunement.

# 2 Cat Pose *or Bidalasana*

Cat Pose teaches you to initiate movement from your center and to coordinate your movements and breath. These are two of the most important themes in asana practice.

The alignment of your center depends on the positioning of your pelvis. Therefore, think of your hip positioning as the center of each pose. This is important because your spine is the most significant line of energy in every pose and because the way your spine elongates from your center depends solely on which way your pelvis is turning. If your sacrum is tilted forward (dog tilt), your spine will project forward before beginning its upward ascent, increasing the curve of your lower back. If your sacrum is tilted backward (cat tilt), your spine will project backward, rounding your lower back.

Every yoga pose involves positioning your pelvis in either "cat tilt," "dog tilt," or "neutral"—or in moving *toward* one of these or the other. In most poses only one of these choices is appropriate.

**Note:** As you read these instructions, *feel* the action being described. Look closely at the photos, imagine yourself doing the pose, and experience it in your body as you read. This will give your muscles, nerves, and cells their first important imprint about how to do the various poses. Then when you actually perform the poses, they will seem familiar, and you will intuitively know what to do. Throughout these instructions, **boldface** type indicates the most essential information. For quick review read boldface only.

**1** **Start on your hands and knees.** Position your hands directly beneath your shoulders and your knees directly beneath the hips. Have your fingers fully spread with the middle fingers pointing straight ahead. Make your back horizontal and flat. Gaze at the floor. This is your "neutral" positioning. When your pelvis is in neutral, your spine will be at full extension, with both the front and back sides equally long.

**2** **Establish a smooth flowing breath and wait for the inner cue to begin.** Consciously produce the ujjayi throat sound and remind yourself that the breath is the life of the pose and the fuel for movement.

**3** As you wait for the inner cue, do not sag into your shoulders (photo 1). Instead, create a line of energy through each arm by pressing *downward* into your hands and lifting *upward* out of your shoulders (photo 2). Go back and forth like this several times to make sure you understand the movement. As you exhale, sag into your shoulders and do the incorrect action; as you inhale, lengthen the arms, lift out of the shoulders and do the correct action.

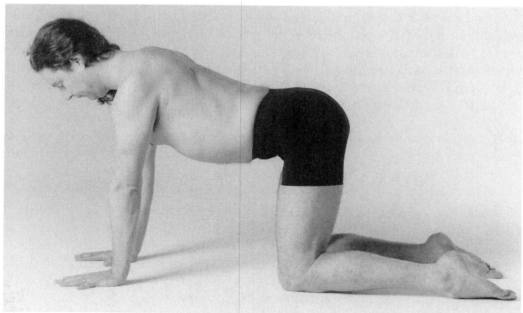

1

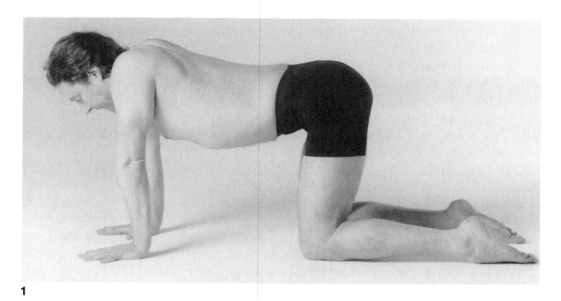

2

## CAT TILT

**4 When you are ready to begin, breathe in deeply. As you exhale, turn your hips into "cat tilt"** (photo 3). Do this by gently pulling the abdominal muscles backward toward the spine, tucking the tailbone (coccyx) down and under, and gently contracting the buttocks. Press firmly downward with your hands in order to stay lifted out of the shoulders, and press the middle of your back toward the ceiling, rounding your spine upward. Curl your head inward. Gaze at the floor between your knees.

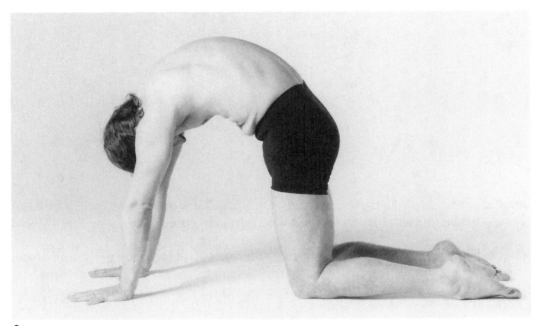

3

**5** Because this is a "closing" movement in which you are reducing lung volume, this movement is done as you exhale. This positioning of your hips (coccyx tucked, sacrum tilting backward) is called "cat tilt." Be here several breaths.

## DOG TILT

**6 As you inhale, turn your hips into "dog tilt"** (photo 4). Do this by releasing the grip of the buttocks, reversing the tilt of your pelvis, and curving your spine into a smoothly arched backbend. The pubic bone will move backward through the legs, the sitting bones will turn upward, and the sacrum will change its angle. Keep the navel backward toward the spine as you do this, and continue pressing downward into your hands to lengthen the arms and stay lifted out of the shoulders. Lift your chest away from the waist, lift your head, slide the shoulder blades

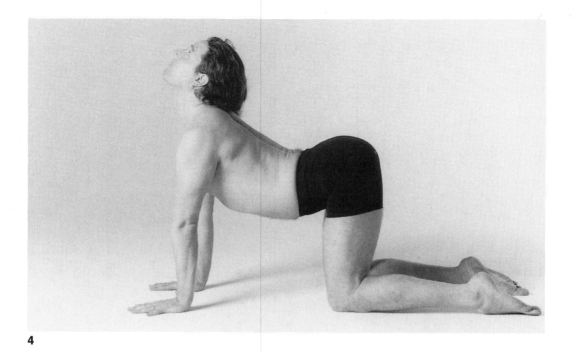

**4**

down your back, and either gaze at a point on the floor in front of you or upward toward the ceiling—or close your eyes and immerse yourself in the way this feels.

**7** Feel the flow of the curve. Increase the curve by tilting your pelvis more and moving the spine deeper into your back, bringing the curve up your back. Do this without sagging into the shoulders. Arch the full length of your spine to its maximum.

**8** Because this is an "opening" movement in which you are increasing lung volume and expanding the chest, this movement is done as you inhale. This positioning of your hips (buttocks spread, sacrum tilting forward) is called "dog tilt." Be here several breaths.

**9** The technique involved in this backward-bending movement is an important action in many of the postures, and you should be careful to learn it correctly. The idea is to curve your spine evenly as you approach your maximum, not to overbend in the lumbar (lower back). Do this by continuing to pull the navel and abdominal muscles backward toward the spine as you tilt the pelvis forward and arch your spine, and then direct the apex of the curve into your upper back and chest—behind your heart—sliding the shoulder blades down your back as you expand your chest and gaze upward.

**10**  **Go back and forth ten times.** As you exhale, turn your hips into cat tilt and press the middle of your back toward the ceiling; as you inhale, turn your hips into dog tilt and arch your spine. Go slowly back and forth, coordinating these two movements with your breathing. Match the speed of each movement with the speed of your breathing. Breathe slowly, smoothly, so your movement is slow and smooth. Let the inhalation begin just prior to the movement into dog tilt and finish just after the movement finishes—so the movement is surrounded by air, cushioned. Let the exhalation initiate the movement into cat tilt and come to an end just after the movement is complete. Pause momentarily after inhaling and exhaling. Keep the entire movement full of air.

**11**  As you move back and forth from cat tilt to dog tilt, sense the breath initiating the movement and the movement originating from your pelvis. Your hips turn first. The movement then flows through your spine and out the crown of your head. Stay smooth. Keep the movement fluid.

**12**  Be sure you understand this: The movement is sparked by the breath, and the first thing to move is your hips. For example, every time you exhale, you naturally draw your lower abdomen inward, backward toward the spine, tucking the coccyx under. Let that initiate the cat tilt action, and then follow through with the full spinal movement. Initiate the dog tilt phase of the pose in exactly the same way, letting the inhalation spark the movement. Understand that the breath fuels the movement and the movement starts from your center.

**13**  **Come back to neutral and relax.**

**14**  Your hips will always be in cat tilt or dog tilt, or moving toward one of these extremes or the other. It is essential that you learn to translate these two simple movements into every pose you do. Know which way your pelvis should be turning, depending on the pose, and always establish correct alignment at your center. Tilting the sacrum backward brings the hips toward cat tilt; reversing this brings the hips toward dog tilt.

**15**  Most backbends will be done with cat tilt, though there are exceptions, because this prevents overbending in the lumbar region of the spine. Forward bending is done with dog tilt because this enables you to hinge forward from your hips without rounding your back.

**16**  Always "think" from your center. Every line of energy and every breath originates here. Your center is the source of movement. The more you move from your center—the more you *feel* from inside and are sensitive—the more your body will tell you how to do the various poses properly. Only what is right can feel right, and cultivating your feeling-sensitivity will help you tell the difference. This is the key in learning to do yoga.

**17**  You are your own best teacher, and by maintaining an inner focus you will best learn how to do yoga. Turn your awareness inward, and let this express itself outwardly. Yoga is not mechanical.

# Benefits: Cat Pose

Spine and back loosener. Stretches front and back of body, frees neck and shoulders. Teaches correct pelvic movements: cat tilt, dog tilt, neutral. During cat tilt, the back muscles elongate and the abdominal muscles contract; during dog tilt, the back muscles contract and the abdomen stretches; in neutral, the spine is at its longest. Stimulates spinal fluid, digestive tract. Improves circulation through spine and core.

## STANDING POSES

# 3 Mountain Pose I & II *or Tadasana I, II*

This is called Mountain Pose because it promotes the experience of stillness, strength, relaxed power, and immovable stability associated with mountains. Remember that experiencing yourself in stillness is the most direct way to experience yourself with clarity. This pose, and coming back to this stillness after other poses, is one of the very best ways of becoming acquainted with stillness.

Tadasana is the most basic pose and is, therefore, the foundation for all others. There are two versions of Mountain Pose. The first, being stationary and passive, involves learning to stand erect, relaxed, and still. The second, being more active, involves learning to stretch and elongate your body from the inside out. Each version has two primary lines of energy radiating outward from your center: one line moving upward through the spine and one line downward through the legs. Your hips will be in cat tilt.

## QUIET MOUNTAIN

**1 Stand with your feet hip-width apart and your arms at your sides.** Look down at your feet and check that they are straight: the inner edges of each foot pointing straight ahead. Spread your toes.

**2** Bend your knees slightly, gently bob up and down a few times, and allow the weight of your body to sink into your feet. Snuggle the soles of your feet into the floor, make your feet heavy, and get grounded. This is easier to do with your legs bent. Experience yourself being supported by the floor.

**3** With your legs still bent, align your center. Bring your pelvis into a soft cat tilt by gently bringing the navel backward toward the spine until the tailbone points straight down toward your heels. The sacrum will become more vertical as the pelvis rotates backward. This is not a strong cat tilt (it's more like neutral), but you are turning your pelvis *toward* cat tilt.

**4** Maintaining the alignment of your center as effort-lessly as possible, slowly straighten your legs (photo 5). Do this slowly so as to keep track of what you're doing. Your feet will become more grounded as you do this, more firmly in contact with the floor because you are pressing straight down into them. Merge each foot into the floor and be sensitive not to let your weight be too far forward or too far backward, or too much toward the inside or outside of either foot. Balance the four directions equally so that each whole foot is engaged, so you have the best possible connection with the floor, with the earth.

**5** Once your legs are straight, maintain the alignment of your center by gently moving the thigh bones back-ward as you delicately press forward with your tailbone. This is another way of saying "Rotate the pelvis back-ward" or "Turn your hips toward cat tilt." Observe how these opposing movements work together to create sta-bility between your upper and lower body.

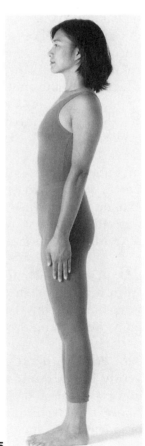

**5**

**6 Close your eyes.** With your eyes closed, lean forward a little and shift your weight to the front of your feet. Notice how the toes grab the floor to prevent a fall. Stay here a moment and experience the strain both in your feet and throughout your body. Then lean backward slightly and shift your weight onto the heels. Feel your toes becoming weightless and lifting from the floor. Stay here a moment and experience the uncertain balance.

**7** Shift your weight forward and backward several times, experiencing the difference, and then look for the balance point at which your weight is equally distributed between the heels and toes—just in front of the ankles. Be sensitive and delicate as you do this. When you find the perfect balance point, settle into it and stand absolutely still.

**8** To achieve perfect balance you must organize your center of gravity (your hips, abdomen, and pelvis) directly above the central point of your base of support (your feet). Find this spot by paying close attention to the inner sensations of balance. When your posture is aligned improperly, you will experience the downward pull of gravity as heaviness. When you are perfectly aligned and balanced, however, you will experience a buoyant lightness and spontaneous, natural uprightness. You will feel expanded, spacious, relaxed, and nearly weightless. Make subtle internal adjustments until you feel this way.

**9** Elongate your core upward through the crown of your head. Your core, your "invisible spine," extends from the tailbone at the bottom to the crown of the head. Feel where this is, then allow your spine and core to release and elongate. Imagine the spaces between your vertebrae expanding, especially in any area where you tend to experience discomfort or pain. As the spaces between vertebrae expand and increase, you will sense a subtle downward pull from the coccyx and a gentle upward movement throughout the length of your spine. Become familiar with this subtle movement.

**10** Allow your chest gently to expand, float, and ease its way upward away from the pelvis. This will elongate the waist and increase the distance between your hips and lower ribs. You are learning to create, or allow, more space in your body. Keep going upward through the crown.

**11** Feel the thoracic area of your spine, behind your heart, and allow it to move gently forward into your back. Feel how this encourages your chest to expand, and experience how this new openness is supported by the strength of your spine. Allow the sternum to rise effortlessly and come forward so the collarbones broaden across the top of your chest. Soften the shoulders back and down, away from the ears, and slide the shoulder blades down your back. Keep your navel backward toward the spine.

**12** Allow your head to float upward off the shoulders. Soften your neck and lower or elevate the chin, as needed, in order to eliminate any strain in your throat. Relax your face, allow a faint smile to emerge, and simply let your arms dangle limply. The more your arms, hands, and fingers relax, the more your neck, spine, and core will elongate.

**13** Be aware again of your feet on the floor and continue letting the weight of your body drop downward into the earth. At the same time, continue rising up-ward through the crown of your head. The weight of your body goes down, and the inner feeling rises up. Experience yourself going up and down at the same time, without going anywhere.

**14** Be very grounded as you sense the spinal release coming upward and out through the crown of your head. This grounded, upward-moving inner feeling is the natural impulse of balanced uprightness. The more you feel it, the more you'll know your balance is correct. Sense the subtle, effortless traction between your head and feet as they move away from one another. Your core now extends the full length of your body, from the soles of your feet at the bottom to the fontanel at the top.

**15** **Relax.** As you relax, you will expand. It's this subtle sense of expansion that effortlessly holds you up and ensures your new alignment.

**16** **Breathe smoothly.** Remember that the breath orchestrates the feeling-tone of the pose. Orchestrate stillness, softness, smooth evenness.

**17** **Be still.** Be motionless. Do not move a muscle. Do not even think. Just be wide awake and aware. How does it feel to be you right now? Be wide open like space, like the sky.

## TALL MOUNTAIN

**1 Stand with your feet together and your palms in prayer position (namaste) (photo 6) in front of your chest.**

**2** Get grounded first. Do this by spreading your toes, distributing your weight equally between the ball of each foot and the heels, and snuggling the soles of your feet into the floor. Allow the weight of your body to sink into your feet, make them heavy. Experience yourself being supported by the floor. Your feet are the foundation of the pose.

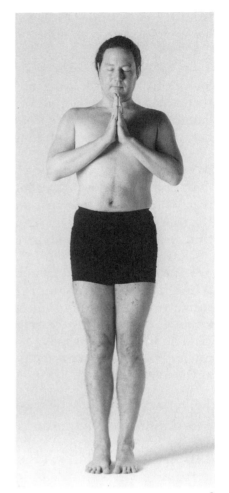

**3** Establish the alignment of your center. Do this by bending your knees slightly first, then tilt your pelvis toward cat tilt by gently moving the navel backward toward the spine, making the sacrum more vertical; there's no need to contract the buttocks.

**4** Establish the leg line. Press your legs straight, being careful not to lose the alignment of your center. Press straight down into the soles of your feet, feeling them merge with the floor, so the energy through your legs moves straight down in the direction they are pointing. You will become increasingly grounded as you do this. Do not hyperextend the legs,

**6**

though, by pressing the knees backward. Press *downward* into the feet rather than *backward* into the knees. Draw the kneecaps up, firm the thighs, and move the thigh bones backward as you press the tail bone foward. Then gently squeeze your inner legs together so your two legs work as one—like a single tree trunk taking root into the earth through the soft soles of your feet. Feel your connection with the floor, the earth. Hold your legs firm throughout the pose. This is the leg line.

**5** This downward-moving leg line will give you a strong sense of stability from which to stretch upward. The more you stretch downward through your legs and sink both feet into the floor, rooting yourself into the earth, the more you will be able to stretch upward, skyward, through your arms.

**6** Breathe smoothly and wait for the inner cue to proceed. As you wait, allow your chest gently to expand, easing its way upward away from the waist. Shrug the shoulder blades down, keep your navel backward toward the spine, and subtly increase the distance between the soles of your feet and the crown of your head. Elongate internally. Elongate your core. The crown of your head will move upward, and your feet will become more grounded. Keep your eyes open, your chin level, and your gaze straight ahead.

**7** When you are ready to proceed, lace your fingers together, turn the hands inside out, and rest them on top of your head with the palms facing skyward. Alternatively, bring your prayer hands on top of your head with the fingers pointing up; that's the direction your hands will be moving. Keep your elbows backward, in line with the ears, so the forearms make a single straight line from elbow to elbow. Relax your neck and shoulders. Exhale.

**8** **Stretch your arms straight up.** As you inhale, slowly move your hands toward the ceiling. Make it feel as though the inhalation were causing the movement, as though your hands are going up *because* you are breathing in. Straighten them about two-thirds of the way, then stop; do not press them fully straight yet. As you exhale, keep your hands where they are and pull your navel backward toward the spine. It feels natural to do this. Inhale again and take the hands higher, and as you exhale, reaffirm the alignment of your center by again pulling the navel backward. Proceed like this until your arms are fully straight.

**9** Feel your two lines of energy: one from your belly downward through the legs, and one from your belly upward through the spine and arms. Immerse yourself in the *feeling* of the lines. Breathe with feeling. There's an energetic feeling-tone to what you are doing. Feel your energy moving vertically up and down through your core, between the soles of your feet and the palms of your hands.

**10** The arm line starts at your belly, remember, not the shoulders. Therefore, in order to establish a good line of energy upward through the arms, lift upward from your belly into your chest and shoulders, from the shoulders stretch upward into the elbows, and from the elbows press your palms toward the ceiling. Squeeze your elbows inward toward one another. Press your arms fully straight. Put some oomph into it. Elongate. But also let it feel as though someone else were pulling you up by your hands and you're letting them—you're dangling—and the full length of your body is slowly increasing. It should feel as though you are ''doing'' and ''not-doing'' at the same time.

**11** Stretch upward through the arms in the direction they are pointing. If they are sloping forward slightly, stretch outward in that direction. It is the outward-upward stretch through the arms that will eventually bring them vertical. This upward-moving arm line will elongate your core, open the chest and shoulders, and energize your arms, head, and hands. Become as long, tall, and thin as possible. Reach for the ceiling, the sky, infinity.

**12** **Come up on your toes and balance** (photo 7). As you exhale, lean forward until your heels hover lightly off the floor. Be sensitive and aware as you do this, feel what you are doing, shift your weight forward slowly. Then flow with your breathing and come up on your toes: As you inhale, press the ball of each foot into the floor and rise higher, and as you exhale, pull the navel backward toward the spine, gently squeeze your inner legs together, and become more firmly grounded. Proceed like this until you are all the way up on your toes. Stay here and breathe.

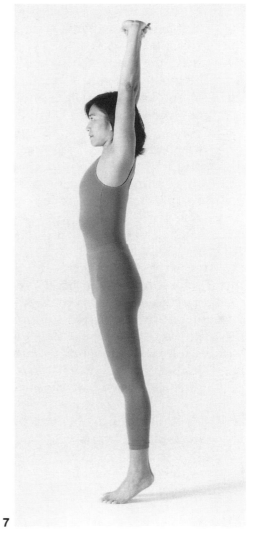

7

**13** The leg line starts at your belly and travels downward through your legs and feet into the earth. Keep your inner legs squeezing together, your ankles gently pressed into one another, and your toes spread. Direct the weight of your body straight down through the inner edge of each leg into the base of each second toe. Press downward into your feet and gently squeeze the legs together. When this is done properly, your legs will feel strong and springy, enthusiastic.

**14** Notice that your kneecaps are pulled up, lifted and tight, without pressing the knees backward. You are pressing straight downward through your legs into the feet, in the direction the legs are pointing, not backward through the knees.

**15** Deliberately increase or decrease the current in your arms and legs until the feeling-tone seems perfect to you—not too much, not too little. Allow it to fluctuate and change as you stay in the pose so that it always feels "most right" to you.

**16** Stay in the pose for about a minute. Bring it to life with your breathing: Stretch up *and* down as you inhale, pushing downward into your feet and upward into your hands, and *release* upward and downward as you exhale, gently pulling the navel backward toward the spine to reaffirm the alignment of your center. Allow your hands to rise effortlessly higher as your feet merge more thoroughly with the floor. Stretch up and down as you inhale, and release up and down as you exhale. Elongate yourself from the inside out.

**17** Try not to wobble. Do this by becoming increasingly grounded. Balance with confidence in a relaxed manner.

**18** Keep your eyes open most of the time, but occasionally test your balance by closing your eyes. This is considerably more difficult.

**19** If you are experiencing excess tension anywhere—in your throat, the back of your neck or shoulders, your lower back, or legs, feet, or calves—make subtle internal adjustments until the tension is diminished. Be as strain-free as possible, yet do what you have to do.

**20** **To come out of the pose, exhale as you lower your heels and bring your palms together in namaste position on your chest.** Be here a few moments with your eyes closed. Then lower your arms, stand quietly, and experience what's happening. Be aware.

# Benefits: Standing Poses

The Standing Poses are big, whole body poses that teach you to move in an even, integrated way. They make the finer, more contortionistic poses possible. Be sure to spend plenty of time with these poses, even as you become more advanced, but especially as a beginner, because they build the strength and endurance necessary to support the increased flexibility that will accrue over time through practice. The Standing Postures help create a balance between strength and flexibility throughout the body by developing both simultaneously, not one at the expense of the other. They especially increase strength, power, and mobility in the feet, legs, and hips, which then become a firm base of support for your spine and torso in other poses. Feet, knees, legs, hips, spine, torso, abdomen, chest, neck, shoulders, arms, and hands, even the fingers and toes, all gain strength and become more elastic with these poses—free of tension, aches, and pains. And because they are somewhat strenuous, they improve blood circulation, stimulate digestion and elimination, build heat for other poses, expulse dullness and depression, and leave you feeling invigorated, refreshed, and light. All of this helps bring the subtle energies of the body into harmonization. Daily life will then seem and be easier. You won't tire as easily. You'll have more energy and enthusiasm, and be more interested in what's going on.

# Benefits: Mountain Pose I & II *or Tadasana I, II*

Mountain Pose is the foundation for all poses. It aligns the body, teaches correct standing, increases awareness, develops a refined sense of balance, and steadies the breath. The basic ideas here translate into all poses.

# 4 Standing Side Stretch *or Ardha Chandrasana I*

The Standing Side Stretch is another pose with two lines of energy radiating outward from your center. One line of energy reaches upward from your belly and outward through the arm, and one line travels downward through the legs. Your pelvis will be in cat tilt. This is a simple pose with a wonderful stretch.

**1 Stand in Tadasana (Mountain Pose) with your feet together.** Have your arms by your sides, gaze straight ahead, and establish a smooth flowing breath as you wait for the inner cue to begin. When you are ready, exhale.

**2 As you inhale, raise the left arm until it is vertical, alongside your ear, with the palm facing inward.** Stretch outward through your arm and hand as you bring it up, circumscribing as large a circle as possible with your fingertips. Keep your left arm alongside your ear throughout the pose. Place your right hand on your right hip.

**3** Feel where the lines of energy are, one up the arm and one down the legs, and then establish the alignment of your center. Do this by pulling the abdominal muscles inward, gently backward toward the spine, so the coccyx (tailbone) points straight down and the sacrum comes to a more vertical alignment—cat tilt.

**4** Establish the leg line. Spread your toes and snuggle your feet into the floor. Lift the kneecaps, tighten the thighs, and gently squeeze your legs together. Press downward through your legs into your feet, become grounded, and take a moment to be very solid and stable. You will not be coming up on your toes in this posture, but create that same springy feeling.

**5** Establish the upward-moving arm line. From your belly, lift upward into your chest, and from the left shoulder, stretch straight upward through the arm and out your hand. Spread your fingers. Keep both shoulder blades tugging down your back, and continue pulling the navel backward toward the spine. Feel the difference between the left side of your body and the right.

**6** Stay in this position for several breaths, clarifying the vertical line upward and downward from your center. Then inhale deeply and increase the current up the arm. Stretch with enthusiasm.

**7** **As you exhale, lean to the right** (photo 8). Turn your head and look down, pressing your hips sideways. This feels wonderful.

**8** Go as far as you comfortably can, then take inventory. Expand the chest away from the waist, slide the shoulder blades down your back, and keep the abdominals pulled backward toward the spine. Squeeze your legs together as you press downward into your feet, and reach enthusiastically outward through your left arm. Stretch through the arm in the direction it is pointing. If your arm is pointing straight up, stretch straight up; if it's at a forty-five-degree angle, stretch outward at a forty-five-degree angle. Follow the lines deeper into the pose.

**9** Keep your body in one plane with the abdomen facing straight ahead. Correct the tendency to sway off-plane by moving the left frontal hip bone forward and the left shoulder backward, so the left shoulder stays directly above the right.

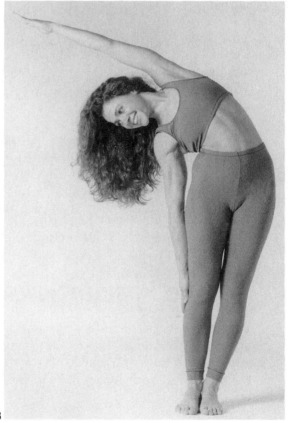

8

**10** Breathe consciously, smoothly, and bring the pose to life with the breath. Increase the stretch through the arm line as you inhale, then exhale as you lean farther into the pose, pressing your hips to the left. Stretch through the shape as you inhale, release through the shape as you exhale. Practice "doing" and "not-doing" within the span of a single breath. Take your time.

**11** Close your eyes, go inward, and experience the pose. Feel what you're doing. Stay relaxed as you increase or decrease the current through your lines. Be as effortless as possible. Relax with the intensity. Wait for the sensations of stretch to diminish somewhat before going deeper. Be here from thirty seconds to one minute.

**12** Do not concern yourself with how far you can or cannot lean to the right. Instead, savor the stretch. Enjoy what's happening. It's exhilarating. You're one long curve of energy.

**13** When you're nearly done, turn your head and gaze upward, spiraling your chest toward the sky, and then accelerate your energy through the pose for a few seconds. Then come out of the pose.

**14** Inhale as you come up. Exhale as you lower your arm.

**15** Stand still for a few moments and savor the aftereffects of the pose. Wait for the inner signal to proceed and then do the other side.

# Benefits: Standing Side Stretch *or Ardha Chandrasana I*

Tremendous side stretch increasing flexibility of spine, arms, and rib cage. Stimulates liver, kidney, spleen function.

# 5 Tree Pose *or Vrkshasana*

The Tree Pose is a one-legged balance pose with three lines of energy radiating outward from your center. One line travels down the straight leg, one line stretches up the spine and out the arms, and a third line moves outward through the bent knee. Your hips will be in cat tilt.

**1** **Stand in Tadasana (Mountain Pose) with your feet together.** Have your arms by your sides, establish a smooth flowing breath, and wait for the inner cue to begin. When you are ready, shift all your weight onto your left foot and balance here where it's easy. Breathe in deeply.

**2** **As you exhale, bring your right foot up, placing the sole of the foot as high as possible on the left inner thigh with the toes pointing down. Bring your palms together into namaste, the prayer position.**

**3** Steady your balance before refining your alignment. There are several aids to this:

a) Spread your toes fully and snuggle your left foot firmly into the floor. Become grounded, merge with the earth, and allow the weight of your body to sink downward into that foot. This is your contact point with the ground, the foundation of the pose. Take root. Be solid. The more you allow your weight to sink into the foot, the more certain your balance will be.

b) Fix your gaze on something that is not moving, then don't let your mind move. Hold that point with your eyes and mind. Maintain a steady, soft gaze and clear focus. This will concentrate the mind, which will facilitate balance.

c) Breathe with awareness. Produce a smooth, even sound; an erratic breath will disturb the balance.

d) Stand with your right knee lightly touching a wall.

**4** Refine your alignment and establish an energy flow through the lines. Ideally, you want the abdominal plane facing straight ahead with the bent knee stretching straight outward to the side, not angling toward the front as is its tendency. The main action of the pose is to flatten the pelvis. The three energy lines work together to help you do this.

**5** Establish the alignment of your center first. Bend the left leg very slightly—this will help you feel more grounded—then gently pull the abdominals backward toward the spine and point the coccyx straight down (toward the left heel) so the sacrum becomes more vertical—cat tilt.

**6** Slowly press the left leg straight without changing the alignment of your center. Press straight down into your left foot, keeping the sole of your foot soft. Root yourself into the earth. This establishes your first line of energy.

**7 Inhale as you raise your arms above your head** (photo 9). Either keep the palms together and stretch upward through the fingertips, or interlace your fingers, turn your hands inside out, and press upward through the palms. Take them up breath by breath, the way you did in Tadasana II, the Tall Mountain. This is your second line of energy.

**8** The arm line originates at your center, remember. Therefore, lift the rib cage away from the waist, elongating the waist, squeeze the elbows inward toward one another, and stretch straight upward through the hands in the direction the arms are pointing. If the arms are sloping forward, direct your line of energy in that direction. It is the outward-upward stretch that will eventually bring them vertical. If the arms are already vertical, try to lift your elbows several inches above your ears and then move them backward behind your ears, still stretching upward. Keep the shoulder blades tugging down your back and continue pulling the navel backward.

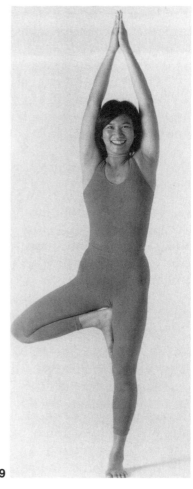

9

**9** Check that the abdominal plane is facing straight ahead. Move the right frontal hip bone forward, if necessary, until it is equal with the left. Also check that your chest is facing straight ahead; if necessary, bring the right side of your chest forward until it is equal with the left.

**10** Establish your third line of energy by stretching outward into the bent knee and moving it backward. Flex your right foot and press the heel into the left inner thigh, stretch the inner side of the right thigh toward the knee, and gently aim the right knee backward. This is the action that will flatten the pelvis. Do this without turning your body, however. Keep the supporting foot, the abdominal plane, and your chest facing straight ahead.

**11** You are now stretching in three directions simultaneously: downward, upward, outward. You are running ''energy'' through the shape.

**12** Breathe deeply, smoothly, and bring the lines to life. As you inhale, press downward into the supporting foot, reach upward through the hands, and stretch outward and backward through the bent knee—filling out the shape you now are. As you exhale, pull the navel backward toward the spine and release outward in all three directions. Be here one minute.

**13** This is a simple pose, but the ability to flatten the pelvis releases tension in this area.

**14** **Exhale as you bring your hands and foot down.** Stand motionless for a few moments, then do the other side.

# Benefits: Tree Pose *or Vrkshasana*

Develops balance, concentration, stability, poise. Strengthens legs and feet. Increases flexibility in hips and knees, opens chest, tones shoulder muscles. Steadies the nerves. Calming.

# 6 Standing Forward Fold *or Uttanasana*

Uttanasana has two lines of energy radiating outward from your center. Your hips will be in dog tilt, and the spinal column will be your primary line of energy. The idea is to elongate the spine outward through the crown of your head as you fold into the pose. This is the basic forward fold. Everything you learn here will be applicable to all forward folds.

There are several excellent ways of practicing Uttanasana. I am including my three favorites.

### DANGLING UTTANASANA

**1** **Stand in Tadasana (Mountain Pose) with your feet hip-width apart.** Look down at your feet and check that they are parallel with one another, that the inner edge of each foot is pointing straight ahead, and that your toes are spread. Snuggle your feet into the floor. Wait until you are ready, then breathe in deeply.

**2** **As you exhale, slide your hands down your legs and fold forward from your hips.** Go slowly. Clasp hold of your elbows and let your head and arms dangle, or clasp your hands around your legs and let your arms slide down the back of your legs (photo 10).

**3** **Relax.** Do nothing. Simply become thoroughly limp. Let go inside and surrender to the pose.

**4** The idea here is to let go of all effort, all resistance to being in the pose, and simply to be thoroughly relaxed. Scan your body at a leisurely pace and mentally encourage your cells, nerves, muscles, and skin, everything, to relax and soften. Release every sense of holding on. Relax your belly, buttocks, back, shoulders, face. Allow your neck to soften, your head to dangle, and your arms to be limp. Especially elongate your core. Hang from your hips. Dangle. Let go, fall. Let go everywhere. *Practice* letting go. The more you let go and release tension, the better you'll get at it. Relax in this bent-over position. Consciously, deliberately surrender.

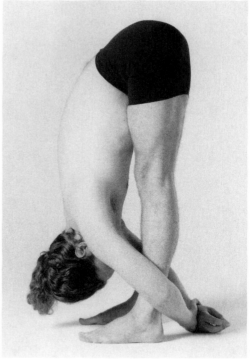

**10**

**5** Especially feel where your spine is, your core, from coccyx to fontanel, and allow the spaces between vertebrae to expand. You'll feel your spine elongate as your core clarifies. Do this by letting go, releasing. You're letting go of tension, contracted energy, pain.

**6** Orchestrate softness with a soft breath. Breathe smoothly in a relaxed, strain-free manner.

**7** If dangling from your hips is too intense, then either bend your knees or place your hands on your shins and brace yourself further up. Bending your legs will reduce strain considerably, and bracing yourself with your arms will prevent you from folding too far. Stay within your comfort zone. Find a place in which you can relax. Be farther up if necessary.

**8** Continue letting go, over and over. Letting go is not something you do just once. As you relax inside and release every sense of tension, your muscles will become less hard, less contracted. Gradually they will soften, lengthen, and you'll find yourself folding deeper into the pose, effortlessly. From there, let go more. Continue letting go, and see what happens. Wherever the stretch is, be there mentally. Soothe any part of your body that is resisting the stretch, holding on due to fear, or unnecessarily tense and clenched. Coax all of yourself to soften and relax. You'll find yourself going deeper when your body is ready for a deeper stretch, not before. You have no say in the matter. This is what makes this technique so safe.

**9** The only "control" is to stay in the pose long enough for a change to occur. Everything else is a let-go and surrender. Stay here as long as five minutes, but do not force yourself to stay longer than feels right. Come out of the pose when you have had enough. Later, it may feel appropriate to challenge your endurance edge by willingly staying in the pose even if you are experiencing some degree of discomfort. This will be voluntary, however, and it will not feel as though you are attacking yourself. It will be attractive and pleasurable.

**10** Occasionally, vary the distance between your feet. It is often easier to relax when your feet are farther apart.

**11** **To come out of the pose, bend your knees and slowly come down into a squatting position.** Be here several breaths, then stand erect in Tadasana, Mountain Pose.

**12** Close your eyes and practice standing perfectly still. Do not move a muscle. Don't even think. But don't *hold* yourself still, either. Relax yourself still. Be as relaxed as you can possibly be, and simply be aware of how you feel. Immerse your awareness in the natural rhythm of your breathing and experience your own unique feeling-tone. Enjoy this part.

## UTTANASANA IN SIX STAGES

**1** **Stand in Tadasana with your feet hip-width apart.** Look down and check that the inner edge of each foot is pointing straight ahead so your feet are parallel to one another. Spread your toes, lift your kneecaps, and stand tall by lifting upward through your spine, chest, and head.

**2** Breathe smoothly, making an even, pleasant sound in your throat as you wait for the inner cue to begin. When you are ready, breathe in deeply.

### STAGE ONE

**3** **As you exhale, hinge forward from your hips and place your hands either on your thighs just above your knees or at the top of your shinbones**

**just below the knees** (photo 11). The idea here is to flatten your back and elongate your spine.

**4** Turn your hips toward dog tilt and feel where your three lines of energy are: one down the legs, one through the arms, and one outward (and eventually downward) through the spine.

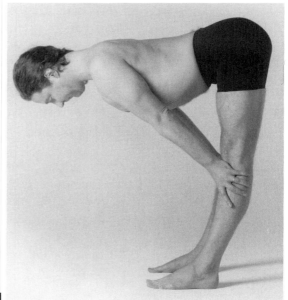

**11**

**5** Clarify the leg line. First, snuggle your feet into the floor and feel your connection with the earth. Make sure you are grounded. Then pull the kneecaps up by tightening the quadriceps (thigh muscles), press both feet into the floor, and turn the sitting bones upward. Roll the thighs inward as you do this, spreading the buttocks apart, and make sure your weight is coming down through the center of each foot—not too far forward or backward, nor toward the inner or outer edge of either foot. These actions will establish and increase dog tilt.

**6** Clarify the arm line. Press your arms straight, making them long, and lift upward with the back of your head and neck. Do not lean into your hands or sag into your shoulders. Lengthen your arms, lift up, and stay lifted. As you do this there will be some weight on your hands in the form of palm pressure, but minimize it.

**7** Elongate your spine horizontally forward. Press backward through the buttocks, and stretch forward through the crown of your head. Do not shorten the back of your neck by lifting your head and looking forward. Softly tuck your chin without tightening the throat, roll the back of your head forward, and shrug the shoulders away from your ears so the shoulder blades slide down your back. You will feel like a turtle sticking its head out of its shell. Gaze at the floor. This is Stage One.

**8** The forward fold is initiated by turning the hips into dog tilt. This segments the body in two opposite directions from your center. The key to folding deeper in this pose, as in all forward folds, is to increase the pelvic rotation toward dog tilt, so you hinge from the hip joints, and to lift the rib cage away from the waist as you stretch forward through the crown of your head. As you direct the stretch outward, your spine will form an indented groove down your back. Check with your fingers to make sure there are no protruding vertebrae.

**9** Your breathing, remember, is the most important aspect of yoga technique. It is the life of the pose. Therefore, savor the air as it flows in and out and listen to the sound you are making. Breathe smoothly, generate the perfect degree of current through your lines, and wait for the initial sensations of stretch to diminish before folding deeper.

## STAGE TWO

**10 Slide your hands to your ankles** (photo 12). When the initial sensations of stretch diminish in Stage One and you notice your elbows wanting to bend, slide your hands farther down the legs.

**11** Fold deeper into the pose slowly, with care, breath by breath. Elongate the spine horizontally forward as you inhale and fold deeper as you exhale. Keep your arms and legs straight.

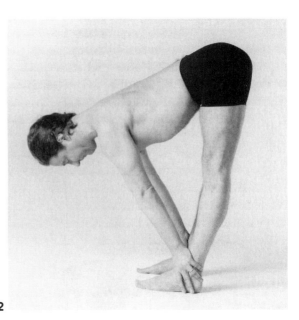

12

**12** When you reach your ankles, check the alignment of your lines once again: Press your feet into the floor and turn the sitting bones up, bringing your lower back down; press your arms straight, making them as long as you can, and lift upward with the back of your head and neck so you're not sagging into the shoulders; then press *backward* through the sitting bones and *forward* through the crown of your head, shrugging the shoulders away from the ears. These three lines work together beautifully.

**13** The better your spinal extension now, the deeper your stretch later. Create the degree of stretch that feels perfect—not too much, not too little. Breathe deeply, keeping it smooth. Wait for the sensations of stretch to diminish some-what at this edge before proceeding further.

## STAGE THREE

**14** **Bend your arms and rest your elbows on your shins** (photo 13). Your hands are still at your ankles. Continue lifting upward with the back of your head and neck, lifting upward out of the shoulders, and attempt to further elon-gate your spine forward in the direction it is now pointing. Flatten your back by turning the sitting bones up and bringing the lower back down, spreading the buttocks sideways away from one another, and then press backward through the buttocks and forward-outward through the crown of your head.

**15** Breathe smoothly. Be here several breaths. Wait for the sensations of stretch to diminish somewhat at this new edge before proceeding deeper.

## STAGE FOUR

**16** **Clasp hold of your elbows and then slide your elbows down the shin-bones toward the ankles** (photo 14). Keep the elbows in contact with your shins, if you can, and do not frustrate yourself by thinking you are not as deep as you should be. Do what you can do. Then stay where you are and breathe, waiting for the musculature to open and the sensations of stretch to diminish. When you can reach your ankles with your elbows, stretch deeper by sliding

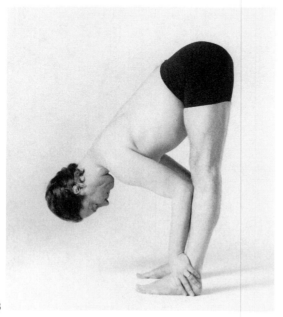

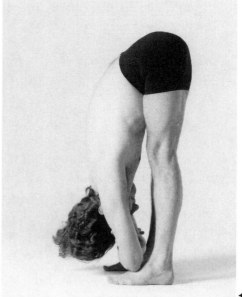

13

14

them across the top of your feet toward the toes. Lower your head and look straight backward through your legs.

**17**  You are now the same shape as Dangling Uttanasana, but you are not limp. You are actively stretching. Be deliberate about this, and gentle. To intensify the stretch, push into your elbows and pull down with your hands.

**18**  Breathe smoothly, deeply. Relax with the intensity. Do and not-do at the same time. Allow the stretch to penetrate.

## STAGE FIVE

**19**  **Bend your knees until your chest and thighs touch, interlace your fingers behind your back, and straighten your arms** (photo 15). Hold a strap if you have difficulty clasping your hands or straightening your arms.

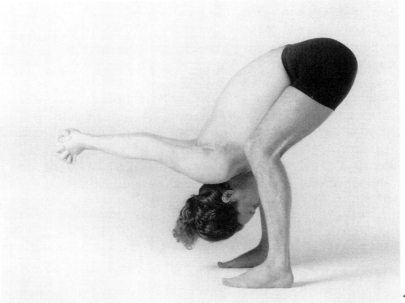

**15**

**20**  Immerse yourself in your breathing and gently go after the stretch. As you inhale, stretch outward through your arms in the direction they are pointing. As you exhale, make your hands heavy and gently squeeze them toward the floor. From there, inhale again and stretch outward through the arms, then exhale and squeeze them toward the floor. Do this with each breath. Immerse yourself in what you are doing. Get involved. Participate. Be here several breaths.

## STAGE SIX

**21** **Slowly straighten your legs** (photo 16). Do this in two parts. First, keeping the arm line active and your hands heavy and, keeping the chest and thighs pressed together, slowly allow your hips to rise toward the ceiling. Let them float upward all by themselves—no effort or doing on your part. Then, gently press both feet into the floor and delicately try to straighten the legs—allowing the chest and thighs to separate, if necessary. Your hips will move upward as your feet press downward. Stretch the sitting bones toward the ceiling. This can be intense, so proceed slowly, with sensitivity. Move your head inward toward your legs as you straighten them, and continue squeezing your hands down.

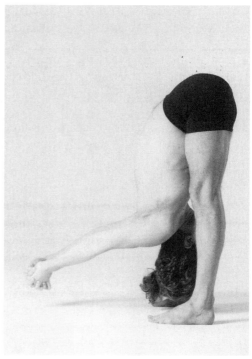

**16**

**22**   Eventually, at this point, your chest will be in firm contact with your thighs, your legs will be straight, and your hands will be touching the floor behind you. Be here several breaths working the arm line outward and down.

**Note:**  These six stages are not easy. They may take years to master. Be patient, therefore, but persistent. Do what you comfortably can; no more than that is necessary.

**23**   To come out of the pose, release your hands from behind your back, place them on your ankles and return to Stage Two: arms straight, legs straight, back flat, gazing at the floor. Be here for a breath or two. Then place your hands on your hips and come to a standing position. Lower your arms.

**24**   You are now in Tadasana, Mountain Pose. Close your eyes and practice standing still. Be aware of your feet on the floor and allow the weight of your body to sink downward. Let the soles of your feet be soft. Be sensitive to your connection with the earth, merge with the floor, become grounded. Then let the crown of your head float upward, without becoming ungrounded, and experience the inner feeling coming upward through your spine, chest, and crown. Chest up, shoulder blades down, navel backward toward the spine. Find the perfect point of balance. This, remember, is where you feel most weightless, light. Be aware of how you feel. Be still. Experience what's happening.

## CHEST TO THIGHS UTTANASANA

**1  Stand in Tadasana with your feet together.** Spread your toes and snuggle your feet into the floor so you feel grounded and secure, unmoving.

**2  Bend your knees, fold forward, and press your chest into your thighs** (photo 17). Clasp your calves, hook your chin over your knees, and use your arm strength to keep your chest in firm contact with the thighs. Stretch the back of your upper arms toward the elbows, press forward with your hands, and squeeze inward (hugging your legs) with your elbows.

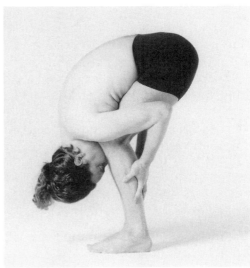

**3**  Center yourself in a smooth flowing breath and wait for the inner cue to proceed. When you are ready, breathe in deeply.

**17**

**4  As you exhale, move your hips toward the ceiling and delicately press your legs *toward* straight.** When your chest begins to separate from your thighs, stop. This is your spot. Do not straighten your legs any further yet. This is where the pose actually begins. Be here several breaths and wait.

**5**  The idea is to start with your chest pressed firmly into your thighs, and then to keep it there as you straighten your legs—rather than the other way around. Your job is to keep the chest and thighs together as you straighten the legs. When you are ready, proceed.

**6**  Straighten your legs a little, then stop; straighten, stop, straighten, stop. Increase the depth of this stretch slowly, edge by edge. Take your time. Do not rush. Stretch downward through the crown of your head, squeeze inward with your elbows, hugging your legs, and with each exhalation, gently press your feet into the floor. This will cause your legs to straighten and your hips to rise. Stay here as you inhale and straighten the legs further as you exhale. When you are able to press your legs fully straight and still maintain the chest-thigh contact, you will be in a very tight forward fold (photo 18), but do not forcibly press your legs straight. Keep your arms active, your chest in firm contact with your thighs, and allow your hips slowly to rise toward the ceiling. Immerse yourself in the breath.

**7** Breathe deeply at your deepest extension for at least five breaths. Breathe from the back of your throat and listen to the ujjayi sound. Make the breath long, smooth, and even.

**8** To come out of the pose, bend your knees and return to a standing position.

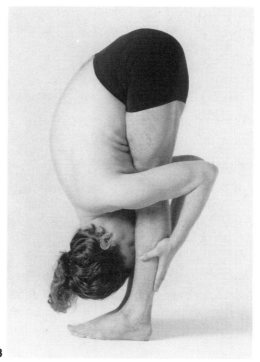

18

**9** You are now in Mountain Pose. Lift your chest, slide the shoulder blades down your back, and gently pull the navel backward toward your spine. Then close your eyes, stand quietly, and relax. Be aware of how you feel. Savor the aftereffects of the pose.

*Question:*   I find these stretches painful in the back of my legs. What can I do?

*Response:*   That means you are too deep. Either come farther up and be in the pose without pain, or bend your legs as much as necessary. Learn to stretch and be in the pose without pain. Get near pain, but do not be in it. If the sensation is too intense, your muscles will contract in order to protect themselves from being overstretched. That means you're going too deep, too fast. Stay within your comfort zone and delicately nudge into your tight areas.

*Question:*   Why do you emphasize locking the elbows in the Six Stage Technique?

*Response:*   Actually, you do not want to "lock" the elbows. You want the arms extended fully straight. If you think of "locking the elbows" when pressing the arms straight, there will be too much emphasis on the elbows, and there will be a tendency toward hyperextension. You want the energy flow to pass freely through the elbows. You do not want it locked up. The same is true with your knees when your legs are straight. You do not want to lock your knees. You want to lift the kneecaps as you press your legs straight in order to enhance the energy flow.

I emphasize the arm extension while making the descent so as better to extend the spinal line outward. Only after you have achieved the outward spinal extension do you let your elbows bend inward. Unless you stretch outward, the lumbar and sacral regions of your spine will never get their full extension. It is this outward stretch that will eventually take you deeper into the pose. Your spine will then be as long and flat as possible. If you curve your head inward toward your knees, your back will round too much. You will feel your energy going out the middle of your back instead of out the top of your head.

**Question:**  If someone is breathing too fast, would you take that as feedback they have gone too deep?

**Response:**  Yes. Fast breathing is only necessary when you are pushing a final edge pretty hard, and it is rarely recommended. It is not recommended for beginners. At any rate, it should be voluntary.

The whole trick is to find a place in the pose in which you can deepen the breath, stretch with sensitivity, and enjoy what you are doing. When that happens, you will relax deeper into the pose. The fastest way to deepen a pose is by going slowly, not by rushing toward the "completed" pose or your deepest extensions. The completed posture is like froth on a wave: It's there, it'll happen, but it is not the important thing. The important thing is to flirt with your physical and mental edges (wherever they are), enjoy the process, and immerse yourself in your now-experience. Being wholehearted rarely means going full-blast. It means generating the feeling-tone and degree of intensity that feels best to you now; sometimes more, sometimes less.

In all these variations, work to your capacity without straining. Stay within your comfort zone. This will change as you become stronger and more flexible. It will also change as you become tired or fatigued. The best way to progress is gradually. Persist. Enjoy what you are doing.

# Benefits: Standing Forward Fold *or Uttanasana*

Stretches entire backside of body, especially legs and lower back. Elongates spine. Increases flexibility. Massages internal organs, tones liver, spleen, kidneys. Increases blood circulation to legs, torso, and brain. Good pose to rest in after strenuous poses.

# 7 Dog Pose *or Adho Mukha Shvanasana*

Dog Pose has two lines of energy radiating outward from your center. The center of this pose, as always, is your pelvis. Your hips will be in dog tilt. The first line of energy moves down the legs and into the feet, the second line travels through your spine and arms into your hands on the floor. The idea in this pose is to form a triangular, pyramidal shape. You'll look like a dog stretching after a nap.

**1**  **Start in Child's Pose with your arms extended straight** (photo 19). Stretch your hands as far away from you as possible. This establishes your hand and knee placement.

**2**  **Keeping your hands where they are, come up onto your hands and knees into a flat-back Cat Pose.** The arm line will not be vertical, but position your hands so they are shoulder-width apart. Have your knees and feet hip-width apart. Snuggle your hands into the floor, fingers spread, and align your hands so each middle finger is pointing straight ahead. Curl your toes under.

**3**  Establish a smooth-flowing breath with the ujjayi throat sound and wait for the inner cue to proceed.

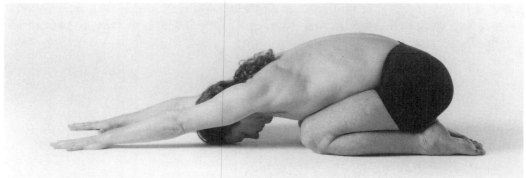

**19**

**4** As you wait for the inner cue, do not sag into your shoulders. Instead, lengthen the arms by pressing downward into your hands and lifting upward out of the shoulders. This simple movement is vital to this pose. When you are ready, exhale.

## STAGE ONE

**5** **As you inhale, turn your hips into dog tilt** (photo 20). Your spine is now arched. Gently pull the navel backward toward your spine to stabilize your pelvis.

**6** **As you exhale, straighten your legs** (photo 21). Pause here a moment and take inventory.

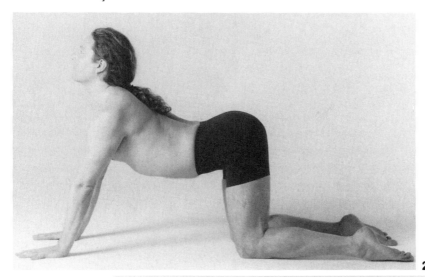

**20**

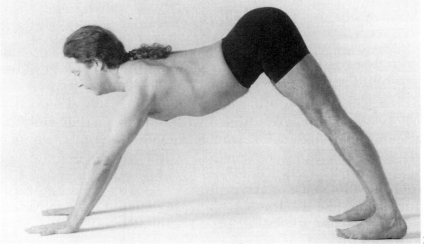

**21**

**7** Your first objective is to arch your spine and establish dog tilt with straight arms and straight legs. Do this by pushing downward into your hands and lifting upward with your head; do not sag into the shoulders and do not retract the head backward into your neck. Lengthen your arms by lifting up. Then turn the sitting bones upward and spread the buttocks sideways away from one another, dog tilt, so the thighs roll inward slightly and the inner thighs move backward, away from you. Lift the kneecaps by tightening the quadriceps, check that your feet are straight, toes spread, and press the heels toward the floor. Make your legs feel springy. Breathe. Be here several breaths.

## STAGE TWO

**8** Your second objective is to establish a straight line through your spine and arms (photo 22). Do this with the breath.

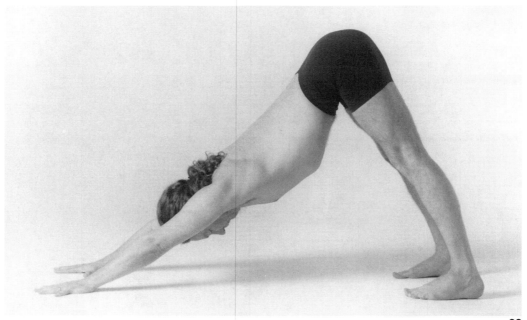

**22**

**9** **As you inhale, press downward into your hands and lift upward out of the shoulders.** Lift your head and torso away from the floor as much as possible; this is "not sagging" or "lengthening the arms."

**10** **As you exhale, move your pelvis backward and upward, bringing your torso toward your legs.** Feel how the groin, the crease formed by your torso and thighs, moves up, away from your wrists.

**11** Do these two movements over and over, breath by breath, until you have achieved a straight line from your hands, through your shoulders, to your hips. With each inhalation, push into your hands to lengthen the arms, lifting upward out of the shoulders, and with each exhalation take the groin deeper, moving the pelvis away from you. Eventually your arms and spine will form a straight line.

**12** The downward-forward push into your hands and the upward-backward movement through the pelvis is the same line of energy; it is a two-directional line. This two-way stretch opens the shoulders and chest, elongates the spine, and flattens the back.

**13** Squeeze your elbows inward toward one another so the arms become fully straight, and press the palm and index finger of each hand firmly into the floor. Do not grip the floor. Press into it.

**14** Press the legs fully straight, tighten the quadriceps, turning the thighs inward toward one another to help spread the buttocks, and press the feet firmly into the floor. This can be an intense stretch, so be sensitive; don't overdo it. Turning the buttocks upward and pressing the heels downward (another two-way stretch) will create a strong pull on the hamstring muscles.

## STAGE THREE

**15** Your third objective, once you have achieved a straight line from your hands to your coccyx, is to deepen the fold at your hips and bow your spine toward the floor. Do this by squeezing your head and chest downward and inward toward your legs (photo 23). Do not attempt this, however, unless you have first estab-

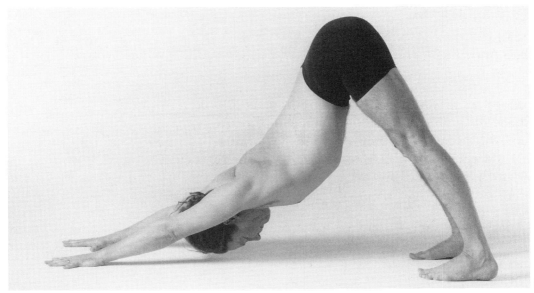

23

lished a straight line through your spine and arms. Let me repeat: Create a straight line from your hands through your shoulders to your hips before attempting to bow your spine.

**16** **As you inhale, press into your hands to lengthen the arms and achieve maximum length from your hands to coccyx. As you exhale, gently squeeze your head and chest toward your legs.** From there, elongate again with the next inhalation, then squeeze your head and chest closer to the floor with the exhalation. Do this over and over: inhale elongate, exhale squeeze. Coordinate your stretching with your breathing. When you cannot increase the stretch any further, stay where you are and deepen the breath.

**17** This is a backbend. So, like the dog tilt phase of Cat Pose, turn the sitting bones upward, move your thoracic (mid) spine deeper into your back, and slide the shoulder blades down your back to help open your chest toward the floor. Keep the navel pulled backward toward the spine and take the groin deep. Eventually, you will have your arms and legs straight, your head on the floor, with your spine forming a smooth graceful curve. Deepen the pose by moving your head closer toward your feet.

**18** Stay in the pose for one minute or until you feel you have had enough. Then bend your knees, come out of the pose, and rest.

## QUARTER DOG

Both Quarter Dog and Half Dog are less strenuous versions of Dog Pose. These variations eliminate the hamstring stretch and enable you to focus specifically on the arm and shoulder stretch.

**1** **Start on your elbows in neutral Cat Pose.**

**2** **Bring your right hand behind your left elbow.** Do not sag into the right shoulder; instead, press downward into your right elbow and lift upward. This action creates space in the shoulder joint. Maintain this increased space for the duration of the pose.

**3** **Stretch your left arm straight.** Spread your fingers, have as much of your palm on the floor as possible, and tighten the left elbow so it lifts away from the floor.

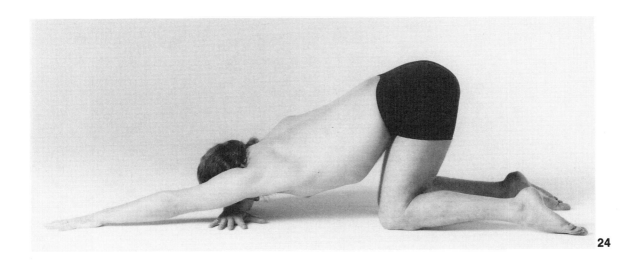

24

**4** **Gently press your hips backward and bring your forehead toward the floor** (photo 24). Your arm and torso will form a straight line, and you'll probably experience a stretch in your left arm, shoulder, or chest.

**5** When this stretch eases up somewhat, lift your head, look forward, and curve your chest toward the floor. This is a lovely stretch. Close your eyes, breathe smoothly, and immerse yourself in the sensations of stretch. Be here half a minute, then change sides.

## HALF DOG

**1** **Start on your elbows in neutral Cat Pose.**

**2** **Stretch both arms straight.** Slide one hand forward, then the other. Have your hands shoulder-width apart, fingers spread, middle fingers pointing straight ahead. Press your arms fully straight so your elbows stay lifted away from the floor.

**3** **Press your hips away from you and bring your forehead to the floor.** Your thighs should be vertical, with your hips directly above the knees. Be here several breaths, being careful not to jam the shoulders.

**4** **Lift your head, look forward, and curve your chest toward the floor** (photo 25). If this bothers your neck, go back to being on your forehead. Close your eyes and breathe smoothly. Immerse yourself in the way this feels. It's lovely. Be here one minute.

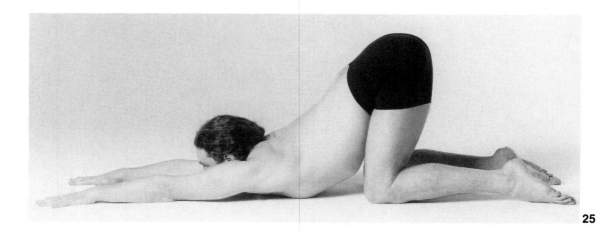

**25**

# Benefits: Dog Pose *or Adho Mukha Shvanasana*

Stretches entire backside of the body, especially the arms, shoulders, hips, hamstrings, calves, and Achilles tendon. Strengthens hands, arms, and upper body, opens the chest, improves breathing. Overall body stretch, removes fatigue, and rejuvenates body. Lengthens spine, rejuvenates discs. Increases circulation to brain.

# 8 Triangle Pose *or Trikonasana*

Triangle Pose has five lines of energy radiating outward from your center. One line of energy travels downward through each leg, one line stretches outward through each arm, and one line moves up the spine and out the crown of your head. One hip will be in dog tilt, the other in cat tilt.

There are many subtleties of stretch and alignment in this pose. We would do well, therefore, to go over them in detail. These subtleties bring out the flavor of the pose and convey a fuller, more accurate portrait of what yoga feels like from the inside.

### PRELIMINARY EXERCISE: *Stepping Apart and Together*

Each of the following Standing Poses involves starting from a centered attitude in Tadasana (Mountain Pose), stepping into the pose, performing the pose, and then stepping out of the pose—back to center and Tadasana. Let's practice stepping apart and together.

**1** Stand tall with your feet together. Become centered and still and deepen your breathing. When you are ready to begin, inhale deeply. As you exhale, bring your palms together in front of your chest in namaste, prayer position (photo 26).

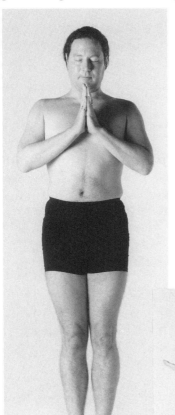

**2** As you inhale, bend your knees slightly and step your left foot to the left, sweep your arms to the sides, and come to full extension (photo 27). Press your legs straight, lift and expand the chest, and stretch outward through the arms. As you exhale, bend your knees slightly, step back to center, and bring your palms together in namaste. That's the movement.

26

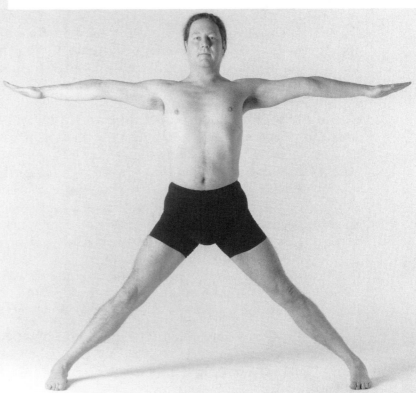

27

**3** As you inhale, again bend your knees and step your feet apart, stepping to the right this time, sweeping your arms to full extension. As you exhale, step back to center. This completes one repetition.

**4** Step apart and together five times. Make the movement smooth. Do not be in a rush, do not be mechanical, and practice coordinating the breath and movement perfectly.

## STAGE ONE

**1** **Stand in Tadasana (Mountain Pose) with your feet together.** Establish a smooth flowing breath and wait for the inner cue to begin. When you are ready, exhale and bring your palms together into namaste position in front of your chest.

**2** **As you inhale, step your left foot to the left and sweep your arms outward until they are horizontal.** Have your feet one leg's length apart and check that your heels are on the same invisible line. Your legs will now form an equilateral triangle with the floor; have them a little wider if you prefer.

**3** **Exhale as you turn both feet to the right.** Pivot on the left heel to turn the left foot inward to a forty-five-degree angle, and pivot on the right heel to turn the right foot outward to a ninety-degree angle. Your heels are still on the same line. Spread the toes of each foot, press both legs straight, and root each leg into the floor through the soles of the feet.

**4** **Take a deep breath in, expanding and filling out the shape that you now are, and as you exhale, stretch into the pose.** Reach outward through the right arm as you gently press your hips to the left (photo 28). Attempt to create a straight line from your right hip to your right fingertips, hinging at your right hip. Then, without losing this length along the underside of your right chest or changing the alignment of your body in any way, lower your right hand to the shinbone and slide it down to the ankle or floor (photo 29). Bring the left arm vertical. This is Stage One. Acclimatize to where you are and breathe consciously.

**5** Remember, the basic idea is to fill out the shape that you now are by breathing smoothly, deeply, and running energy through the lines. Take inventory. Feel your way through the pose, keeping the following actions in mind:

a) First, spread your toes to the maximum, snuggle your feet into the floor, and become grounded. Keep the soles of your feet soft so they can merge with the floor. Balance the inner and outer ankles so your ankle joints are strong. Do not be weak or wobbly in your ankles, and do not allow them to fall or collapse inward or outward. You'll know this is happening if you are experiencing exces-

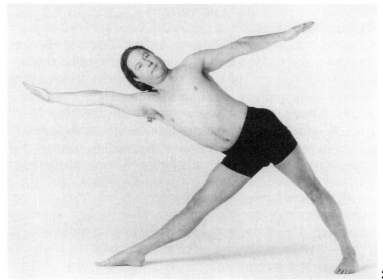

28

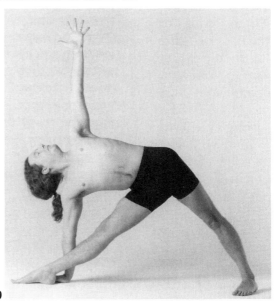

29

sive weight or pressure toward either the inner or outer edge of either foot. Merge the whole sole of each foot evenly into the floor, and make your ankles strong so the base or foundation of the pose is solid, secure.

b) Strengthen and energize the leg lines. First, establish the left leg line by tightening the left buttock and pressing downward into the left heel so the leg becomes fully straight. This action places the left hip and buttock in cat tilt, which causes the left frontal hip bone to roll up, opening and broadening the pelvis. Become grounded down the back leg, then keep that leg strong throughout the pose. Clarify and increase the line of energy down the right leg by, first, *feeling* the sole of your foot on the floor, then pushing downward through the leg, into the foot, so the leg becomes straight, strong and grounded. Be aware not to push backward into the knees, but downward into the feet—in the direction the legs are pointing. Draw both kneecaps up, tighten the quadriceps, and turn both knees outward, aiming the line of energy toward the outer edge of the left foot and the inner edge of the right. When your leg lines are grounded and strong, your spine will more easily elongate outward from your center.

c) Establish the alignment of your center. You'll find that this is already beginning to happen simply by virtue of having strengthened and clarified the leg lines. As you run energy down the right leg and push your foot into the floor, the hinge at your right hip will deepen. Doing this will deepen the hinge at the top of your right leg and place the right hip and buttock in dog tilt. Deepen the hinge as much as possible, roll the right outer thigh backward, bring the right side-ribs down, and press the right sitting bone away from you in the direction of your left foot. Then, without losing dog tilt and without losing the deep hinge, pull the abdominals in and gently draw the navel backward toward the spine. Your left hip is in cat tilt, the right in dog tilt.

d) Establish the line of energy down your right arm. Snuggle your palm into the floor or firmly hold your ankle, then press downward through the arm from the shoulder so your head and torso lift away from the floor. Lengthen the right arm so you are not sagging into the supporting shoulder. This is the same action described in Cat Pose.

e) Lengthen your spine and core in the direction it is pointing—outward through the crown of your head. Lift the rib cage away from your waist and expand your chest so the front of your body slides up your front. Shrug both shoulders away from your ears and slide the shoulder blades down your back, so you feel the back of your body sliding down your back. Continue pulling the navel backward toward the spine. Then delicately move the whole backside of your body forward toward the front, as though you were a sail on a boat and the wind were gently filling you out from the rear—and you're letting it. Rotate your chest toward the ceiling, reach upward and outward through the left arm, and gaze through your fingertips into infinity.

f) Endeavor to align your whole body in one plane over the invisible line between your heels. Position the left hand directly above the left shoulder so your arm is vertical, align the left shoulder directly above the right, and especially try to bring the tailbone and crown of your head over the line.

**6** Breathe with feeling, and clarify the five energy lines. Feel them radiating outward from your center, establish the perfect intensity of current, be as effortless and relaxed as possible, and breathe smoothly, deeply. Continue lifting upward from your belly into the chest, use your breathing to help you do this, then stretch outward through your arms as you press downward into your feet. As your feet press into the floor, notice how this increases the lift into your chest, and as your chest lifts and expands, sense the increased freedom through the arms.

**7** Take your time establishing these lines, immerse yourself in a smooth flowing breath, and pay attention to the experience you are having. Be here about half a minute, five or six deep breaths.

## STAGE TWO

**8** **As you exhale, take the top arm backward.** Try to make the left arm horizontal with the palm upward (photo 30), but do not lose the integrity of the pose. Keep the foundation of the pose strong, the hinge deep, the left buttock tight, the abdominals in, and maintain the lift through the chest. Keep your head and chest turned upward, and gaze outward through the left arm at the fingertips. Press downward into your feet, stretch your hands away from you, and gently fill out and expand the shape you now are. Breathe smoothly, deeply. Be here several breaths.

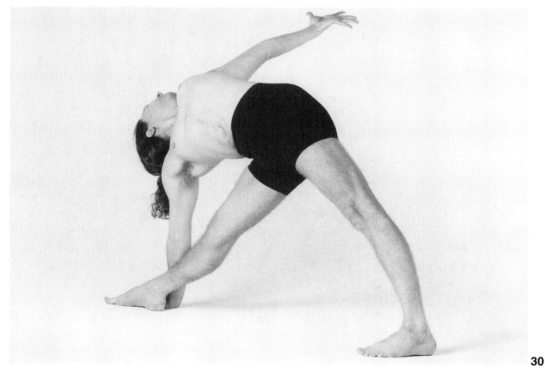

30

**9** The left arm line, remember, originates at your center. To clarify and energize the left arm, first lift from your belly into the chest, and then stretch outward through the arm in the direction it is pointing. Increase the energy flow through both arms. Press both hands away from you. If any part of the pose weakens, do not take your arm further. Observe how everything is connected.

**10** **Fold the left arm down behind your back, and catch hold of the right thigh with your left hand** (photo 31). Take a moment to wriggle your left hand in as deeply as you can. The pose now has four lines of energy. The top arm, now entwined behind your back, works to enhance the spinal rotation and is no longer a separate line. This is Stage Two.

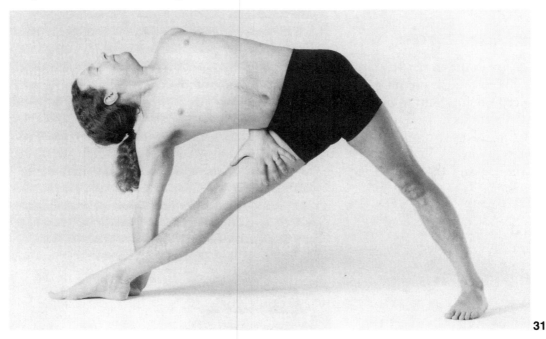

31

**11** Use your breathing to refine your alignment. First, gently pull the abdominals in, backward toward the spine, then inhale and expand the chest. The rib cage will actually lift away from the waist, giving you room with which to twist. As you exhale, roll the left shoulder and elbow backward, spiral your chest toward the sky, and gaze upward. Roll both shoulders backward as you do this, and be sure to pull both shoulder blades down your back. Ease your way into your maximum spinal rotation. Wriggle your left hand in deeper when you can.

**12** Run energy through your lines, gradually fill out the shape of the pose, and gently wind the pose tighter. Look for parts of the pose that are compressed or deflated, and try to inflate them. Increase or decrease the current in your lines until the feeling-tone of the pose is perfect. Gaze upward most of the time, but feel free to turn your head and look downward should you be so prompted.

**13** Endeavor to align your whole body in one plane. Your hips should not jut backward, nor your head forward. Everything should be over the line between your two feet, especially the tailbone and crown. Feel where your lines are and how they radiate outward from your center. Keep them filled with air. Stay in this position one minute. Breathe smoothly.

**14** Do not be concerned with how deep you are or aren't. Do be concerned with the overall feeling-tone. This is a beautiful pose. Orchestrate the breath, the stretch, and the intensity of the lines so everything feels perfect.

**15** To come out of the pose, exhale as you release the left hand from the right thigh, straighten the arm, and bring it forward and around until it is alongside your left ear with the palm facing down. Bringing your arm to the front like this will relieve any discomfort in the arm or shoulder from being held behind your back so long.

**16** **Inhale as you come up.** Turn your feet straight.

**17** **Exhale as you step back to center.** Bring your palms together in front of your chest in namaste, prayer position.

**18** Now perform the pose on the other side. Inhale as you sweep your arms and step your feet apart, right foot to the right. Exhale as you turn both feet to the left. Inhale as you fill out the shape, and exhale as you stretch into the pose. Proceed slowly, feelingly, through the stages.

**19** When you are finished, come back up, step your feet together, and lower your arms to your sides. Close your eyes and stand quietly. Be relaxed. Experience your feeling-tone and absorb the effects of the pose in stillness.

# Benefits: Triangle Pose *or Trikonasana*

Increases strength and flexibility of the feet, legs, hips, and back. Opens the chest, elongates the spine, relieves backache, strengthens neck. Improves digestion and elimination.

# 9 Bent Knee Side Stretch *or Parshvakonasana*

**1** **Stand in Tadasana (Mountain Pose) with your feet together.** Center yourself in a smooth flowing breath and wait for the inner cue to begin. When you are ready, inhale, then exhale as you bring your palms together in namaste.

**2  As you inhale, step your feet apart.** Step your left foot to the left, sweeping your arms to the sides. Both arms and legs are now straight. Check that your heels are on the same line.

**3  As you exhale, turn both feet to the right.** Pivot on the heels as you turn the left foot inward to a forty-five-degree angle and the right foot outward to a ninety-degree angle.

**4  Inhale deeply.** Fill out the shape that you are. Press both legs straight, lift the chest upward, and stretch outward through the arms.

## STAGE ONE

**5  As you exhale, bend your right knee until it forms a right angle, rest your right elbow on the knee, and bring the left arm alongside the left ear with the palm facing down** (photo 32).

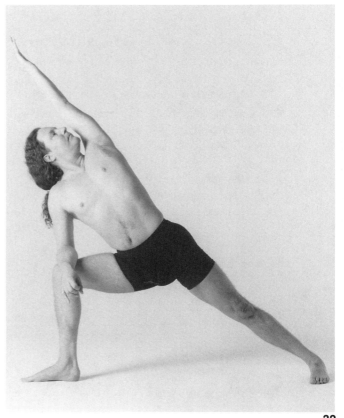

**6** Adjust the distance between your feet, if necessary, until the right knee forms a right angle. Make the thigh horizontal, level with the floor, and the shinbone vertical, so the heel is positioned directly below the knee. If your feet are too close together or too far apart, your right knee will not form a square. Remember this distance. This is your spot.

**7** Establish the alignment of your center before clarifying the lines. Pull the abdominals in and gently contract the buttocks, just enough to tilt the sacrum toward cat tilt.

32

**8** The tendency here is to sag into the right shoulder. Instead, press downward into the right elbow and lift upward out of the shoulder. Then, keeping the abdominals in, inhale and expand the chest as you reach enthusiastically outward into the left hand. Lift your rib cage away from the waist, spread your fingers, and reaffirm this action with each breath. This is Stage One. Feel where your lines are.

**9** Imagine an invisible line on the floor from one heel to the other. Check that your right knee is directly over this line, and then bring the right sitting bone forward until it also is directly above this line. Gently nudge the right knee backward with your right elbow to achieve this alignment.

**10** Tighten the left knee. Lift into the chest. Stretch through your lines. Breathe. Be here several breaths.

## STAGE TWO

**11** **Take the left arm backward and catch hold of the right thigh** (photo 33). Reach outward through the arm as you take it back, being alert to not collapse into the right shoulder. Continue pressing downward into the right elbow, nudging the knee away, as you entwine the left arm.

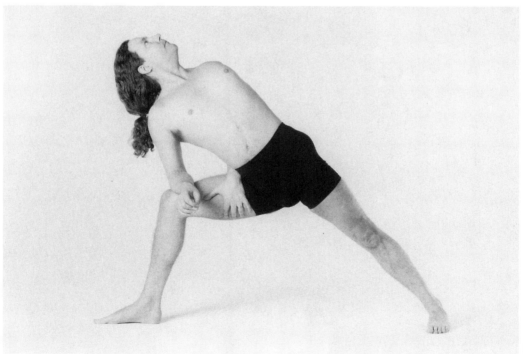

33

**12** With each inhalation, lift and expand the chest away from the waist, and with each exhalation, spiral your chest toward the sky. Pull gently with your left hand, and squeeze the left elbow and shoulder backward to help rotate the chest. Roll both shoulders backward as you do this, sliding the shoulder blades down

your back. Strive to achieve maximum chest expansion in this stage before proceeding. Be here several breaths.

## STAGE THREE

**13** **Bring your right hand to the floor in front of the leg** (photo 34). Retain
the chest expansion you achieved in Stage Two as you come down onto your
right hand, and continue breathing consciously with the ujjayi throat sound.
Make the breath long and deep with a smooth even sound.

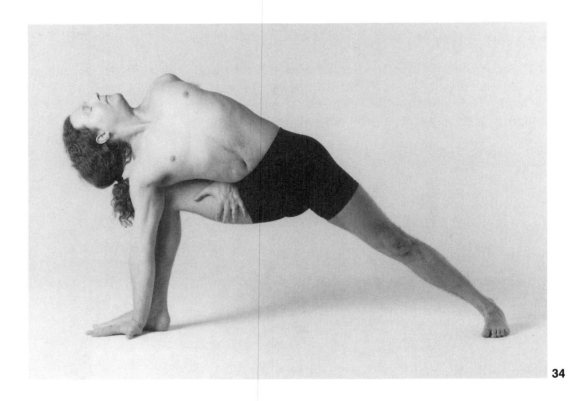

34

**14** Reaffirm the alignment of your center. Pull the abdominals in, lengthen
your lower back, and gently contract the buttocks. Squeezing the buttocks will
encourage the right knee to move and stay backward, away from the shoulder.
Lengthen the right inner thigh toward the knee.

**15** Stretch downward into the right hand and snuggle your palm into the floor,
lengthening that arm so you have maximum height. The higher you are, the
more space you'll have with which to rotate the chest. Pull with the left hand,
squeeze the elbow backward, and gaze upward. Be here several breaths.

## STAGE FOUR

**16** **Release the left hand from the thigh, straighten the arm, and bring it forward and around until it is alongside your left ear with the palm facing down** (photo 35). Tighten the left knee, tighten the left elbow, and reach outward through the left arm in the direction it is pointing. Run energy through your lines. Be relaxed as you do this, but stretch fully. Be here several breaths.

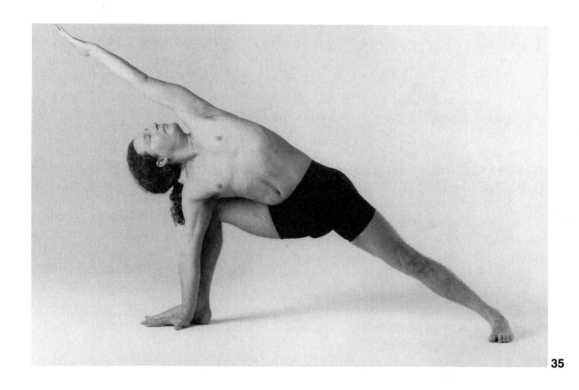

35

**17** **To come out of the pose, inhale as you come up, turning your feet straight, and exhale as you step your feet back to center.** Bring your palms together in namaste position on your chest.

**18** Pause for a few moments before doing the second side. Wait for the inner cue. Then inhale and step your feet to the right, exhale as you turn your feet to the left, and proceed through the stages.

**19** When you are done, come back to Tadasana (Mountain Pose). Close your eyes, stand quietly, and be aware of how you feel. Do not skip this part. Be thoroughly relaxed. Feel the energy you are made of.

# Benefits: Bent Knee Side Stretch *or Parshvakonasana*

Increases strength and flexibility of thighs, legs, hips, and back. Opens chest. Stretches side waist and lateral rib cage areas. Strengthens arms. Excellent for digestive and eliminative systems.

# 10 Warrior Pose I *or Virabhadrasana I*

**1** **Stand in Tadasana (Mountain Pose) with your feet together.** Center yourself in a smooth flowing breath and wait for the inner cue to begin. When you are ready, exhale and bring your palms together in namaste.

**2** **As you inhale, sweep your arms to the sides and step your left foot to the left.** Have your feet the same distance apart as Parshvakonasana, the Bent Knee Side Stretch, so that when you bend your right knee, it forms a right angle.

**3** **As you exhale, turn your feet and body to the right.** Turn the left foot inward to a forty-five-degree angle, the right foot outward to ninety degrees, and then swivel your hips and chest to the right until you face the right foot. Your arms are still extending outward from your sides.

**4** **As you inhale, raise your arms above your head** (photo 36). Be smooth as you do this. Draw the abdominals backward toward the spine first, then reaching outward through your arms, inhale as you raise the hands high above your head, bringing the palms together if you can. Feel your upper arms rotating outward as your arms go up, shoulder blades sliding down your back. If you cannot bring your palms together, then simply continue reaching outward-upward through your arms in whatever direction they are pointing. Lace your thumbs, squeeze the elbows inward toward one another, and energize straight upward through the arms and fingertips. Lift the chest away from the waist. Become as long, tall, and thin as possible. This feels wonderful.

**5** Snuggle your feet into the floor, become grounded, and then press downward through your legs into your feet. Press the whole sole of each foot firmly into the floor, but aim the leg line into the outer edge of the left foot and the inner edge of the right foot. Bring the left frontal hip bone forward so the abdominal plane faces forward, then try to keep your hips squared to the front as you move into the pose.

**6** Be in this preparatory position several breaths. When you are ready to proceed, inhale and turn your head upward (photo 37). Gaze through your fingertips into infinity.

**7** **As you exhale, bend your right knee until it forms a right angle** (photo 38). Aim your knee directly toward your toes and sit down until your thigh is horizontal, level with the floor. The thigh bone should be straight, not angling in or out. This usually requires lengthening the inner thigh toward the knee, so the knee moves in the direction of the little toe, and bringing the buttock in so the right sitting bone is directly over the line between your heels. Once your alignment is correct, lengthen the inner core of the thigh toward the knee. This is the pose. Be grounded.

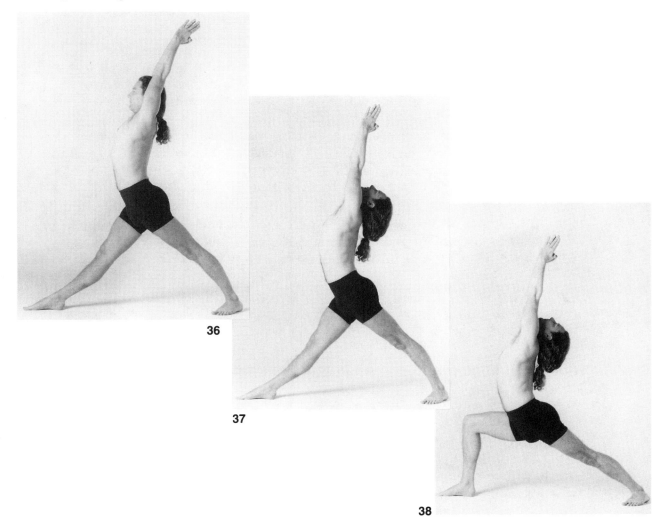

36

37

38

**8** Take inventory. Tighten the left quadriceps, keep the left foot firmly grounded, and continue nudging the left frontal hip bone forward so the abdominal plane and chest face forward toward your right leg. Continue pulling the navel backward toward the spine, attempt to achieve maximum lift and expansion in the chest, and reach straight upward through the arms. Stretch with enthusiasm. Press the sternum, or breastbone, forward. Inflate deflated areas.

**9** Breathe fully, deeply, without strain. Use your breathing to fuel and energize your lines, then increase the current through your lines and fill out the shape of the pose. Fill out your energy field. Express beauty. Reach to your comfortable maximum, yet be as effortless and relaxed as possible. Do what you have to do. This can be intense, so be at your maximum extension for a comfortable length of time only. Do not overdo it. A few seconds may be enough at first. Keep your gaze steady.

**10** If your body is asking for a stronger stretch, curve backward. Pull the abdominals in first, then inhale and stretch straight upward through your arms in the direction they are pointing, and as you exhale, move your hands backward an inch or two. Reach upward again as you inhale, making your arms longer, and take the hands farther back as you exhale. This is a backbend, so move your spine forward into your back and bring the curve *up* your back. Lift up from underneath the sternum, behind the heart, and gently curve your head backward, keeping your neck soft. Gaze straight backward into infinity.

**11 To come out of the pose, inhale and straighten your right leg, bringing your head to normal alignment and turning your feet to the front. As you exhale, sweep your hands into namaste and step back to center.**

**12** Repeat the pose on the other side. Step to the right this time, turn your feet to the left, then proceed through the pose. Do not be mechanical. Be inspired. Breathe. Flow.

**13** The practice, remember, is to merge and participate and be fully involved with what you are doing. Therefore, breathe with feeling and stretch with sensitivity. Immerse yourself in the pose. Be here now in the pose. It will teach you if you listen, feel, and are attentive.

**14** When you are finished, step back to center, lower your arms, and stand quietly with your eyes closed. Be relaxed. Be aware. Practice standing motionless with no holding anywhere. Enjoy how you feel.

# Benefits: Warrior Pose I *or Virabhadrasana I*

Strengthens legs, back, shoulders, and arms. Develops strength, stability, and stamina in the entire body. Increases flexibility in the front groins, hips, back, and shoulders. Opens chest. Beginning of backbending poses. Strengthens energy in body.

# 11 Warrior Pose II *or Virabhadrasana II*

**1 Stand in Tadasana (Mountain Pose) with your feet together.** Center yourself in a smooth flowing breath and wait for the inner cue to begin. When you are ready, exhale and bring your palms together in namaste.

**2 As you inhale, sweep your arms up until they are horizontal and step your left foot to the left.** Your feet should be the same distance apart as in Parshvakonasana and Virabhadrasana I. Again, your feet should be far enough apart so that when you bend your knee, it forms a right angle. Check that your heels are on the same line.

**3 Exhale as you turn your feet to the right.** Pivot on the heels as you turn the left foot inward to a forty-five-degree angle and the right foot outward to a ninety-degree angle. Press both legs straight and root your feet into the floor.

## STAGE ONE

**4 As you inhale, raise the right arm until it is vertical, alongside the right ear.**

**5 As you exhale, stretch into the side bend** (photo 39). Slide your left hand down the left thigh. Gaze downward.

**6** Breathe deeply and stretch with feeling. Run energy through your lines. Both legs are straight, both arms are straight, and your center is in cat tilt. Be here several breaths, reaching outward through the right arm in the direction it is pointing. When you are ready to proceed, breathe in deeply.

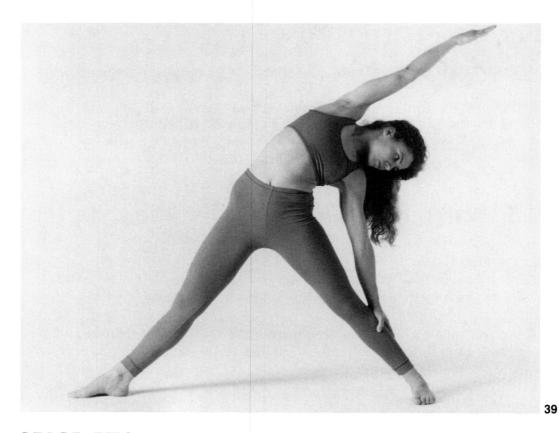

39

## STAGE TWO

**7 Exhale as you bend your right knee until it forms a right angle** (photo 40). The tendency here is for the right knee to angle inward and the right buttock to jut out backward. Instead, bring the right knee, right sitting bone, and tailbone over the line between your feet. Aim the right knee directly over the toes, lengthening the right inner thigh toward the knee. Be grounded and firm.

**8** Pull the abdominals in, lift the chest away from the waist, and reach outward through the right arm in the direction it is pointing. Remember, the arm line starts from your center; therefore, stretch from the waist, then from the ribs, then from the shoulder, toward the elbow, all the way out through the fingertips.

**9** Be aware of the shape you are, run energy through your lines, then turn your head and gaze upward, spiraling your chest toward the sky. Stretch with feeling. Breathe deeply. Be in the pose half a minute.

**10 To come out of the pose, straighten your right leg, turn your feet to the front, and step back to center.**

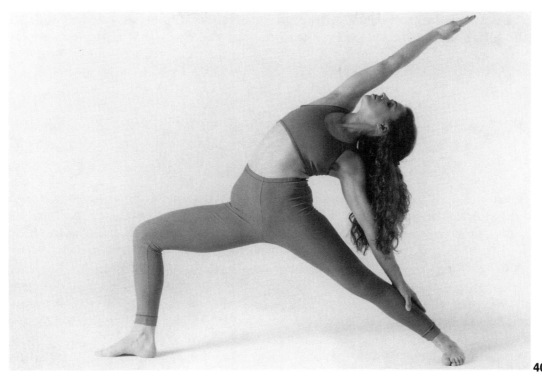

**40**

**11** Do the pose on the other side. Step to the right, turn your feet left, then proceed through the stages. When you are finished, stand quietly and be aware of how you feel.

# Benefits: Warrior Pose II *or Virabhadrasana II*

Opens groins and hip joints, stretches the inner thigh muscles, strengthens buttocks, legs, quadriceps, arches of the feet, abdominals, shoulders, and arms. Opens chest, improves breathing. Increases circulation throughout body.

# 12 Half Moon Pose *or Ardha Chandrasana II*

**1 Stand in Tadasana (Mountain Pose) with your feet together.** Center yourself in a smooth flowing breath and wait for the inner cue to begin. When you are ready, exhale and bring your palms together in namaste.

**2** **As you inhale, sweep your arms to the sides and step your left foot to the left.** Have your feet one leg's length apart and check that your heels are on the same line. As you exhale, turn both feet to the right, the left foot inward to a forty-five-degree angle and the right foot outward to a ninety-degree angle. Inhale deeply, lifting your chest and stretching outward through the arms.

**3** **As you exhale, stretch into Triangle Pose.** Be in Stage One several breaths. Then entwine the top arm behind your back, Stage Two, and be here several breaths.

**4** **To move into Ardha Chandrasana, Half Moon, first turn your head down and look at the floor. Bend the right leg, slide the left foot closer to the right foot, place your right hand on the floor about a foot away from your right foot, and lean onto your right hand and foot until your left foot leaves the floor** (photo 41). You are now balanced on the right hand and foot.

**5** **Keeping the right leg bent, inhale as you raise the left leg until it forms a straight line with your torso.** Keep the left leg straight as it rises.

**6** **As you exhale, slowly press the right leg straight** (photo 42). Press the right foot straight down into the floor. Merge your foot with the floor. You'll become more grounded as you do this and the left foot will rise higher. Keep the left leg and torso in line. Lengthen the right arm with the next inhalation—this will lift you away from the floor somewhat—then rotate the chest upward as you exhale. This is the pose. For now, keep looking down.

**7** Feel the shape that you now are, breathe, and take a moment to acclimatize and steady the balance. Then begin to circulate energy through your lines and refine the pose.

**8** You are balanced on your right hand and foot, and there are certain sensations in your hand and foot associated with the balance. Feel the palm of your hand and the sole of your foot on the floor and try to keep the sensations steady. If you keep them steady you won't lose the balance. Snuggle your hand and foot into the floor, merge with the floor, keeping the palm of your hand and the sole of your foot soft, sensitive. Simultaneously, lengthen the right arm and lift upward. The more you lift, the easier it will be to rotate the chest. Lift upward out of the right shoulder, keeping the right hand grounded, then gently squeeze the left elbow and shoulder backward to spiral your chest toward the sky. Pull gently with your left hand.

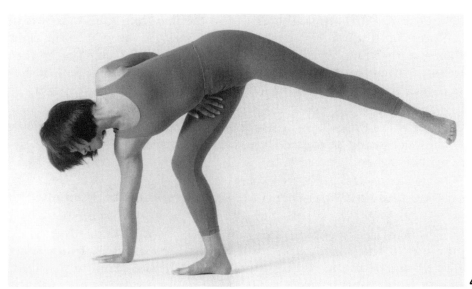

41

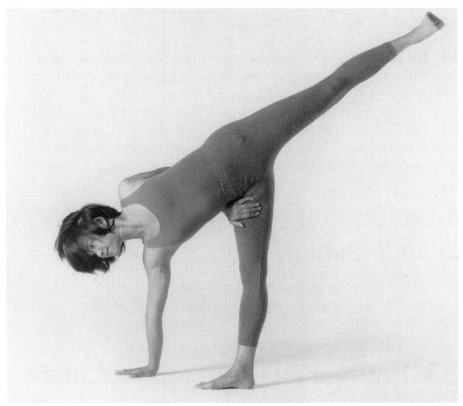

42

**9** Feel where your feet are—the right foot is on the floor and the left foot is in the air—then press both feet away from you. Press straight down into the right foot—you'll become even more grounded as you do this—and stretch the left foot away from you. Flatten the pelvis by rolling the left hip up. Try to align the left hip directly above the right hip, and the left shoulder directly above the right.

**10** At first, gaze at the floor. Stare at a spot and do not let your attention move. Once your balance is steady, turn your head to look forward and eventually upward. This is tricky at first.

**11** This is a beautiful pose. Your energy is moving vertically, horizontally, and circularly.

**12** **To come out of the pose, exhale and bend your right leg. Touch your left foot to the floor near the right foot, step back to the original position, and bring your right hand to your right ankle or the floor. As you inhale, straighten the right leg and spiral your chest upward.** This has a nice feeling to it. You are now in Stage Two of Triangle Pose again. Center yourself here for a moment.

**13** **Exhale as you release the arm, bringing it forward and up alongside your left ear. Inhale as you come up and turn your feet straight. Exhale as you step back to center.**

**14** Perform the pose on the other side and then stand motionless. Again, don't miss this part. Immerse yourself in the way you feel. Savor the way you feel. Practice not thinking as you stand quietly. Be relaxed.

# Benefits: Half Moon Pose *or Ardha Chandrasana II*

Develops balance, coordination, leg and buttock strength, and tremendous flexibility in the legs and hips. Frees the rib cage and shoulders, opens the chest, improves breathing.

# 13 Pyramid Pose *or Parshvottanasana*

**1** **Stand in Tadasana (Mountain Pose) with your feet together.**

**2 Bring your hands up behind your back in reverse namaste, the prayer pose:** Start with your fingertips together behind your back, pointing down, then turn your hands inward and bring them up. Acclimatize to this position for a few moments as you gently expand the chest away from the waist, roll the shoulders and elbows backward, and press the palms together. Wriggle your hands higher when you can. The higher you get them, the more comfortable this will be. If you cannot bring your hands into reverse prayer, then either hold your elbows behind your back, clasp your wrists, or rest your hands on your hips. Wait for the inner cue to begin. When you are ready, exhale.

**3 As you inhale, step your left foot to the left until your feet are one leg's length apart.** Your legs will now form an equilateral triangle with the floor. Your feet can be farther apart if you wish.

**4 Exhale as you turn your feet, hips, and chest to the right.** Pivot on your heels as you first turn the left foot inward to a forty-five-degree angle and then the right foot outward to a ninety-degree angle. Then turn your hips and chest to face the right leg.

**5** Bring the left frontal hip bone forward until the abdominal plane is squared to the front and your chest faces the right foot. Straighten both legs, pull the kneecaps up by tightening the quadriceps, and snuggle the whole sole of each foot firmly into the floor. Make sure you are grounded.

**6 As you inhale, curve your head and chest upward** (photo 43). Lift the chest, press the sternum upward, and get round. Gently tug the shoulder blades down your back and keep the navel pulled backward toward your spine.

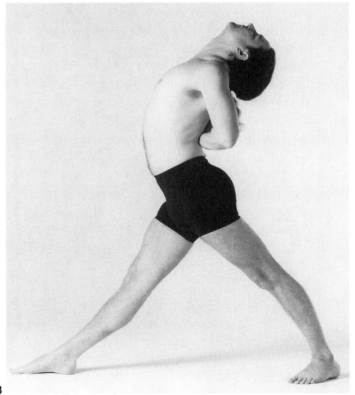

43

**7 As you exhale, fold forward** (photo 44). Bring your whole torso down onto the right leg—or as close to that as you can. Lead with the chest initially, moving the sternum forward so you stretch out over your leg, then gently tuck the chin, lengthen the back of your neck, and bring your forehead to your shinbone. Elongate your spine outward through the crown of your head as you fold into the pose. Keep moving the fontanel away from you.

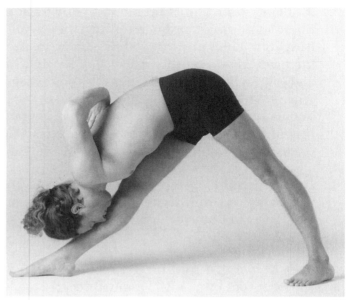

44

**8** Breathe smoothly, acclimatize to the stretch, then refine your alignment. You'll feel the stretch in your hamstrings, but the work is that of keeping your sacrum level by making sure your pelvis stays squared to the front and then fully elongating your spine. Press the right sitting bone backward and bring the left frontal hip bone forward so your sacrum stays level—do not allow the left shoulder or hip to tilt upward—then press backward and up through both sitting bones as you elongate your core. Extend your torso forward away from the pelvis.

**9** If your back is dome-shaped, rounded, even if the sacrum is level, then your pelvis has not rotated sufficiently forward toward dog tilt. If that's the case, come up a bit, press both sitting bones backward to increase dog tilt, and try to lengthen your spine. The longer you get, the flatter you'll be. Then fold into the pose again.

**10** Lift the elbows, expand your chest, and slide the shoulder blades down your back toward the waist.

**11** Breathe smoothly, stay grounded, and continue elongating your core. Keep your feet firmly rooted into the floor as you try to achieve maximum extension from your tailbone to the crown of your head. Immerse your awareness in the various sensations of stretch and the smooth flow of breath. Do not tighten up. Relax with the intensity. Breathe through it. Be here about a minute.

**12** **Inhale as you come up.** Then turn your feet, hips, and chest to the left and repeat the pose on the other side for an equal length of time. When you are finished, step back to center, release your hands, and stand quietly in Tadasana. Close your eyes and savor the way you feel.

# Benefits: Pyramid Pose *or Parshvottanasana*

Tremendous leg, back, and shoulder stretch. Increases flexibility of hips, spine, shoulders, and legs. Strengthens legs. Tones abdominal organs. Develops balance and stamina. Improves circulation throughout the body, especially the head.

# 14 Revolved Triangle Pose *or Parivrrta Trikonasana*

**1** **Stand in Tadasana (Mountain Pose) with your feet together.** Establish a smooth flowing breath and wait for the inner cue to begin. When you are ready, breathe in deeply. As you exhale, bring your palms together in namaste position in front of your chest.

**2** **As you inhale, sweep your arms outward until they are horizontal and step your left foot to the left.** Have your feet one leg's length apart and check that your heels are on the same line.

**3** **Exhale as you turn your feet and body to the right.** Pivot on your heels, turning the left foot inward to a forty-five-degree angle and the right foot outward to a ninety-degree angle. Check that your heels are on the same line, then turn your hips and chest to face the right leg and foot. Your arms are still extending out to the sides. Take a breath.

**4** **Exhale as you fold forward. Place your left hand on the floor on the outside edge of the right foot and bring the right arm up until it is vertical** (photo 45). Nestle the left wrist in snugly against your ankle, and conform the outer edge of your hand to the outer edge of your foot. If you cannot be on your palm, be on the ball of your hand or fingertips. This is the pose.

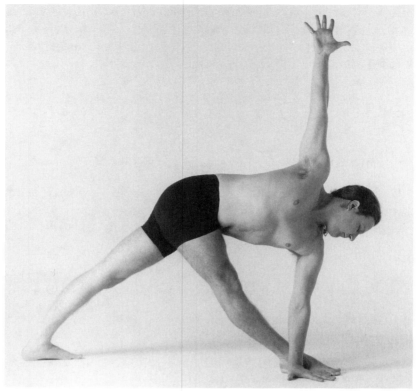

**45**

**5** Establish the leg lines. Spread your toes, snuggle the soles of your feet into the floor, and press each leg fully straight, taking root into the floor. Aim the line of energy toward the outer edge of the left foot and the inner edge of the right foot. Get grounded.

**6** Establish the left arm line. Press the left hand firmly into the floor, lengthen the arm, and lift up as high as possible. This is the same movement you learned in Cat Pose: Don't sag into the shoulder. Maintain this height throughout the pose.

**7** Elongate and rotate the spine. Do this by moving the right hip away from you as you lift the chest away from the waist. This is an important movement in this pose. You're creating length through the waist and opening the chest. To get the correct feeling for how to do this, place your right hand on your right hip and gently press the hip away from you. You'll feel your spine and chest wanting to elongate out of the waist.

**8** Elongate the spine horizontally outward in the direction it is pointing, moving the tailbone and crown of the head away from one another. Press the right foot firmly into the floor to assist in pressing the buttocks away from you and, at the same time, elongate the spine by pressing the crown away.

**9** The important actions in this pose are: 1) establish strong leg lines and root your feet firmly into the floor; 2) press the left palm down and lift up out of the shoulder; 3) turn the right hip away from you; and 4) elongate and rotate the spine. At first, think of these as separate actions and do each of them very specifically, over and over, until they are firmly ingrained in your awareness. Then do them simultaneously, all four at the same time, so the pose comes alive and feels like one multidimensional action. Because of your alignment and positioning, these actions will encourage the spine into a long, tight, spiraling twist. Gently rotate the chest more up—bit by bit, not suddenly.

**10** The right arm stretches skyward and the hands move away from one another—one straight up and one straight down. This will create more space in the area of your rib cage and chest, which allows for greater spinal extension and rotation. Move the hands away from one another, and elongate outward through the crown of your head as you twist and rotate your spine.

**11** Gaze at the floor first, then straight ahead, then toward the ceiling. Change when necessary.

**12** Be relatively still in the pose. Keep these actions happening, but increasingly make them more mental than physical. Relax with the intensity as you increase the energy flow and deepen the twist. "Do" and "not-do" at the same time.

**13** Breathe with feeling—sometimes deeply, sometimes more shallowly. Always breathe with the vigor and depth that feels most right. Be in the pose for one minute.

**14** **To come out of the pose, inhale and come up, turning your feet to the front. Exhale as you step back to center.**

**15** Repeat the pose on the other side. Stay for an equal length of time. Then stand motionless and savor the effects of the pose.

# Benefits: Revolved Triangle Pose *or Parivrrta Trikonasana*

Tremendous leg stretch and spinal rotation. Strengthens legs, increases flexibility in hips, frees rib cage, making for improved breathing and greater self-confidence. Relieves back tension. Tones abdominal organs. Frees energy through spine and core. Improves balance and concentration.

# 15 Standing Spread Leg Forward Fold *or Prasarita Padottanasana*

**1 Stand in Tadasana (Mountain Pose) with your feet together.** Pause for a moment as you center yourself in the breath and wait for the inner cue to begin. When you are ready, exhale, bringing your palms together in namaste.

**2 As you inhale, sweep your arms outward until they are horizontal and step your feet apart.** Spread your legs four or five feet apart. Check that your feet are parallel with one another and that the inner edge of each foot is pointing straight ahead.

### STAGE ONE

**3 As you exhale, fold forward and place your palms on the floor directly below your shoulders** (photo 46). The arms are now vertical. Spread your fingers and have the middle finger of each hand pointing straight ahead.

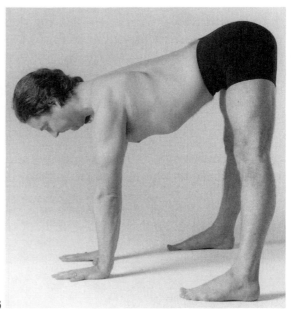

46

**4** Press your hands firmly into the floor, lengthen the arms, and lift up out of the shoulders. Again, this is the same movement you learned in Cat Pose: Don't sag into the shoulders. Gaze at the floor and keep the back of your neck long.

**5** Snuggle the soles of your feet into the floor, then press both legs straight. Pull the kneecaps up, contract the quadriceps, and turn the knees and thighs inward toward one another; the buttocks will spread as you do this. Then press your feet firmly into the floor and turn the sitting bones up: dog tilt. You now have maximum height both in the shoulders and hips.

**6** Make your back flat, lengthening the spine horizontally forward in the direction it is now pointing. Do this by moving the tailbone and crown of the head away from one another. Press backward through the sitting bones as you stretch forward through the fontanel. Be sure to maintain the lift out of the shoulders as you do this and continue turning the sitting bones up.

**7** Be here about half a minute, breathing smoothly. When you are ready to proceed, inhale deeply.

## STAGE TWO

**8** **As you exhale, walk your hands forward** (photo 47). Keep your arms straight and palms flat as you move your hands forward a foot or two. Then lift upward out of the shoulders, press forward into your hands, and stretch backward through the sitting bones to bring your head down. Try to bring your forehead to the floor. You are now in a position similar to Dog Pose, except your legs are wide apart.

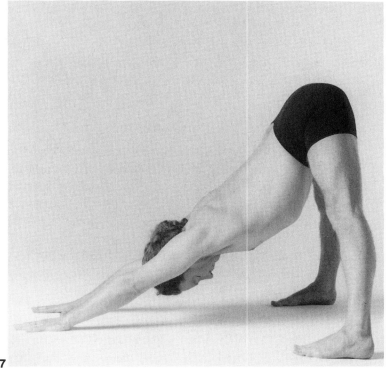

47

**9** Breathe smoothly. Form a smooth curving line from your hands, through your arms and spine, to the tailbone. Keep your pelvis over the line between your feet, not forward or backward. Be here about half a minute.

## STAGE THREE

**10** **Walk your hands backward through your legs** (photo 48). Keep your hands shoulder-width apart and your fingers spread. Walk your hands far enough backward so that when you bend your elbows, they form a square with the forearms vertical and the upper arms horizontal. Bring the elbows toward one another until the upper arms are parallel with one another and the forearms are parallel with one another. Snuggle your palms into the floor.

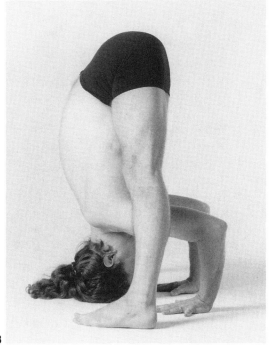

**48**

**11** Deepen the stretch by stretching into the elbows, pressing them away from you, as you simultaneously press your hands firmly forward on the floor—as though you were trying to slide the floor forward—without actually allowing your hands to move. Stretching into the elbows and pressing forward with the hands will take you deeper through your legs.

**12** Roll the buttocks over your head. Bring your hips forward until they are over the line between your two feet. From the side, your hips will appear to be directly above your feet.

**13** Lengthen your spine in the direction it is now pointing: straight down. Gaze backward through your legs, and direct the crown of your head toward the floor. If your head touches the floor, bring your feet closer together.

**14** Breathe smoothly. Bring the pose to life.

## STAGE FOUR

**15** **Bring your hands behind your back and clasp them, straighten the arms, then gently squeeze your hands downward toward the floor** (photo 49). With your inhalations, stretch outward through the arms in the direction they are pointing; lengthen your arms by moving your shoulders toward the hands. With your exhalations, make your hands heavy, squeezing them gently downward toward the floor. Be firm yet gentle as you do this. Orchestrate this action perfectly, making it the perfect mix of doing and not doing: Do what you have to do, yet also be relaxed. Be here several breaths.

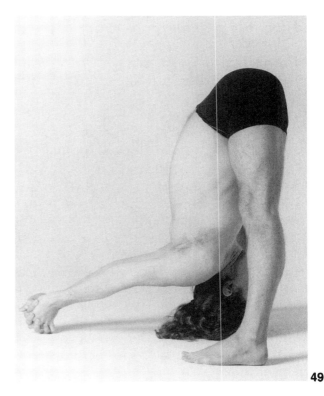

**49**

**16** **To come out of the pose, first release your hands. Then inhale as you come back up and exhale as you step your feet back to center.** Stand quietly. Enjoy the way you feel.

# Benefits: Standing Spread Leg Forward Fold *or Prasarita Padottanasana*

Tremendous stretch to hamstring and adductor (inner thigh) muscles. Strengthens legs, feet, and ankles. Spinal traction relieves upper body tension, elongates spine and core. An alternative to Headstand, increasing blood flow to the brain. Removes fatigue at end of standing pose sequence.

# 16 Standing Pose Flow

The Standing Pose Flow is a series of standing poses linked one after another, all performed on the right side first and then the left. It's an excellent way to practice the standing poses once you've learned them, flowing from one to the next. In the following sequence you will stay in each asana approximately half a minute. Once you have the flow memorized, practice going through it intuitively, staying in each pose as long or as little as the inner feeling dictates. Make the practice that of staying in each pose the perfect length of time. When the inner feeling says, "Move on to the next pose," or "Stay here a little longer," do so. Later you can order the poses differently, add or delete poses, or make up your own sequence. The idea at the moment is to stay in each pose the perfect length of time and flow from one to the other.

**1 Stand in Tadasana (Mountain Pose) with your feet together.** Center yourself in a smooth flowing breath and wait for the inner cue to begin. When you are ready, breathe in deeply. As you exhale, bring your palms together into namaste (photo 50).

**2 As you inhale, sweep your arms until they are horizontal and step your left foot to the left** (photo 51). Spread your legs four or five feet apart so that when you bend your knee, it makes a square.

**3 As you exhale, turn the left foot inward forty-five degrees and the right foot outward ninety degrees.** Pull the kneecaps up, tighten the quadriceps, and push downward into your feet. Become grounded.

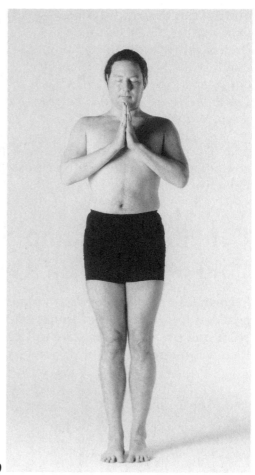

**50**

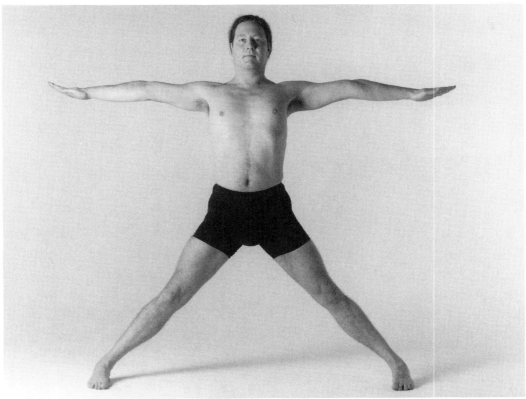

**51**

**4** **As you inhale, sweep the right arm up alongside your ear, lowering the left hand to your left thigh.** Pull the abdominals in, lift your chest, and stretch straight up through the right arm. Energize the vertical line through your arm.

**5** **As you exhale, lean to the left, sliding your left hand down the left leg** (photo 52). This is Stage One of Virabhadrasana II, Warrior Pose II. Reach outward through the right arm, turn your head, look down, and stretch sideways. Be here half a minute, breathing smoothly. When you are ready to proceed, breathe in deeply.

**6** **As you exhale, bend your right knee until it forms a square** (photo 53). Aim the knee directly over the toes. Pull the abdominals in, expand the chest as you inhale, then exhale and spiral your chest toward the ceiling. Reach outward through the right arm *from your center* and gaze into the sky. Experience yourself as a strong curve of energy. Be here half a minute. When you are ready to proceed, inhale deeply and accelerate the stretch.

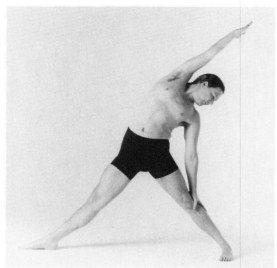

**52**

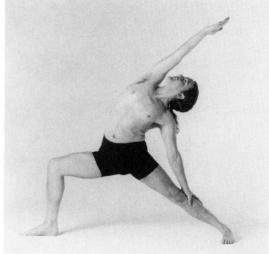

**53**

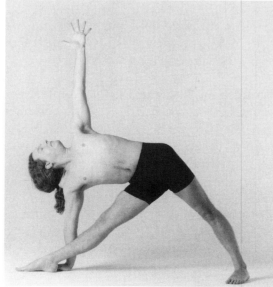

**54**

**7** As you exhale, stretch into Trikonasana, Triangle Pose (photo 54). Keep the length you achieved on the right side of your body as you come into the pose. Bring your right hand to the right ankle or floor, make the left arm vertical, and gaze upward. Breathe. Be here half a minute. When you are ready to proceed, inhale deeply and accelerate the stretch, increasing the current through your lines.

**8** Exhale as you take the left arm behind your back (photo 55). This is Triangle Pose, Stage Two. Take a moment to wriggle the hand in and catch the right thigh. Pull the abdominals in, breathe upward into your chest to lift the rib cage away from the waist. and as you exhale, rotate your chest toward the sky. Gaze upward. Be here half a minute.

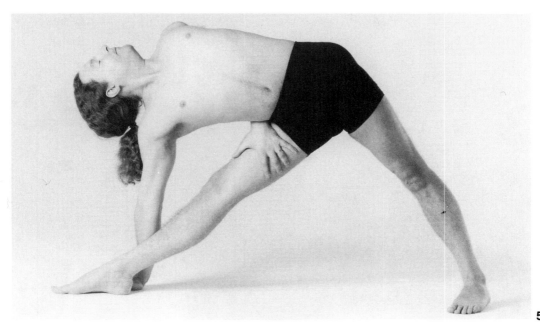

55

**9** Flow into Ardha Chandrasana II, Half Moon Pose (photos 56, 57). First, turn your head and look down. Exhale as you bend your right leg and slide the left foot closer to the right. Place your right hand on the floor, lean until your left foot leaves the floor—you are now balanced on your right hand and foot—and then inhale and float your left foot upward until the leg and torso form a straight line. Exhale as you slowly straighten your right leg, pressing the right foot straight down into the floor. Inhale and lengthen the right arm—your head and body will lift upward away from the floor—then exhale and roll your left shoulder and elbow backward, spiraling your chest toward the sky. Continue looking down. Be here and breathe, half a minute.

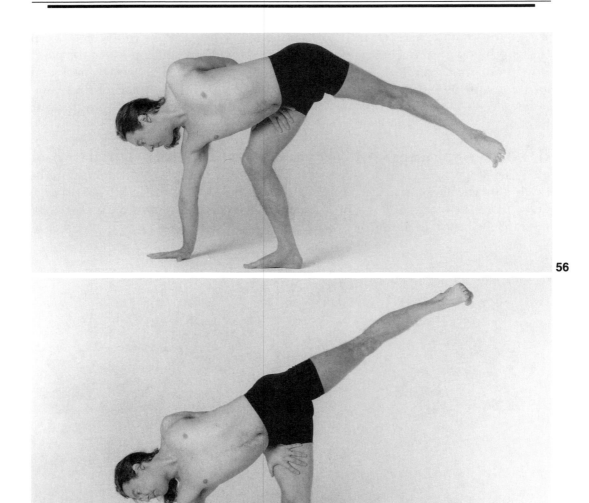

56

57

**10** **As you exhale, come down into Stage Three of Parshvakonasana, the Bent Knee Side Stretch** (photo 58). Bend your right leg, touch the left foot to the floor near the right foot, then step back to your original wide-stance position. Bring the right arm in front of the right leg and bend the right knee until it forms a right angle. Your left arm is still behind your back. Pull the abdominals in, lift upward into the chest, and rotate your body toward the sky. Gaze upward. Breathe smoothly, half a minute.

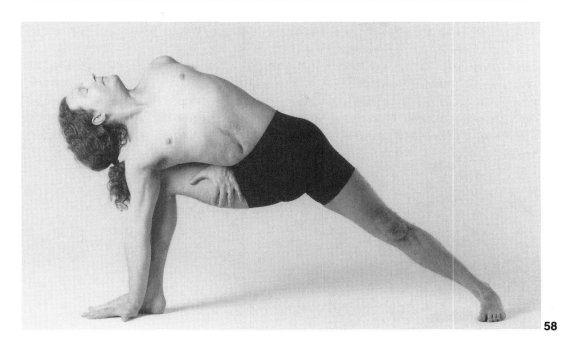

**58**

**11** **Release the left arm**. Bring it forward, up, and around until it is alongside your left ear with the palm down (photo 59). This is Parshvakonasana, Stage Four. Move the left hand and foot away from one another. Gaze upward. Be here half a minute.

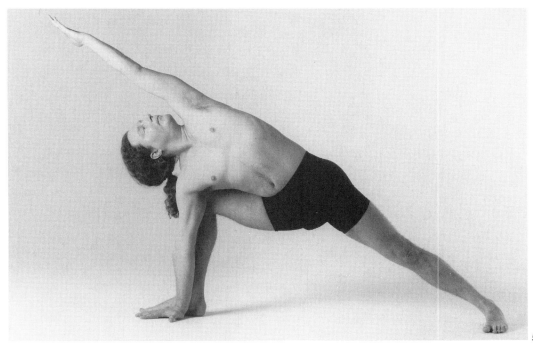

**59**

**12** **Flow into Virabhadrasana I, Warrior Pose.** Inhale as you sweep the left arm up, straightening the right leg. Exhale as you turn your body to face the right foot. Your arms are extending outward from your sides. As you inhale, sweep your arms up until they are vertical, bring the palms together, and turn your head to look upward (photo 60). Exhaling, bend your right knee, and come into the pose (photo 61). Pull the abdominals in, lift your chest, and gaze through your fingers. Reach enthusiastically upward. Be here half a minute, breathing smoothly.

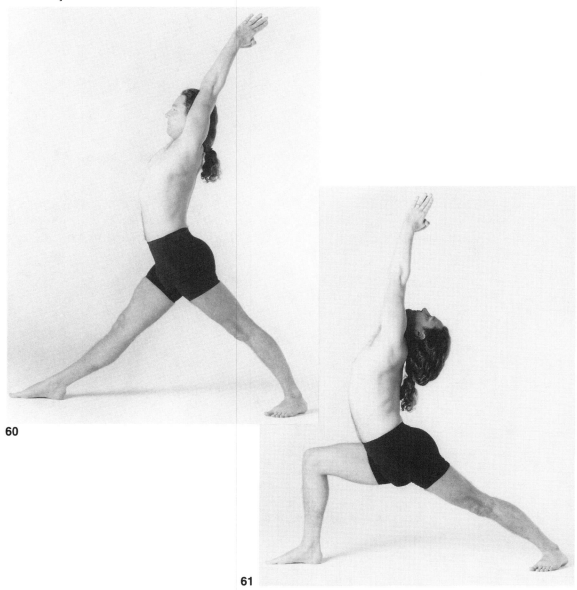

60

61

**13** As you exhale, sweep your arms to the sides and fold forward into this variation of Parshvottanasana, Pyramid Pose (photo 62). Straighten the right leg and walk your hands forward away from you, fingers pointing forward, palms flat. Rest your face on your shinbone. Be here and breathe, half a minute.

**14** Walk your hands backward toward the left foot into this variation of Parshvottanasana, Pyramid Pose (photo 63). Keep your arms straight, palms flat, and your fingers pointing away from you. Breathe smoothly. Let the stretch penetrate. Be here half a minute.

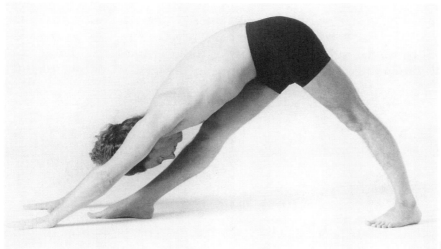

**62**

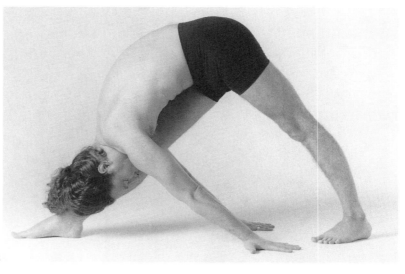

**63**

**15** Bring your left hand to the outside edge of your right foot, sweep the right arm up, and rotate into Parivrrta Trikonasana, the Revolved Triangle Pose (photo 64). Gaze downward at your left hand some of the time, then turn your head upward and gaze toward the right hand. Breathe smoothly. Be here half a minute.

**16** Turn to the front (photo 65). Come into Stage One of the Standing Spread Leg Forward Fold, Prasarita Padottanasana. Turn your feet to the front and place your hands on the floor directly below the shoulders. Press the arms straight, make your back flat, and gaze down. Breathe.

**17** Walk your hands forward into Stage Two of Prasarita Padottanasana, Standing Spread Leg Forward Fold (photo 66). Press forward into your hands and stretch backward through the sitting bones to bring your head down. Endeavor to form a smooth curve through your arms and spine.

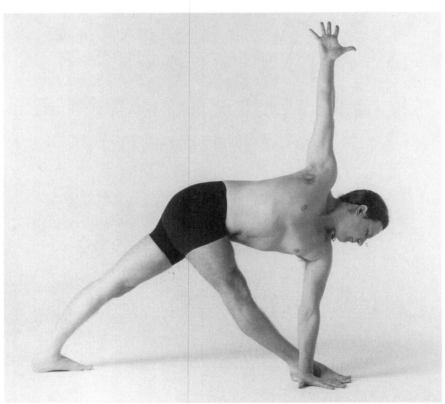

**64**

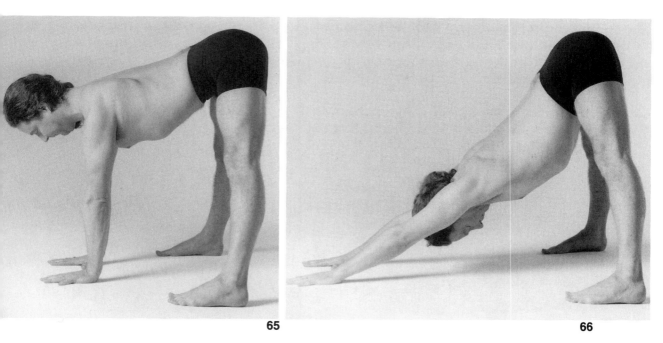

65                                                      66

**18** **Walk your hands backward through your legs and fold forward, Stage Three of Prasarita Padottanasana** (photo 67). Have your palms flat, fingers forward, then bring the elbows inward toward one another until the upper arms are parallel. Stretch the crown of your head straight down toward the floor. Breathe smoothly.

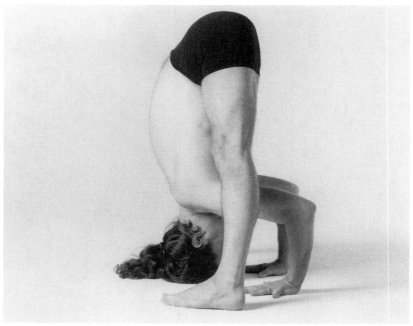

67

**19** **Bring your arms around behind you into Stage Four of Prasarita Pa-dottanasana** (photo 68). Clasp your hands, straighten the arms, then elongate your arms before gently squeezing them downward toward the floor. Be here several breaths.

**20** **Release your hands, sweep your arms to the sides, and as you inhale come up. Exhale as you step your feet together.** Bring your hands together in namaste (photo 69).

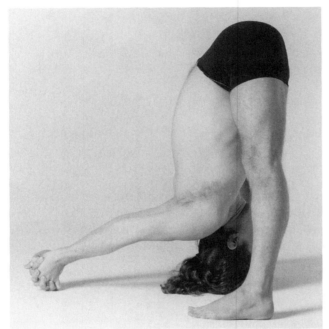

**68**

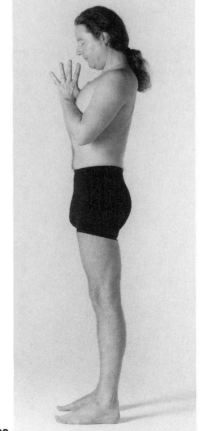

**69**

**21** **Lower your hands and stand quietly.** You are now in Tadasana, Mountain Pose. Close your eyes, breathe smoothly, and be aware of how you feel. Be motionless without holding yourself still. Be relaxed.

**22** Now do the flow on the other side: Step to the right, turn your feet to the left, and then sweep the left arm up and flow. Be in each pose an equal length of time. Then stand quietly and experience the way you feel.

# Benefits: Standing Pose Flow

Builds strength and stamina, increases flexibility. Benefits of all standing poses.

## SUN SALUTATIONS

# 17 Sun Salutations *or Surya Namaskar I, II, III*

There are many variations of the Sun Salutation, Surya Namaskar. I am including my three favorites. The Half Salute is a warm-up and preparation for the others. The Jumping Back version involves stepping or hopping backward and then lowering yourself into Crocodile Pose; this version is fairly strenuous and is especially good for developing upper body strength. The Lunge Salutes are less strenuous and involve stepping back into a Lunge.

### SUN SALUTATION I: HALF SUN SALUTE

**1 Stand in Tadasana (Mountain Pose) with your feet together or hip-width apart.** Take a moment to get centered, ready. Breathe smoothly, making the ujjayi throat sound, and wait for the inner cue to begin. When you are ready, exhale and bring your palms together in namaste, the prayer position (photo 70).

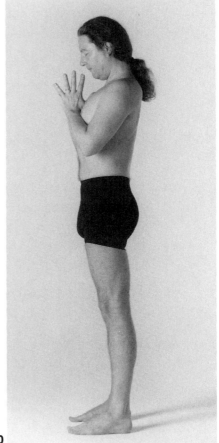

**70**

**2** **As you inhale, sweep your arms above your head** (photo 71). Make this movement smooth. Coordinate it perfectly with your breathing.

**3** **As you exhale, sweep your arms to the sides and hinge forward from your hips.** Reach outward through your arms as you fold, fingers spread. Do not be in a rush. Be smooth. Place your hands alongside your feet with the fingertips and toe tips in line and bring your head inward toward the legs (photo 72).

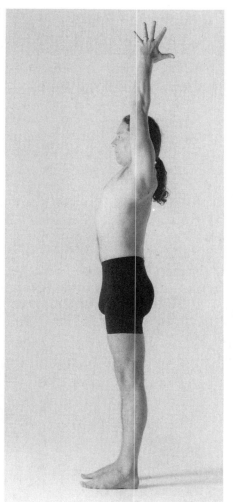

71

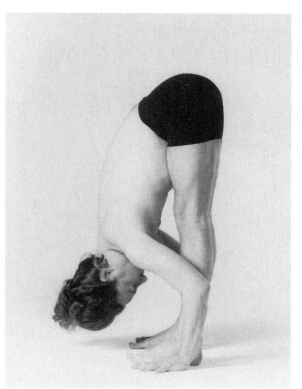

72

**4**  **As you inhale, come halfway up** (photo 73). Elongate the spine horizontally forward, make your back flat, and keep your gaze downward. Your hips will be in a strong dog tilt with your feet pressing down and your sitting bones turning up. Come up as high as necessary in order to flatten your back; if your fingers need to leave the floor, allow them to do so.

**5**  **As you exhale, fold forward into Uttanasana, the Standing Forward Fold** (photo 74). Press your palms flat, move your shoulders toward your elbows, and attempt to slide the floor forward with your hands, without moving them. This will take you deeper into the pose. Bury your face in your legs.

**6**  **As you inhale, sweep your arms to the sides and come back up** (photo 75). You are now in Tadasana with vertical arms. Pull the abdominals in, lift the chest, and reach upward. Stay grounded.

**7**  **Sweep your arms to the sides as you exhale, bringing your palms together in front of your chest into namaste position** (photo 76).

That's one round. Do four to six repetitions.

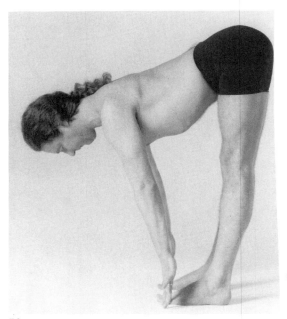

73

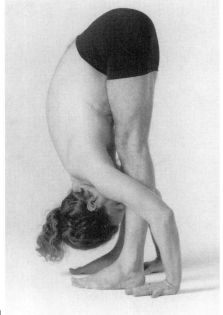

74

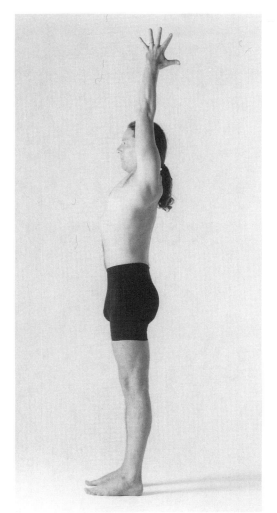

75

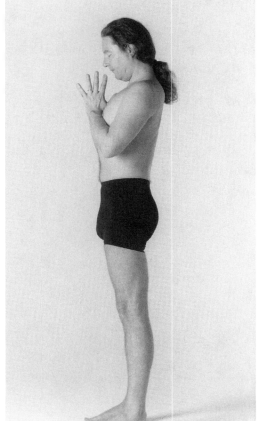

76

## SUN SALUTATION II: JUMPING BACK

**1** **Stand in Tadasana with your feet together or hip-width apart.** Get centered as you wait for the inner cue to begin. When you are ready, exhale, bringing your palms together in namaste position (photo 77).

**2** **As you inhale, sweep your arms to the sides and up above your head** (photo 78). Have your fingers spread and reach outward through your arms as you bring them up. Make the movement smooth. Coordinate it perfectly with the breath. Feel the path your hands trace through space.

**3** **As you exhale, sweep your arms to the sides and hinge forward from your hips** (photo 79).

**4** **As you inhale, come halfway up** (photo 80). Make your back flat. Come up as high as you need to flatten the spine. Allow your fingers to leave the floor if necessary.

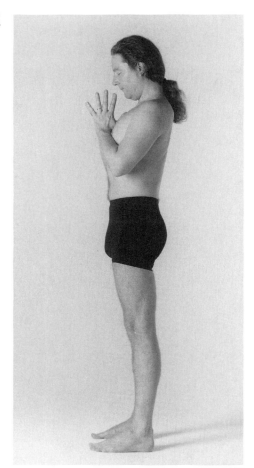

**77**

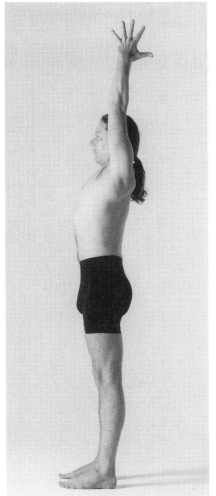

78

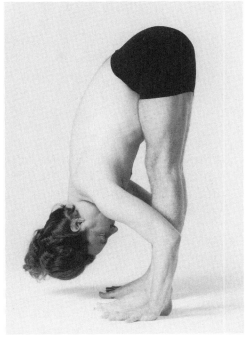

79

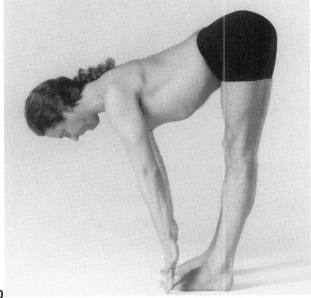

80

**5** **As you exhale, bend your knees, hop backward, and slowly lower yourself into Crocodile Pose** (photo 81). Hug inward with your elbows, keep the abdominals in, and lower yourself down until you are two inches off the floor. Try to not touch the floor. This is similar to a push-up. This movement will develop tremendous upper body strength.

**6** **As you inhale, press into Cobra or Upward Facing Dog Pose and gaze toward the ceiling.** Take your pick about which backbend to do. In Cobra your pelvis and legs remain on the floor; in Upward Facing Dog (photo 82) you're supported by your hands and the tops of your feet only, and your pelvis and knees will be off the floor. Pull the abdominals in, be strong in your legs, and gaze upward. Be here two breaths.

**7** **As you exhale, turn your toes under, dip into Crocodile Pose again, then press into Dog Pose** (photo 83). Omit the dip if that is too strenuous for you at the moment and, instead, move directly into Dog Pose. You will have sufficient strength to do this soon enough. Proceed gradually. Be in Dog Pose three deep breaths.

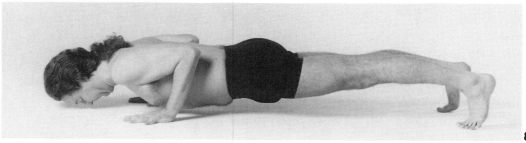

**81**

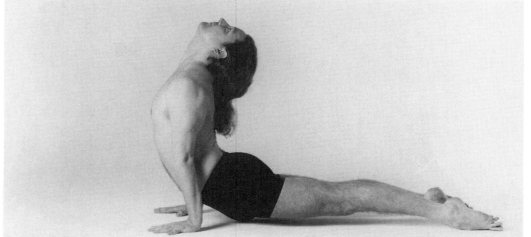

**82**

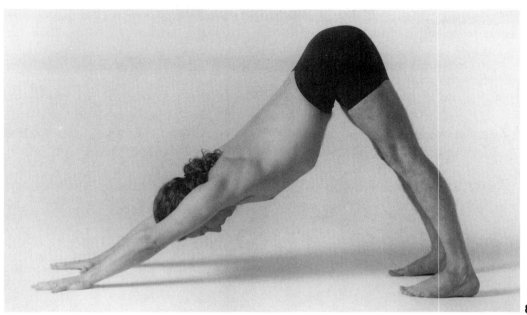

**83**

**8** **As you inhale, lift your head and look forward between your hands. Bend your knees slightly and, as you exhale, hop forward.** Land lightly with your fingertips and toe tips on the same line.

**9** **As you inhale, straighten your legs and come to flat back** (photo 84). Gaze downward toward the floor.

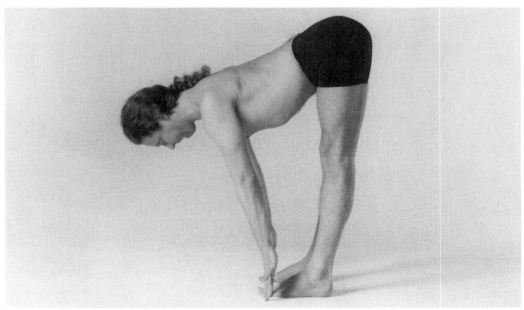

**84**

**10** As you exhale, fold into Uttanasana Standing Forward Fold (photo 85). Reach deeply with your hands.

**11** Sweep your arms to the sides, make your arms long, and as you inhale, come to a standing position with your arms vertical (photo 86). Bring your palms together, fingers spread.

**12** As you exhale, sweep your arms to your sides, bringing your palms together in front of your chest in namaste position (photo 87).

That's one round. Perform one to twelve rounds, according to your capacity.

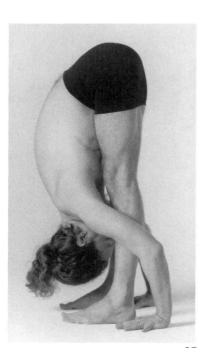
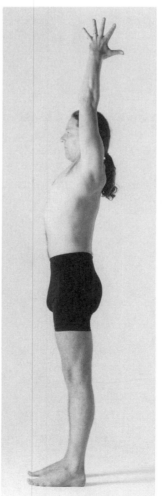
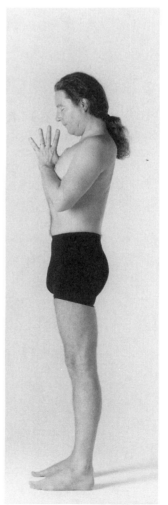

85                                86                                87

# SUN SALUTATION III: LUNGE SALUTES

**1 Stand in Tadasana with your feet together.** Wait for the inner cue to begin. When you are ready, exhale and bring your palms together in namaste (photo 88).

**2 As you inhale, sweep your arms to the sides and up** (photo 89). Make the movement smooth and coordinate it perfectly with your breathing.

**3 As you exhale, sweep your arms to the sides and hinge forward from your hips** (photo 90). Reach outward through your arms as you fold, keep your fingers spread, be smooth. Feel the wind go through your fingers. Place your hands alongside your feet with the fingertips and toe tips in line.

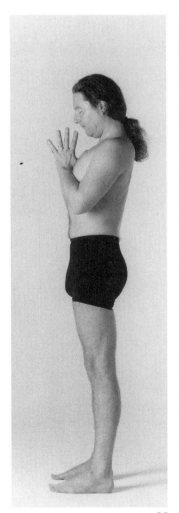

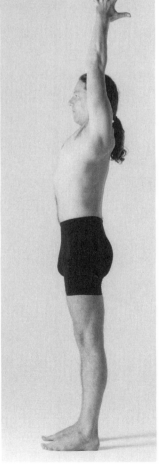

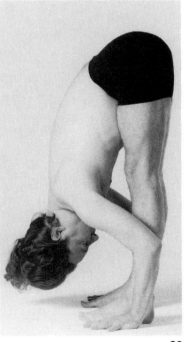

88  89  90

**4** As you inhale, come **halfway up** (photo 91). Elongate the spine horizontally forward and make your back flat. Come up as high as necessary in order to flatten the spine.

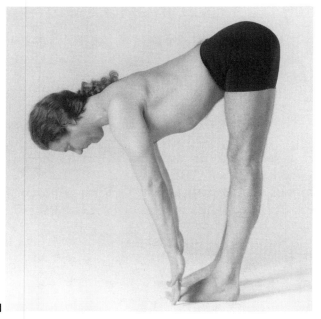

**91**

**5** Exhale as you step back with your right foot and come into Lunge position (photo 92). Bend your right knee to the floor and point your toes.

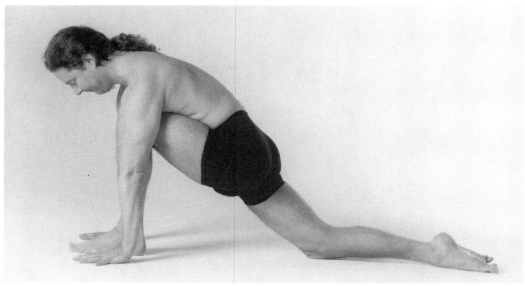

**92**

**6** Inhale as you sweep your arms forward and up above your head (photo 93). Press your hips down as your arms reach up. Keep your hands shoulder-width apart, your fingers spread and palms facing forward. Coordinate this movement with your breathing. Time it perfectly. Be smooth, fluid. Breathe smoothly.

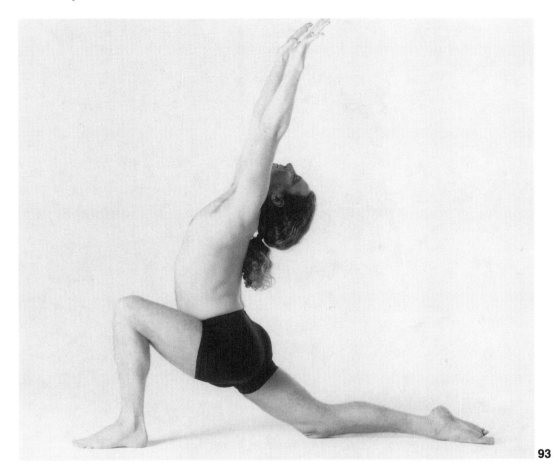

93

**7** **As you exhale, reach forward, placing your hands on the floor in their original position, step back with your left foot, and slowly lower yourself to the floor as you finish the exhalation** (photo 94). Rest your pelvis on the floor and point your toes.

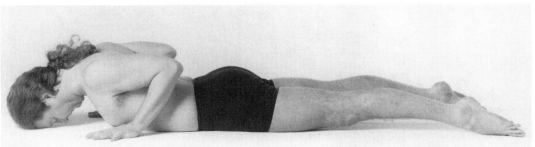

94

**8** **As you inhale, press into Cobra and gaze upward** (photo 95): Shrug the shoulders down away from the ears, hug inward with your elbows, press forward with your chest, making it round, and turn your head and gaze upward.

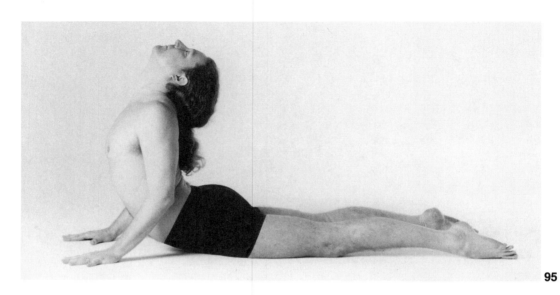

95

**9** **As you exhale, flow into Dog Pose** (photo 96). Be here three deep breaths.

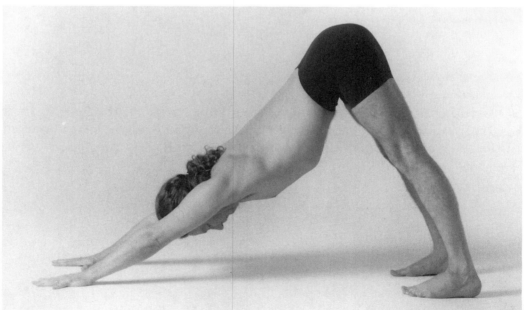

96

**10** On the fourth inhale, lift your head and look forward between your hands. As you exhale, step forward with your right foot. You are in Lunge position again, except now the right leg is forward. The leg you stepped backward with is the leg you now step forward with.

**11** As you inhale, sweep your arms above your head (photo 97). Press the hips down as your arms go up.

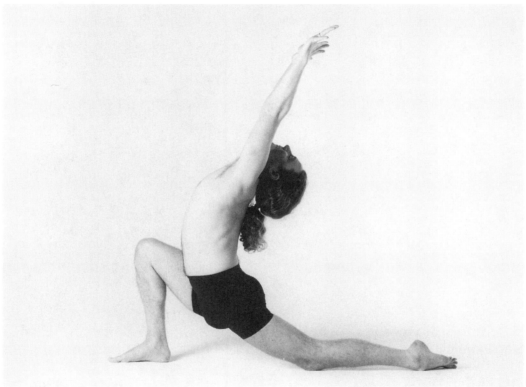

**97**

**12** As you exhale, reach forward with your hands, place them on the floor straddling the right foot, and step forward with your left foot. Your feet are now together, straddled by your hands.

**13** Inhale as you press the arms and legs straight and come halfway up (photo 98). Flatten your back, dog tilt, gaze downward.

**14** Exhale as you fold forward (photo 99). Take your head inward toward your legs, reach deeply with your hands, and flatten your palms to the floor.

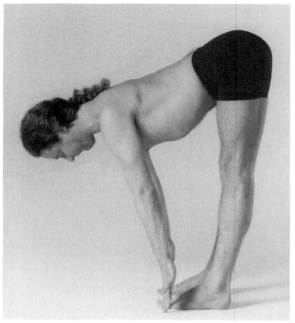

98

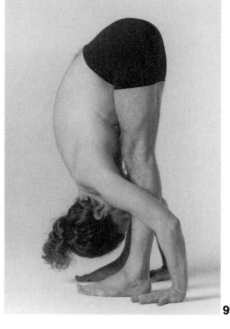

99

**15** Inhale as you sweep your arms to the sides and up above your head as you come back to a standing position (photo 100).

**16** Exhale as you sweep your arms to the sides and bring your palms together in namaste (photo 101).

That's round one. Remember, the leg you step backward with into the Lunge is the leg you then step forward with after Dog Pose. Do the second repetition with the other leg; that is, step backward and then forward with the left leg. Do several repetitions on each leg, alternating.

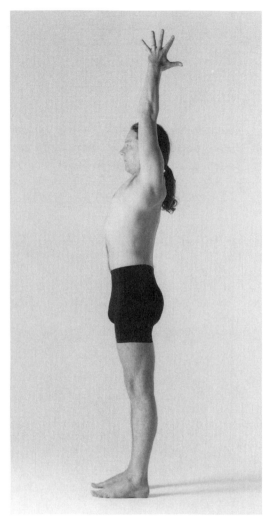
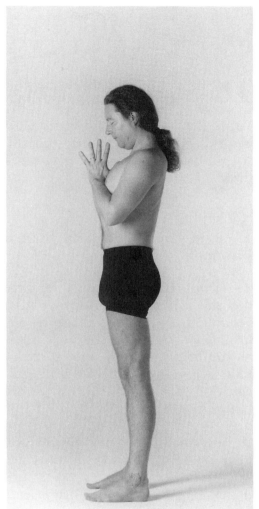

**100**                                                                                          **101**

# Benefits: Sun Salutations

Sun Salutations are exhilarating and enjoyable. They develop strength, flexibility, grace, speed, alertness, stamina, and coordination. They stimulate the abdominal organs, wake up the spine, build heat for the practice, and unleash held energy. Arms and wrists strengthened. Back strengthened, chest opened. Movements co-ordinated with breath increase awareness of breath and flow. Excellent whole body exercise.

## SHOULDERS AND HIPS

# 18 Shoulder Stretches

The following eight shoulder stretches are excellent for loosening the shoulders and restoring lost movement to the whole upper body. Practice them daily for several weeks and notice the changes. You will need a long strap for the first three.

### ONE

**1 Sit in any comfortably erect position. Clasp hold of the strap and straighten your arms.**

**2 As you inhale, sweep your arms forward and up until they are vertical** (photo 102), **and exhale as you bring them down behind you. Inhale as you bring them up again, and exhale as you return to starting position.** Go back and forth like this five times.

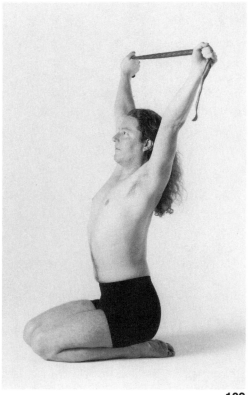

**3** Coordinate this movement with your breathing, making the movement smooth. Make sure the strap is sufficiently long and your hands sufficiently far apart, so that you can keep your arms straight. If you cannot keep your arms straight, lengthen the strap.

**4** The idea is to circumscribe as large a circle as possible with your hands as they go up and over. Therefore, at every given moment you are stretching outward through your arms in the direction they are pointing.

**102**

**5** **Bring your arms behind you** (photo 103). Keep the abdomen in, your chest expanded, and arms straight, and allow the stretch to penetrate for ten or fifteen seconds. Relax with the intensity as you run energy through the arm lines. Breathe smoothly. Then return to starting position.

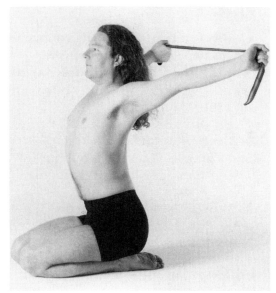

**103**

## TWO

**1** **Shorten the strap so your hands are approximately twenty-four to thirty inches apart.** Adjust the distance to suit your need.

**2** **Raise both arms up, bringing the right arm alongside the ear, and swivel the left arm around and down behind you** (photo 104).

**3** Inhale as you energize upward through the right arm, and exhale as you reach outward through the left arm and pull down with the hand. This is a fantastic stretch. Breathe smoothly and create the degree of intensity you find pleasurable. Be here several breaths, then change sides.

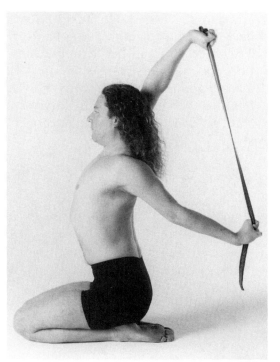

**104**

## THREE

**1** **Shorten the strap until your arms are parallel with one another and your hands are shoulder-width apart.** Pull outward with your hands until the strap is taut.

**2** **Take your arms up** (photo 105). Get as long as you can from your navel to your hands. Be here a few moments.

**3** **Slowly bend your arms** (photo 106). Pull hard on the belt as you slowly bring it down behind your head until it touches the back of your neck. Keep the abdominals in, your chest lifted, and firmly squeeze the elbows backward—and continue pulling the strap taut. Then slowly take the strap back up again, straightening the arms. Try to feel every subtle change of sensation. Do not be surprised if the strap starts jiggling. It's a long way up. This is more difficult than you'd think. Do this several times, then release the strap.

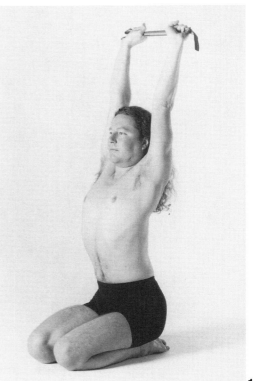

105

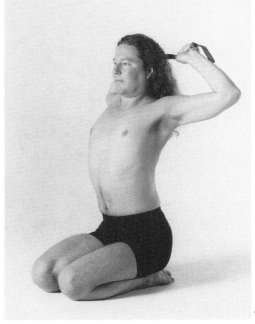

106

# FOUR

**1** **Clasp your hands behind you, straighten your arms, then lift your hands as high as you can** (photo 107). Roll the shoulders backward, gently squeezing the shoulder blades together, and expand your chest by lifting it up and pressing it forward. Pull straight backward through your arms in the direction they are pointing. Be here several breaths.

**2** **Bring your interlaced hands to the left side of your waist** (photo 108). Pull the abdominals in and lift the chest, then roll both shoulders backward as you squeeze the elbows inward toward one another and press forward with your hands. Breathe deeply and expand your chest, deliberately pressing it forward through the shoulders. Be here several breaths, then change sides.

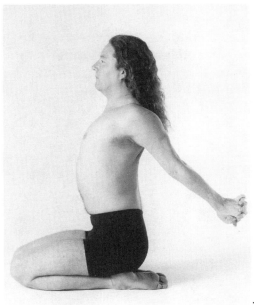

**107**

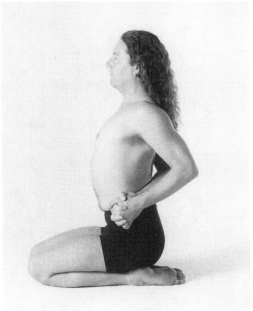

**108**

## FIVE

**1 Stretch the left arm straight up, then bend your elbow and bring your hand down behind your back. Clasp the left elbow with your right hand** (photo 109). Find the groove of your spine with your left fingertips.

**2** Keeping your abdomen in, backward toward the spine, and your chest lifting and expanded, use your right hand to pull the left elbow behind your head. Maneuver your fingertips down the groove of the spine, gently squeeze the right elbow comfortably far backward, and allow the stretch to penetrate for half a minute. Breathe smoothly. Change sides.

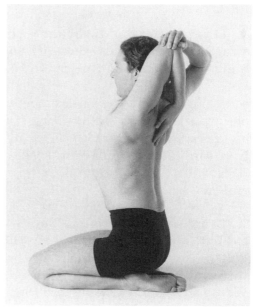

**109**

## SIX

**1 Place the back of your right hand on your lower back, then wriggle it up your back as far as it will comfortably go.** Pause here, acclimatize for a moment, then wriggle it farther up.

**2 Stretch the left arm straight up, bend your elbow so your hand comes down behind your back, and clasp your hands** (photo 110). Move the left elbow away from your head and elevate your chin slightly. Stretch straight up into the left elbow, straight down into the right elbow, and attempt to move both elbows backward—chest up, shoulder blades down, navel backward toward the spine. Be here half a minute, breathing smoothly, then switch sides.

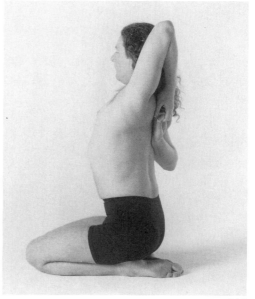

**110**

## SEVEN

**1 Entwine your arms and bring your palms together** (photo 111). Turn your palms until they are straight. Be here half a minute, then entwine them with the other arm on top.

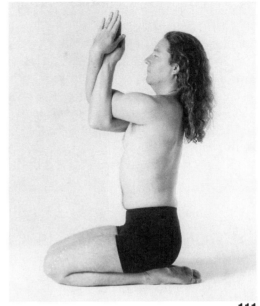

**111**

## EIGHT

**1 Bring your hands into prayer position behind your back** (photo 112). Start with your fingertips together, pointing down, then turn your hands inward and bring them up into prayer position.

**2** Bring the abdominals in, lift and expand the chest, then roll the shoulders backward. Move the elbows backward so the shoulder blades flatten into your back, and gently press your palms together. Wriggle your hands higher when you can. The higher you get them, the more comfortable this will be. Be here several breaths.

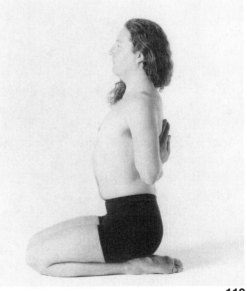

**112**

# Benefits: Shoulders and Hips

Increased strength and mobility of hips and shoulders is an important factor in the correct performance of the poses. These hip and shoulder openers increase shoulder mobility, releasing tension and blocked energy in the arms, shoulders, upper back, and neck, freeing the chest and improving lung capacity; as well as increasing mobility in the lower back, hips, pelvic region, knees and ankles. These are tremendous tension relievers, thereby improving circulation throughout the body, especially between arms and torso, and legs and torso. Improves posture. Improves all-round flexibility. You'll find yourself being more comfortable in your body as a result of these stretches.

# Benefits: Shoulder Stretches

Increase range of motion in shoulders. Release tension in arms, shoulders, chest, upper back, and neck. Strengthen arms. Excellent for those with rounded shoulders, collapsed chest, tense neck.

# 19 Lotus Pose *or Padmasana*

In my hierarchy of poses, I consider Padmasana, Lotus Pose, the most important. Shavasana, Relaxation Pose, is second, and everything else comes after that. All poses are equal, actually—whichever pose you're doing is the most important one—but I like to think of it in this way because the Lotus Pose (if you can do it comfortably) is such a perfect meditation posture. It's a position in which you can sit perfectly straight and be absolutely still, relaxed, comfortable, and alert.

Most people cannot do Lotus Pose the first time they try, or the second. It is important, therefore, to pursue the pose gradually, in stages, and to work at it patiently and consistently over a sustained period of time. If you pursue it properly you should be able to sit in Lotus within a year, probably sooner. It may take you longer. You may never get it. In any case, work it slowly, carefully, gently. A year is not a long time.

You should *never* experience pain in your knees as you do these exercises. If you do, stop what you are doing. Pain is an indication that something is wrong. The knees can be injured when the hips or ankles, usually the hips, are not rotating as much as they should and the knees overrotate in the attempt to achieve the pose. What's needed, therefore, is increased range of motion in the hips and ankles. The following preparatory poses are designed for just this purpose. They will help loosen and mobilize your hips, knees, and ankles—each of which plays an important role in a correctly performed Padmasana. But be patient, take your time, proceed intelligently, and do not force the issue. Do not be impatient. Simply persist. Gentle persistence is the key. Do the exercises regularly.

Here are the basic instructions for Padmasana:

**1** **Sit on the floor in an easy crossed-leg pose.**

**2** **Clasp hold of your left foot with both hands and bring it high onto the right thigh, up into the groin. Bring the right leg over the left and place the right foot in the left groin** (photo 113). This is the full Lotus Pose. Do not be discouraged if you are unable to do this yet. Even if you can, a few seconds may be enough at first.

**3** **Uncross your legs and try it on the other side.** To avoid becoming confused about which leg goes where, remember that the leg you uncross first is the first leg to cross on the second side.

The basic instructions are simple. To make it possible, however, practice the preparatory poses:

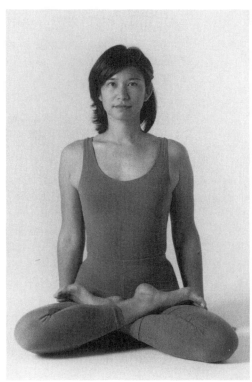

113

## LOTUS PREPARATIONS

### ONE ON YOUR BACK

**1** **Lie on your back with your legs bent and both feet flat on the floor.**

**2** **Place the side of your right foot on your left thigh near the knee.** Make the right shinbone horizontal. Flex the right heel, allowing it to protrude slightly off the left leg, and move the right knee away from you.

**3** **Clasp hold of the left knee with both hands** by bringing the legs toward you, reaching through the window formed by your right leg and left thigh with your right hand, and clasping it around the left knee or thigh with your left hand (photo 114). Put a pillow under your head if your neck or shoulders feel uncomfortable. Your head should be in line with your spine.

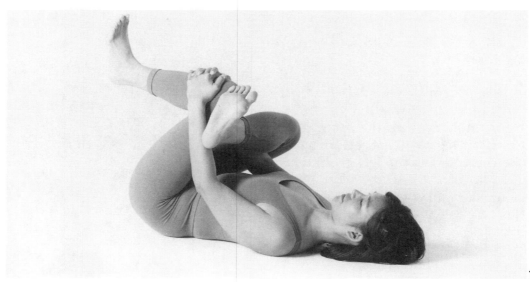

**114**

**4  Pull gently.** Pull the left thigh toward your chest as you simultaneously press your sacrum and lower back into the floor. Keep both feet flexed, your toes spread, and pull with your hands until you create a stretch in the right hip and buttock. Flatten the shoulder blades into the floor as you do this, making your chest round. When you cannot pull the leg in any tighter, stay where you are, maintain the action of the pose, and relax with the intensity of the stretch. Savor the way this feels. Pull the leg in tighter when the sensations of stretch diminish somewhat. Be here about a minute, breathing smoothly.

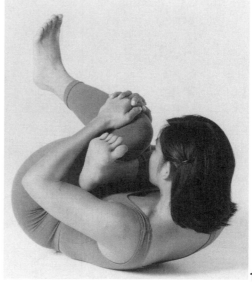

**5  Lift your head, curl your lower back up off the floor, and touch your nose to the left knee** (photo 115). Be here fifteen or thirty seconds, then lie flat on your back again.

**115**

**6 Clasp the right foot and pull it down into the left groin.** Snuggle it in deeply, being careful not to make any sudden movements that may cause you to strain the knee unintentionally. Be delicate as you wriggle it in.

**7 Gently push the lotus, or crossed, knee away from you** (photo 116) by placing your right hand on the right knee and gently pressing. Hold the right foot where it is, if necessary, with your left hand. If this stretch is difficult for you, then this is exactly what you need. Proceed cautiously. Do not be aggressive and do not create even the slightest hint of strain in your knee. The best way to proceed is slowly. Therefore, push gently, firmly. Apply pressure for five or ten seconds, then ease off the stretch and repeat one or many times. This is an especially good position in which to work this stretch because your back is on the floor and therefore can easily remain straight. The opening you receive when your back is flat is consistent with the opening necessary to sit comfortably erect.

**8** Release the right leg, then repeat all of this with your left leg.

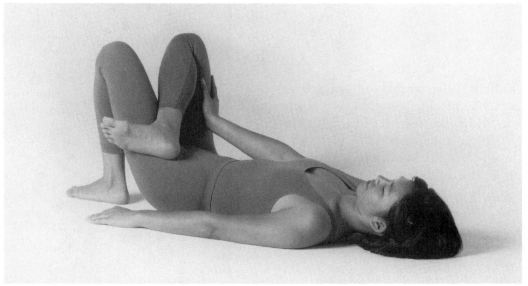

**116**

## TWO SITTING UP

**1 Sit on the floor in Sukhasana, the easy crossed-leg pose.**

**2 Place the right foot in the crook of the left elbow and cradle the leg in your arms.** Bring the right arm around the right knee and clasp your hands (photo 117). Flex the right heel, lift the right foot up until the right shinbone is horizontal, level with the floor, and then gently pull the leg inward toward your chest. Bring your leg toward your chest and your chest toward your leg, aiming the stretch into the right hip and buttock. Endeavor to sit erect as you do this, relaxing the shoulders downward and elongating your spine upward. Press the sitting bones firmly down into the floor, and move the crown of your head toward the ceiling. Elongate your spine upward as you inhale, and pull inward with your arms as you exhale. Be here several breaths, anywhere from half a minute to a minute.

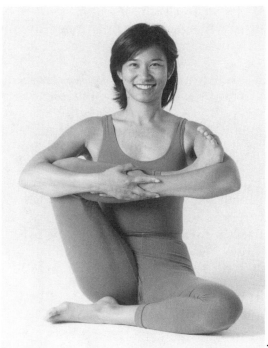

**117**

**3** **Bring the right leg into Half Lotus** by placing the right foot in the left groin, the crease formed by the left thigh and torso, then wriggling the left foot forward until it snuggles under the right knee (photo 118). The right leg is now in a tight Half Lotus and the left shinbone is horizontal. Wriggle the buttocks backward, then sit erect.

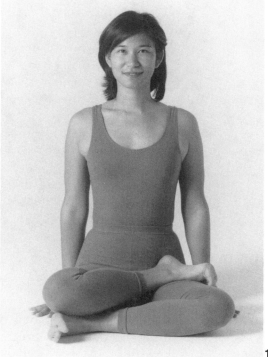

**118**

**4** If the right knee cannot rest comfortably on the left foot, proceed cautiously. Gently press the right knee down with your right hand. Hold this stretch for a few moments, then release the pressure and repeat. Do this several or many times. Do not bounce your knee up and down.

**5** **Lean forward**; place your hands by your hips and slowly tip forward. Do not be in a rush. Melt forward. Wait for the sensations of stretch to diminish before folding deeper. Then slide your hands forward, keeping your arms straight, and go in the direction of resting your forehead on the floor. Be here one minute, then perform each of these steps with the other leg.

**6** **Now place one leg on top of the other so both shinbones are horizontal.** Sit erect for a few breaths. Then wriggle your hips backward so you are on the frontal edge of the sitting bones, pull the buttock muscles sideways and back, and slowly lean forward (photo 119) until (eventually) your forehead rests on the floor. Be here a minute or two. Change legs. Enjoy the way this feels. This is a wonderful pose.

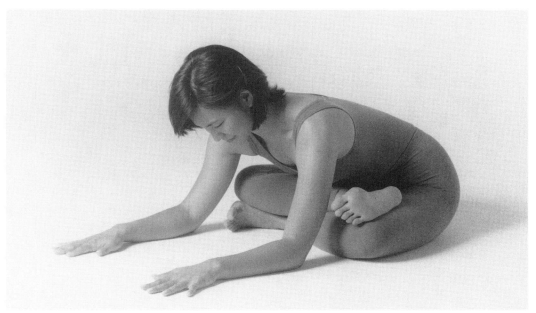

**119**

## HALF LOTUS POSE OR ARDHA PADMASANA

**1** **Sit on a zafu (Zen meditation pillow) or rolled blanket in Sukhasana, the easy crossed-leg pose. Catch hold of the right foot and ankle with both hands, holding the foot from underneath, and bring it up into the left groin** (photo 120). Sit erect with your chest up and shoulders relaxed.

**2** Change legs and do the pose on the other side. This insures that you develop the hips equally. Be aware of the inclination to sit more frequently with your right leg on top, if that's what's easy for you, and endeavor instead to spend equal time on each side. Create a balance.

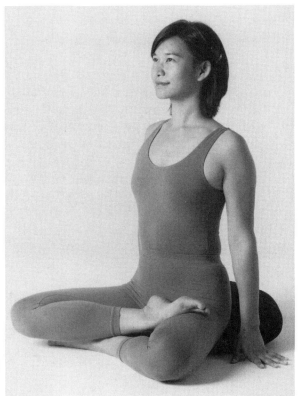

**120**

## LOTUS POSE—ONCE YOU'RE IN IT

**1** Once you've crossed your legs, lean forward slightly and wriggle the buttocks backward until you are on the frontal edge of each sitting bone. You are now in extreme dog tilt. Then bring your torso erect and gently align your center *toward* cat tilt. Delicately bring the navel backward toward the spine until you sense the sacrum is nearly vertical and you are on the tips, rather than the frontal edges, of each sitting bone. Your center is now in "neutral." Your back will not be totally straight. Allow a natural lumbar curve.

**2** From this perfectly aligned "neutral" center, allow the weight of your body to sink into the floor. Become grounded through the sitting bones and perineum, rooted into the earth. Take a few moments to do this. Then feel where your core is, your invisible spine, from the perineum at the bottom to the crown of your head at the top, and allow your core gently to elongate. As you do this, open the crown of your head by relaxing your scalp muscles and let it float upward—

without becoming ungrounded. You'll feel as though you are going up and down at the same time, without going anywhere. Let your pelvis drop down, out from underneath you. Allow your rib cage and chest to float upward away from the waist. Relax the shoulders, sliding the shoulder blades down your back, and gently keep the navel backward toward the spine. Rest your hands where they are comfortable, palms up or down. This usually requires moving them backward several inches so the upper arms are vertical and the elbows are aligned directly below the shoulder joints. If the elbows are forward of the shoulders, your shoulders will round and eventually ache. Balance your head perfectly on top of your spine and be sensitive to the overall feeling-tone of how you are. Look for the balance point where you feel most comfortable, most weightless, and therefore most perfectly balanced. The straighter you are, the less structural strain you'll experience. Make subtle internal adjustments until your alignment feels best.

**3** Your sacrum must be nearly vertical for your spine to be perfectly balanced; not tilting forward too far and not tilting backward. Actually, it will angle forward a little, but it will *feel* vertical. This is because the relationship between your sacrum and spine is fixed and constant. The spine comes straight out of the sacrum. If the sacrum is tilting backward toward cat tilt, your spine will project backward before coming up; this will cause your ribs and chest to sink, and you'll sag into a slump that puts strain on your back, shoulders, and neck. If the sacrum is tilting forward toward dog tilt, your spine will project forward before coming up, making an excessive arch in the lower back that also creates strain. But there is a natural curve in your lower back that you want to maintain, and this is a function of having the alignment of your center in "neutral" with the sacrum just slightly tilting forward, about ten degrees. Some people tend to sit with too much dog tilt; most people are in excessive cat tilt. Especially in Half Lotus, for example, before it opens up sufficiently, one knee may be quite high—and if your knees are higher than your hips, your sacrum will be forced backward, causing you to slump. Sitting on a zafu or folded blanket can correct your alignment, making it easier to sit erect. Look into a mirror, have a friend check your alignment, and become familiar with the inner feeling of being fully erect and perfectly balanced.

**4** Close your eyes, breathe softly, and experience what's happening right where you are. Sit erect without being rigid, be statue-still, unmoving, and consciously practice releasing tensions. Allow your awareness to scan through your body at a leisurely pace and deliberately let go of every discernible tension. Relax everywhere. Expand. Become more spacious. Experience improved energy flow. You'll feel like a gently billowing cloud.

**5** Have in mind the image of a plant, for your spine and body "grow" upward from your firm and grounded connection with the earth and "bloom" into expression much like a plant. Plants do not have muscles to hold themselves up. They're held up by the water they receive from the earth and sky. The water flows into the cells of the plant, they fill and expand, and this gentle expansion is what holds the plant in full expression. The plant then instinctively grows toward the light. When there is insufficient water, however, plants wilt and become limp. Pretend you are a plant that has just been watered. Feel yourself being fed, nourished, allow yourself to relax and expand, effortlessly—no muscles and no straining—and instinctively, like the lotus flower, open gently, bloom, and bathe in the light. The light is right there, here. The sun is shining. Just open yourself to it. Let it in. Receive. And thereby gently express the meaning of the pose. Be you in gentle, full expression.

**Question:**   What are some advantages of Lotus Pose?

**Response:**   First of all, being able to sit in the Lotus posture is not a sign of spiritual advancement. It is, however, the most stable sitting position for meditation. Lotus makes it easy to sit straight. In fact, it's difficult to sit in Lotus and not keep your spine erect. For me, however, it took about two years after I was able to do the Lotus before I could sit in it comfortably.

Once you are able to cross your legs Lotus-fashion, you'll find that, besides being the perfect meditation posture, it opens up enormous possibilities in terms of what you can do in other poses. If you look at your body as an instrument and certain postures as scales, the Lotus Pose can be considered one of the key scales for opening your body and learning to "play" beautifully. With Lotus you'll discover you now have the means with which to open yourself more fully, and that simple forward bends and twists, for example, are transformed into highly efficient, powerful, advanced stretches when done with your legs in Lotus.

Bodies are funny. Lotus will be easy for some people and difficult for others. Keep in mind, therefore, that the degree of flexibility you now possess or the speed at which you progress is not what matters. If you do the preparatory exercises properly and if you sit in Half Lotus frequently, alternating your legs, you will eventually be able to sit comfortably in Lotus. But sitting in Lotus is not the important point. What's important is the knowledge you gain in terms of how to open your body and keep it opened. The yoga lies in how sensitively you nudge your edges and tight areas toward greater openness. The postures are the tools you use for this.

The most important feature of Padmasana is its utilization for motionless sitting, centering. Sitting motionless in Lotus is the most effortless way to expand your energy field, to decompress. It's a way of learning to be consciously relaxed and undefended, instead of unconsciously fearful, contracted, and defensive. When you relax, you expand—and this is good for you on all levels. Your physical health will improve because your energy is flowing better. Your bodily fluids will flow better, you'll *feel* better, and your new outlook on life will give rise to mental clarity, spontaneous optimism, and peace of mind. You will then experience life differently. You'll have a new experience of who you are—and as your sense of identity changes, everything will seem to change. Padmasana is an extremely restful pose, deserving of every effort to attain it.

# Benefits: Lotus Pose *or Padmasana*

Increases mobility and releases tension in hips, legs, knees, ankles. Strengthens back. Improves posture. Improves circulation between legs and torso. Increases circulation in lumbar area and abdomen, thus increases circulation to abdominal organs. Extremely restful position. Best meditation posture.

## BACKBENDS

# 20 Hero Pose *or Virasana*

The Hero Pose is one of the basic sitting postures, also excellent for meditation. The internal rotation of the upper legs and knees is opposite to the movement involved in Lotus Pose; as such, it both loosens the hips, knees, and ankles in preparation for the Lotus and acts as a mild counterpose. The Hero is also the starting position for several forward bends, backward bends, and twists.

**1 Start on your hands and knees as in Cat Pose.** Have your knees hip-width apart so the thighs are parallel with one another, and separate your feet until they are slightly wider than your hips. Check that your feet are pointing directly backward, not turning in or out.

**2 Sit between your feet** by first supporting yourself with your hands and then slowly lowering your hips to the floor (photo 121). If you are unable to sit comfortably, or if you feel any pain in your knees, elevate your hips by placing a

folded blanket or zafu (Zen pillow) beneath you. Use this support until you
experience a feeling of ease (this may
take several months). Eventually you
will be able to sit between your feet with
no discomfort with your buttocks
firmly on the ground.

**3** Sit tall. Counteract the tendency to
slump by adjusting the buttock muscles
sideways and back with your hands,
and tilting the pelvis slightly forward so
you are positioned on the frontal edge
of each sitting bone. Then draw the abdomen backward toward the spine and
delicately adjust your hips toward cat
tilt to establish neutral alignment of
your center, your pelvis making a
ninety-degree angle with the thighs.
You are now on the tips of the sitting
bones.

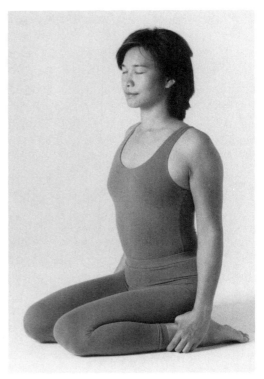

**121**

**4** Rest your hands in your lap, on your thighs, or on your ankles, then close
your eyes. With your eyes closed you'll be better able to sense inwardly for the
perfect alignment. Elevate and free your chest, relax the shoulders back and down
away from your ears, then lift or lower your chin until your head feels perfectly
balanced, weightless on top of the spine. Breathe smoothly, settle in to where you
are, and let the weight of your body sink down into the earth as the inner feeling
rises. Become more and more grounded, increasingly relaxed and undefended,
and feel yourself gently expanding. Be still. Feel the energy you are made of. Feel
the peace within you. Sit quietly for at least a minute.

**5** For some people this position is exceptionally easy, for others it is one of the
most frustrating. Proceed slowly if you experience any difficulty. Be careful not
to strain your knees. Do not be impatient, be persistent—gently. Practice this pose
frequently.

**6** Occasionally, secure a strap around your thighs so they stay parallel. This
will enable you to relax your legs without losing their proper alignment. The
strap, however, is a training wheel. Use it sparingly.

**7** Remember, the purpose of yoga practice—and motionless sitting in particular—is to experience the truth about what you are. It's about the wave experiencing itself as it is and thereby experiencing its inherent ocean nature. Every specific wave is the entire ocean in specific expression, and the peace of the ocean's depth is its peace—available to be experienced. Each one of us is an individually unique expression of the one and only divine Self, God's infinite Self-Expression. And like the wave, we can never get away from our source. The wave is what it is because of what the ocean is. Therefore sit quietly, relax everywhere, immerse yourself in the easy flow of breath, and feel what's happening right where you are. Be effortlessly attentive. Feel the peace within you, the peace of Mind.

# Benefits: Backbends

Backward Bends are exhilarating, strengthening, opening, and exploratory. Of course, forward bends are exploratory also, as are all poses. You're opening and going into areas of yourself that have probably never been opened. Backbends, though, are exploratory in the sense that you really feel as if you're moving into the unknown, into uncharted territory, probably because you can't see where you're going.

Backbends are especially tremendous poses, however, because they encourage a sense of emotional openness and confidence. They gently open the chest, abdominal organs, pelvic region, and the whole front side of the body—the tender, vulnerable side. The chest is where the heart chakra is located. Many of us are closed down and defended in that area, either from a lack of love or from past hurts. The pelvic region is where the sex chakra is located, and many of us have contracted and pulled back in that area. We attempt to protect ourselves emotionally by closing down, pulling back, contracting our bodies, and thereby forming a protective shield or barrier. Closing down is not healthy, though. It's part of what makes you feel more separate psychologically, and it constricts and restricts vital energy flow, which will inevitably cause you to feel more depressed than you would otherwise, more fearful, less vital, and less alive. Not to mention the fact that most of us sit in a somewhat cramped or collapsed position much of the day, anyway—either at a desk, while driving or eating, or in front of the TV—which not only impairs the functioning of the lungs and abdominal organs, but causes the spinal vertebrae to push backward out of healthy alignment.

Backbends open these closed areas, thereby releasing blocked energy while simultaneously building the strength needed to stay open. Strong back muscles, developed with backbends, make it easy to sit and stand erect all day long, so you are alert and comfortable more of the time. Backbends give you energy because they release tension and blocked energy in your chest and pelvic regions as well as through the ankles, knees, quadriceps, abdominal organs, upper back, neck, shoulders, and arms. They are rejuvenating. They encourage youthfulness by keeping the spine supple.

# Benefits: Hero Pose *or Virasana*

Stretches feet, ankles, knees, thighs, hips. Relieves fatigue in the legs. Improves circulation and posture. A very comfortable sitting position, excellent for meditation. Be sure to prop yourself up on a folded blanket or zafu if you are unable to sit on the floor. If you experience any strain in your knees at any time, come out of the pose and prop yourself up further before trying it again.

# 21 Reclining Hero Pose *or Supta Virasana*

**1  Sit in Virasana, Hero Pose.** Be sure you are comfortable here before proceeding. Occasionally, secure a strap around your thighs so they stay parallel.

### STAGE ONE

**2  Lean back on your elbows** (photo 122). First lean back on your hands, then, lifting your hips an inch or two off the floor, rotate the pelvis backward (cat tilt), letting the abdomen fall backward toward the spine as you tuck the coccyx under. Maintain this alignment of your center as you lower your hips to the floor and come all the way down onto your elbows. Keep your head up, fingers touching toes.

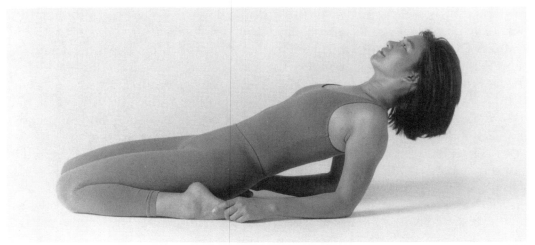

**122**

**3** Be in this position and acclimatize to the sensations of stretch. Breathe smoothly. Wait for the sensations to diminish somewhat before proceeding. If the stretch here is already too intense, then straighten your arms and lean on your hands instead of your elbows; gradually over a period of weeks or months, work your way toward being able to rest on your elbows.

## STAGE TWO

**4** **Lift your hips off the floor.** Pull the abdominals down as you do this, stretching the tailbone toward the knees and bringing your pelvis into a strong cat tilt—hips up, belly down, stretching toward the knees. This action strengthens the buttocks and lower back and will probably create a fairly intense stretch on the front of the thighs. Create the perfect degree of intensity—not too much, not too little. Do not sag into the shoulders. Press downward into your elbows and lift your chest. Hold your hips in this position for several breaths.

**5** **Lie on your back:** Retaining the alignment of your pelvis in cat tilt, lower the buttocks to the floor, slide your elbows apart, and come all the way down onto your back (photo 123). Rest your arms by your sides or under your head like a pillow. This is the pose. Breathe smoothly. Be here anywhere from thirty seconds to five minutes.

**6** When you sense that it is almost time to come out of the pose, lace your fingers, turn the palms inside out, and reach your arms over your head to the floor. Pull the abdominals down as you stretch the knees and hands away from one another. Be here several breaths, running energy through the shape that you now are, then come up.

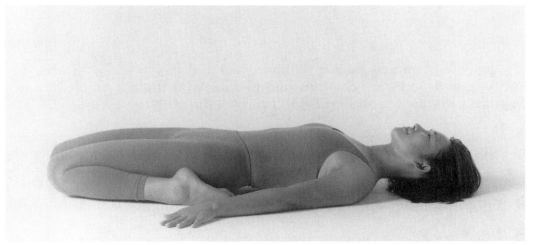

# Benefits: Reclining Hero Pose *or* *Supta Virasana*

Excellent quadriceps, groin, and psoas (the deep vertical muscle in front of your hip) stretch. Very relaxing. Excellent preparation for backbending poses.

# 22 Locust Pose *or Shalabhasana*

The Locust Pose is an excellent back strengthener. It is especially recommended before doing poses that require extreme flexibility simply because it builds the strength needed to support the flexibility that will accrue over time.

### STARTING POSITION

**1** **Lie facedown on the floor with your arms alongside your body, palms and forehead down** (photo 124).

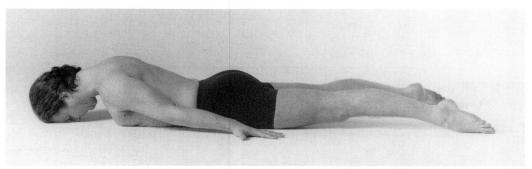

**124**

**2** Align your center by pulling the abdominal muscles inward, contracting the buttocks, and pressing your hips and pubis firmly into the floor. This will lengthen your lower back and establish your hips in cat tilt.

**3** Create a line of energy through the legs. Do this by pressing the top of your feet into the floor, tightening the thighs so your knees leave the floor, and stretching outward through the legs in the direction they are pointing.

**4** Roll the shoulders up, away from the floor.

**5** Establish a smooth flowing breath and wait for the inner cue to begin.

## LOCUST ONE

**1 As you inhale, lift your upper body away from the floor** (photo 125). **As you exhale, lower your upper body to the floor.** Do this slowly, five or ten times. Do not be mechanical and do not be in a rush. Be smooth. Synchronize the movement with the breath, making the breath long so the movement is slow. Keep your hands and feet on the floor.

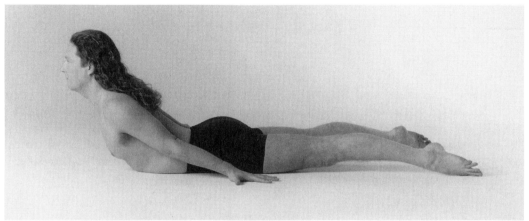

**125**

**2** As you do the repetitions, do not retract your head backward into the neck by looking forward. Tuck the chin, gaze downward, and elongate and lift upward with the back of your neck. Do not create tension in your throat as you do this or draw your chin in excessively—but establish maximum length on both the front and back sides of your neck. Direct the stretch forward and outward through the crown of your head. Keep the shoulders rolled up and back.

## LOCUST TWO

**1 Inhale and lift your upper body away from the floor** (photo 125). Stay here a comfortable length of time, approximately fifteen seconds. Be motionless and breathe smoothly.

**2 Raise your legs** (photo 126). Elongate them in the direction they are pointing and follow the line of energy outward and up. Your legs do not have to be together, but press them straight. Tighten the knees, spread your toes, and press the feet away from you. Stay here another fifteen seconds. Be relaxed without losing the action of the pose.

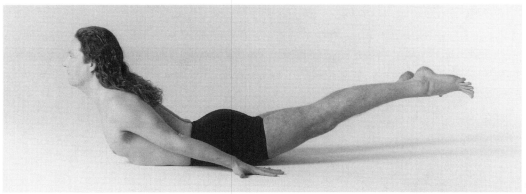

**126**

**3** **Lower your forehead and upper body to the floor** (photo 127). Keep your legs elevated. Continue breathing smoothly. Stay here another fifteen seconds.

**4** **Lower your legs.** Turn your head to the left and relax. Repeat several times, turning your head in the opposite direction when resting between repetitions.

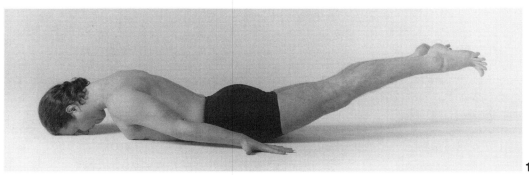

**127**

# Benefits: Locust Pose *or Shalabhasana*

Tremendous back, buttock, and leg strengthener. Improves digestion, elimination.

# 23 Cobra Pose *or Bhujangasana*

This pose is one of the classics.

**1  Lie facedown on the floor with your hands alongside the chest in a push-up position** (photo 128).

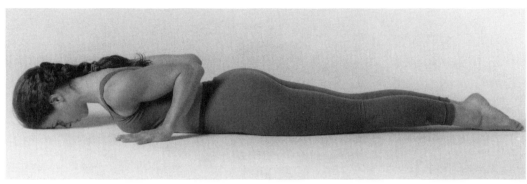

**128**

**2**  There are three standard hand placements for Cobra. The first placement, and most difficult, is with your hands by your lower ribs so your forearms are vertical and the wrists form a right angle with the floor. The second placement (shown in photo 128) is with your hands farther forward, fingertips in line with the top of the shoulders. Most people start the pose here. The third standard hand placement is with your hands even farther forward so that both forearms are flat on the floor. The farther forward your hands are, the easier the pose will be; the farther back they are, the deeper the stretch. Try each of these, sense the differences, and determine which is right for you. In each of these variations, spread your fingers fully and have the middle fingers pointing straight ahead.

**3**  Align your center first: Pull the abdominal muscles inward, contract the buttocks, and press your hips and pubis into the floor. Do this firmly, but not excessively. This initial action lengthens your lower back and aligns your pelvis in cat tilt. Then create a line of energy down the legs by pressing the tops of your feet firmly into the floor, tightening the thighs, and stretching straight backward through your legs and feet. Roll the shoulders up, away from the floor, and be on your forehead. Except for the hand placement, this initial alignment is similar to the starting position for Shalabhasana, Locust Pose.

**4**  The tendency here is for the shoulders to roll down toward the floor and the elbows to splay outward. Instead, move the elbows inward toward one another so the shoulders roll up away from the floor, and shrug the shoulders backward, away from the ears, toward the elbows. This action will open your chest, lengthen the back of your neck, and make your upper arms parallel with one another. You'll feel the skin on the back of your upper arms moving toward the elbows. Sustain this action throughout the pose and continue hugging inward with the elbows. Snuggle your palms into the floor.

**5** Establish a smooth flowing breath and wait for the inner cue to begin before proceeding. When you are ready, exhale.

## STAGE ONE

**6** **As you inhale, raise your torso away from the floor. As you exhale, come down.** Go up and down slowly, coordinating the movement with your breathing. Do this at least five times.

**7** As you go up and down, do not use your arm strength. This will force your back to work and thereby develop tremendous spinal strength, one of the main benefits of this pose. Retain the alignment of your shoulders and arms, however. Hug inward with your elbows and continue shrugging the shoulders away from your ears. This will protect your neck and spine and help keep your chest expanded.

**8** Be especially attentive to slide your shoulder blades *down* your back and to contract your upper back muscles as your torso leaves the floor. Doing this will help bring the curve into your upper back, out of the lumbar, thereby evenly spreading the curve through your entire spine. Be aware also to keep the back of your neck long and your gaze toward the floor. Do not retract your head backward into the neck by looking forward. Land lightly on your forehead when you come down.

## STAGE TWO

**9** **Inhale and come up as far as you comfortably can without using your hands.** Check your alignment. Breathe smoothly.

**10** **Curve deeper into the pose** (photo 129). Lift your torso farther away from the floor by gently pressing your palms down. You are now using your arm strength, and this is fine, just minimize it. Exercise your back.

**11** Come up slowly, a little at a time. Do not rush to your deepest extension, and do not press your arms fully straight yet. Proceed slowly. Wait for your body to let you in. And as a general rule, until you become more skilled, do not let your navel leave the floor. This restriction will help insure correct alignment, safe performance of the pose, and make your back strong and flexible.

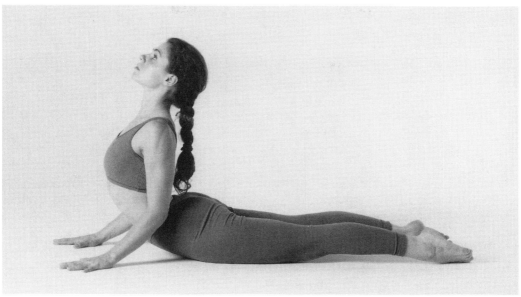

**129**

**12** Press gently into your edges and tight areas. Become rounder and rounder. Do this by again snuggling your palms into the floor and then gently, firmly *pulling* with your hands. Pull as though you were attempting to slide the floor backward underneath you, but do not actually move your hands. Pull with your hands, curve your head and look upward, and press your chest *forward* through the shoulders. Doing this will not cause you to come farther up into the pose, but it will tighten the curve where you already are. Move the thoracic spine, behind your heart, deep into your back.

**13** Notice how the apex of the curve moves down your back as you move deeper into the pose: upper back, middle back, lumbar. Allow this to happen. It's natural. But once you're in the pose, and especially when you are pulling with your hands, try to bring the apex of the curve *up* your back again. Spread the curve evenly throughout the full length of your spine by expanding your chest forward through the shoulders.

**14** Experience yourself as a strong arc of curving energy. Climb into the curve, extend and tighten the curve, and follow the energy flow deeper into the pose. Get round. Also be as effortless and strain-free as possible. Savor the stretch.

**15** Eventually you can go ahead and press your arms fully straight, if you can keep the shoulders down while doing so; otherwise, keep them bent. If you cannot keep your shoulders down as you straighten the arms, then you've gone too far—in which case, bend your arms and back out of the pose a little. The idea here is not to "straighten the arms." The idea is to strengthen your back and curve the spine evenly.

**16** Bring your head to normal alignment at any time.

**17** Sometimes breathe deeply, other times softly, and always generate the perfect degree of intensity and current throughout the pose—not too much, not too little. It's subjective. Stay with your now-experience to know what's right.

**18** If you choose to have your eyes open, turn them upward and gaze through your eyebrows so the energy through your eyes pulls you deeper into the stretch. If you have your eyes closed, stretch mentally in that direction.

**19** Stay as long or as little as you want, somewhere between fifteen seconds and two or three minutes. Some of the time curve your head backward, and some of the time bring it to normal alignment. When you sense it's nearly time to come out of the pose, curve your head backward (or not) and accelerate your energy for a few seconds. Go faster. This feels fabulous. Then release the pose.

**20** **Come down slowly.** Keep your elbows inward toward your body and land lightly on your forehead. Even here, though, come down slowly, incrementally, not all at once. Do not be in a rush to get out of the pose. Come down a little, stop, and then *pull* with your hands for a few seconds to intensify the curve. Then roll down a little farther, stop, and again pull with your hands to intensify the curve. The apex of the curve is moving up your back as you approach the floor. Take your time. Press into as many different areas as you can to exercise the full length of your spine.

**21** Repeat the pose two or three times, then turn your head to the side and relax. Enjoy the way you feel.

# Benefits: Cobra Pose *or Bhujangasana*

Tremendous chest opener. Increases strength and flexibility of spine, arms, back. Breaks up tension in back, shoulders, neck. Stimulates thyroid, kidneys, adrenals. Improves digestion, elimination, reproduction, lung capacity. Safe precursor to other, more strenuous backbends.

# 24 Bow Pose *or Dhanurasana*

## PREPARATION POSE

This preparation pose for Dhanurasana, the Bow, is an extremely effective back strengthener that trains your legs and spine to move properly. The idea is to move your feet straight upward.

**1** Lie facedown on the floor with your arms alongside your body, palms down. Bend your legs until the shinbones are vertical, and bring your feet together. Keep your feet together so they move as one.

**2** As you inhale, lift your upper body away from the floor as far as you comfortably can; as you exhale, move your feet straight up an inch or so. Maintain this position as you inhale, then take the feet higher as you exhale. Move your feet straight up, little by little, breath by breath—keeping the shinbones vertical. Do this until you cannot lift them any higher, then turn your head upward and gaze at the ceiling (photo 130). This pose is surprisingly difficult. It requires tremendous strength to be relaxed as you hold this position. Breathe smoothly. Be here several breaths, then relax.

In Bow Pose you'll do exactly what you just did, leg energy moving upward, except you'll be holding your ankles. The idea is to pull yourself taut like a bow.

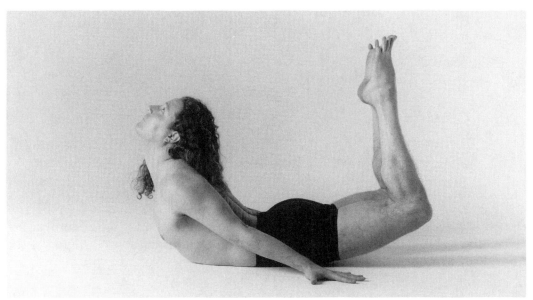

**130**

**1** **Lie facedown on the floor, bend your knees, and clasp your ankles.** In this position establish starting alignment: Pull the abdominals in, pressing the pubis into the floor; roll the shoulders up, away from the floor; and be on your forehead. When you are ready to proceed, exhale.

**2** **As you inhale, raise your upper body away from the floor.** Raise yourself to your comfortable maximum. Be here several breaths, readying yourself, then breathe in deeply.

**3** **As you exhale, move your feet straight up.** Go an inch or so, then stop; stay here as you inhale, reaffirming the chest lift, then exhale and take your feet farther up. Proceed like this until you cannot lift your feet any higher—little by little, breath by breath—then curve your head upward and gaze into the sky (photo 131).

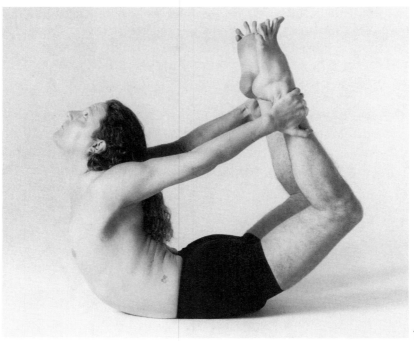

**131**

**4** Do not rock forward or backward. Position yourself on your abdomen, between the pubis and lower ribs, and attempt to lift your chest and thighs off the floor. Keep your arms straight. Do the lifting with your legs and spine.

**5** This is a beginner's pose, but it is definitely not easy. When you reach your deepest extension, stay where you are and be as relaxed as possible. Attempt to be strain-free, yet continue lifting your head and chest as you energize the upward leg line.

**6** Be in the pose a comfortable length of time, anywhere from five seconds to one minute. When you are almost done, take a deep breath in and, as you exhale, accelerate for a few seconds: Stretch your feet straight up, look up between your eyebrows, and go faster. You'll like this.

**7** Repeat the pose two or three times, then release your ankles and rest in Child's Pose.

# Benefits: Bow Pose *or Dhanurasana*

Brings tremendous strength and elasticity to back and spine. Stretches chest, shoulders, abdominals, thighs, and increases strength of back, buttocks, legs. Tones abdominal organs. Stimulates kidneys, adrenals.

# 25 Single Leg Pigeon Pose *or Ekapada Rajakapotasana*

The Single Leg Pigeon Pose is an excellent hip opener and lovely backbend. It gives an intense stretch to the hips, buttocks, and thighs, as well as the spine and chest, and will therefore restore movement to these areas. This pose will especially improve your Lotus and Splits, and prepare your spine for more advanced backbending poses.

**1 Start on your hands and knees as in Cat Pose.**

### STAGE ONE *LIE FORWARD*

**2 Bring your right knee forward between your hands, alongside the right wrist, lower your hips to the floor, and extend your left leg straight back behind you.** The right shinbone should be at about a forty-five-degree angle with the right heel positioned directly beneath the left frontal hipbone. Slide your hands forward and lie flat (photo 132).

**3** As you hold this position, roll the left frontal hipbone downward toward the right heel until the sacrum becomes level, and turn the left outer thigh down until the front of the left leg faces the floor.

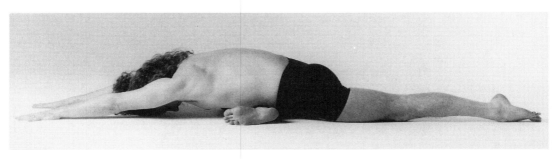

**132**

**4** Make sure there is no pain in your knee; if there is, something is wrong. Fix it by making subtle intuitive alignment changes until you are no longer experiencing pain. Direct the stretch into either your right hip and buttock or your left thigh and groin, not the knee.

**5** Breathe smoothly. Let the stretch penetrate. Be here one minute.

## STAGE TWO  *ON ELBOWS, TOE TURNS UNDER, STRAIGHTEN LEG*

**6** **Come up on your elbows** (photo 133). Have your elbows shoulder-width apart with the elbows directly below the shoulders. Align the forearms so they are parallel with one another, spread your fingers, and have the middle fingers pointing straight ahead.

**7** Gently press the elbows, forearms, palms, and fingers *down* into the floor and lift effortlessly upward out of the shoulders.

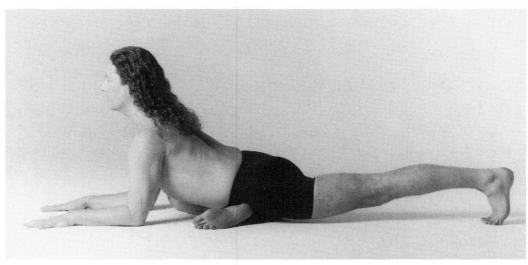

**133**

**8 Turn your left toes under and straighten the leg.** Be as effortless and strain-free as possible as you do this. Keep the current in the back leg steady. Be here about half a minute.

## STAGE THREE  *ARCH BACKWARD*

**9 Point your toes and place the top of your left foot on the floor again. Bring your hands back to their original placement, equal with the right knee.**

**10 Come up into a position similar to Cobra Pose.** First, hug inward with your elbows and shrug the shoulders away from the ears, then lift your body away from the floor using your arm strength as little as possible. Press your arms *toward* straight without allowing your shoulders to hunch upward near the ears. If having your arms straight causes you to hunch your shoulders, compressing your neck, then either bend your elbows or move your hands farther forward.

**11** Acclimatize to this stretch for a few moments, then refine it. First, pull the abdominals in, navel backward toward the spine, and move the shoulders backward. Then lift the rib cage upward away from your waist, lengthening the waist, lengthening your arms, and lifting upward out of the shoulders. Lift and fully expand your chest. Notice how the inhalations help you do this. Be here sufficiently long to achieve maximum height, then inhale deeply.

**12 Arch backward** (photo 134). As you exhale, press forward with your shoulder blades and arch backward. Go up and over, like a fountain, letting your head curve back last. Form a smooth, graceful curve with your spine.

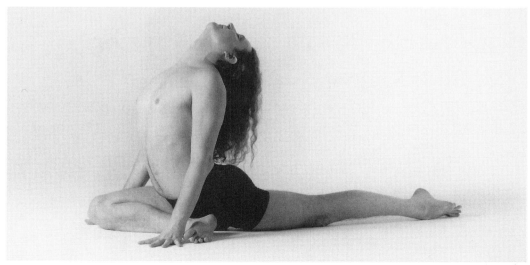

**134**

**13**  Increase the curve by moving your spine deeper into your back and moving the apex of the curve *up* your back, behind your heart. Bring your hands farther back if you can. Roll your chest more and more upward, moving the shoulders more backward, and slide the shoulder blades down your back as you press them forward. Let it feel as though someone else is gently pushing you from behind your back, giving you support and helping you achieve maximum, gentle openness.

**14**  As you hold this position, continue rolling the left frontal hipbone downward toward the right heel so the abdominal plane is squared to the front, and continue turning the left outer thigh down until the front of the left leg faces the floor. Endeavor to have the whole front side of your body facing forward. It may take you a while before you are able to do this. Simply persist—gently.

**15**  Strengthen the line of energy down the left leg by pressing the leg fully straight. Press the top of your foot firmly down into the floor, sustain a strong, steady current, and stretch backward through the leg in the direction it is pointing. Sink your hips downward, making them heavy so you feel grounded.

**16**  Bring your head to normal alignment at any time, but endeavor to keep the chest lifted, fully expanded, and arched throughout. Have your eyes open some of the time, gazing backward wide-eyed into infinity, and some of the time close your eyes and immerse yourself in the *feeling* of the pose. Find the alignment that feels perfect to you now, feel how your energy is flowing through the shape, and gently radiate the meaning of the pose.

**17**  Breathe softly, deeply. Be here one minute. Release the pose when you receive the inner cue to do so, and repeat on the other side.

# Benefits: Single Leg Pigeon Pose *or Ekapada Rajakapotasana*

Chest opener, back strengthener. Improves flexibility in hips, thighs, legs. Makes Lotus easier and safer.

# 26 Fish Pose *or Matsyasana*

The Fish Pose is an excellent way to open the chest and stretch into the upper spine without collapsing or overbending in the lumbar spine. Use your spinal strength to lift the rib cage out of the waist, then translate this simple movement into other more difficult backbends.

There are three leg variations in the Fish: extended straight, folded back in Hero, and crossed in Lotus. The three stages described below are the same regardless of which leg variation you choose.

## STRAIGHT LEG FISH

### STAGE ONE

**1 Sit on the floor with your legs extended straight.** Lean back onto your hands, fingers pointing backward.

**2** Press the legs fully straight and roll the knees inward toward one another until your kneecaps face the ceiling. Bring the inner edges of your feet together, spread your toes, and press forward through the ball of each foot. The idea here is to make both legs work as one.

**3 Curve your chest upward.** First, gently pull the abdomen backward toward the spine and roll the shoulders backward, expanding the chest. Then use your inhalations to help lift the chest upward away from the waist. Push downward into your hands through the ball of each index finger, and move your spine forward deep into your back, especially behind your heart, to help move the chest forward through the shoulders. Be here several breaths, lifting and expanding the chest.

**4 Curve your head backward** (photo 135). Inhale deeply as you emphasize the upward expansion through the sternum, then exhale as you press your shoulder blades and chest forward and curve your head backward. Don't scrunch your neck. Keep your neck soft, press upward through the base of your throat, and stretch outward through the chin. Become round. Savor the way this feels. Gaze into infinity. This is a wonderful stretch. Be here several breaths.

**5** The idea here is to expand the chest fully, making it both vertically and horizontally round. Make your torso vertically round from your pubis to your chin by pressing the hands firmly down into the floor, lengthening the arms, and stretching the chest, throat, and chin up and back; become horizontally round

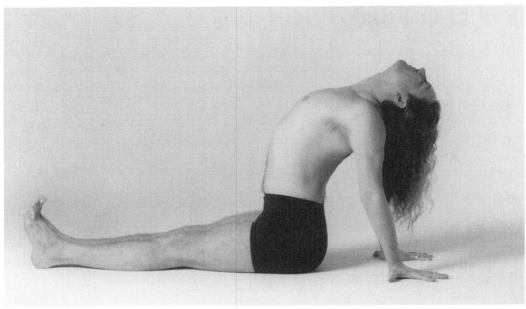

**135**

from shoulder to shoulder across the front of your chest by pulling both shoulders backward as you press forward and upward through the sternum. Move your spine deep into your back. And bring the apex of the curve upward so the entire spine carries the arc. Pretend it's first thing in the morning and stretch!

**6** Breathe deeply, with feeling. Let each breath inspire the pose. Be here half a minute.

**7 To come out of the pose, bring your head to normal alignment, then relax.**

**8** Do all of this very consciously, being very aware of what you are doing. Be *with* what you are doing; participate, get involved, don't hold back. Merge so thoroughly with your now-experience that the normal division between you and the pose dissolves and no longer exists. This division will vanish when you immerse yourself fully in your conscious experience of the pose and are totally involved in what you are doing.

**9** Remember, learning to practice with awareness is not for the physical benefit alone. This is mind training, sensitivity cultivation, skill in action. Do not do yoga mindlessly. The more mindful you are—the more present you are—and the more fully you participate in the practice, the more fully you'll experience your union, your joining, your yoga—the better you'll be guided by the inner feeling.

## STAGE TWO

This stage is nearly identical to the first. Here, however, you will be on your elbows instead of your hands. This minor change will tighten the curve considerably and produce a deeper backbend.

**10** **Lean onto your elbows with the hands pointing forward, fingers just touching your hips.**

**11** **Curve your chest upward.** Use your inhalations to expand the chest and lift the rib cage upward, as before. Keep your head up. Take several breaths here.

**12** **Curve your head backward** (photo 136). As you exhale, press your chest forward and curve your head backward. Become round. Press downward into your elbows, upward through your chest, and outward through the chin. Squeeze your head inward toward the buttocks. Your head is not yet on the floor. Breathe. Press the shape open from inside the shape. Expand from the inside out.

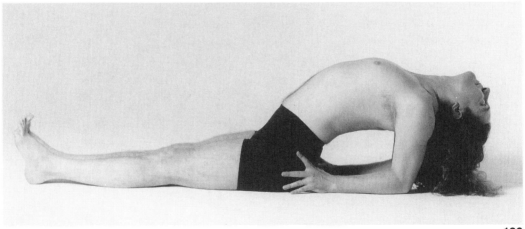

**136**

## STAGE THREE

**13** **Slide your elbows sideways and come down onto the top of your head.** Bring your head in toward your seat as close as possible. Continue pressing upward through your chest.

**14** Lace your fingers, turn the palms inside out, and take your straightened arms over your head (photo 137). Create a line of energy outward through the arms. As you inhale, straighten the elbows and push outward through the hands; as you exhale, squeeze your hands toward the floor. Be here for several breaths.

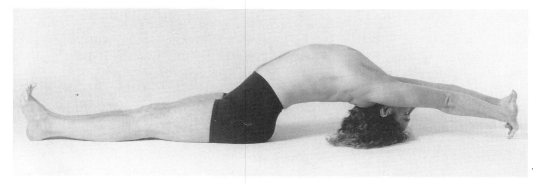

**137**

**15** Clasp hold of your elbows, then gradually stretch them toward the floor (photo 138). The secret is to stretch outward through the elbows before squeezing them down: Press into the elbows as you inhale, squeeze them down as you exhale.

**16** To come out of the pose, release the stretch and recline on your back.

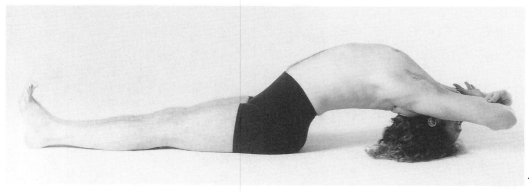

**138**

## FISH IN HERO

### STAGE ONE

**1 Sitting in Virasana, Hero Pose, lean back on your hands.** When you are ready, exhale. Roll your shoulders backward and pull the abdomen inward toward the spine.

**2 Curve your chest upward.** Use your inhalations to lift the chest away from the waist. Continue rolling your shoulders backward as you press downward into your hands, expanding the chest forward through the shoulders. Acclimatize here with your exhalations.

**3** **Curve your head backward** (photo 139). Press downward into your hands, upward through your chest, and outward through the chin. Become round.

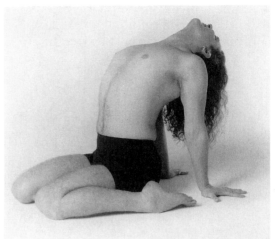

**139**

**4** Breathe deeply, filling the pose with air. Bring your head to normal alignment when you have had enough, and move into the second stage.

## STAGE TWO

**5** **Come down onto your elbows.** Catch hold of your toes, press upward through your chest, and again curve your head backward. Use the breath to expand the shape that you are. Become round.

## STAGE THREE

**6** **Slide the elbows out and come down onto the crown of your head.** Bring your head in as close to the buttocks as possible, then lace the fingers, turn the palms inside out, and take the arms over your head, as before. Create a line of energy outward through the arms. As you inhale, press the hands away from you, and as you exhale, squeeze your hands toward the floor. Be here for several breaths.

**7** Clasp hold of your elbows. As you inhale, stretch outward through the elbows, as you exhale, squeeze them toward the floor.

## LOTUS FISH

This variation is the same except your legs are folded into Padmasana, Lotus Pose.

**1** Lean back on your hands first, then your elbows, then the top of your head. Be in each stage for several breaths.

**2** After you have completed the two arm variations, catch hold of your feet with your hands (photo 140). Pull with the hands, press the elbows toward the floor, and puff upward through the chest, stretching outward through the chin.

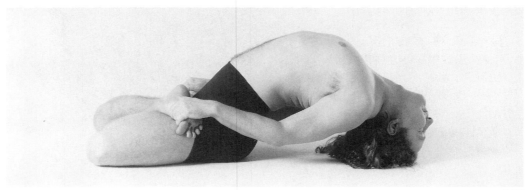

**140**

# Benefits: Fish Pose *or Matsyasana*

Excellent chest expander. Breaks up tension in middle and upper back, stretches chest, shoulders, neck. Counterpose for Shoulderstand and Plow. The action you learn here should be translated into all the backbending poses.

# 27 Camel Pose *or Ustrasana*

**1** **Kneel on the floor with your hands on your hips** (photo 141). Align your knees and feet so they are hip-width apart, then glance at your thighs. Because they are hip-width apart, they should be vertical and parallel with one another. Glance at your shinbones. They should also be parallel with one another. Point your feet straight back. Spread your toes.

**2** Kneel tall for a moment before proceeding. Elongate your core and get grounded. Go upward into the crown of your head and stretch downward through the thighs into your knees. Merge your knees, shinbones, and feet into the floor so that the crown of your head and your knees move away from one another—straight up and straight down. As you do this, gently allow your chest to lift upward away from the waist, move the elbows toward one another until the upper arms are parallel, and delicately bring the navel backward toward the spine.

**3** Then, keeping the tops of the thighs backward so the thighs stay vertical, press firmly forward with your sacrum and tailbone and squeeze your legs (thighs) inward toward one another. Your legs will not actually come together as you do this, your thighs will remain parallel, but by squeezing inward and thus utilizing and increasing the power in the lower half of your body, you establish and strengthen the foundation of the pose—and that's important. You squeeze inward with the lower half of your body so the upper half can bloom upward and over into the backbend. The more powerful your legs are, therefore (without being excessive), the more support you will have in the pose. Do not move your thighs beyond vertical yet. This action opens the groin and helps protect your lumbar spine. Notice also how this action aligns your center and firms the buttocks.

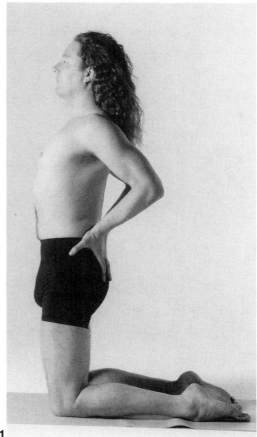

**141**

**4** The idea is to create a dynamic balance in your center by pulling backward with the tops of the thighs and abdominals, pressing forward with the sacrum and tailbone, and squeezing inward with the legs. Doing this will encourage your core to elongate. You'll feel your chest wanting to wriggle upward more, lengthening the sides of your waist—so go ahead and wriggle a little, lift your chest fully, then check that the shoulders are still relaxing down. Breathe smoothly. Wait until you are ready.

**5** **Arch backward** (photo 142): As you inhale, lift and fully expand your chest, and as you exhale, pull the shoulders backward, press the shoulder blades forward, and arch backward. Your thighs will move forward beyond vertical to balance the weight of your trunk going backward; allow this to happen, but minimize it. Keep your head up for the moment. Continue squeezing inward with your legs.

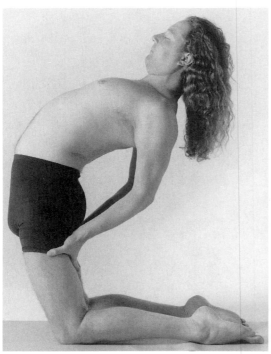
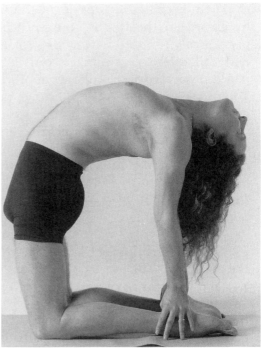

142                                                    143

**6** **Clasp your heels** by sliding your hands down the back of your legs, then reaching for your feet (photo 143). If you cannot reach your feet, come out of the pose and try it again—this time with your toes turned under.

**7** Acclimatize to the stretch, bringing your hips backward if you are experiencing any compression in your lower back. Start easy. Start from comfort. Do not rush to your deepest extension. Wait for your body to signal its readiness before deepening the pose. Breathe smoothly, readying yourself.

**8** Increase the curve. First, as you inhale, lift the chest straight up, away from the waist, roll the shoulders backward, and push downward through your arms. Lengthening the arm lines will considerably assist in lifting and expanding the chest. Then, as you exhale, and starting from the area of your lower back, delicately press your spine forward into your back, feeling the apex of the curve flow up your back. Go up and over. Become round. Bloom your chest toward the ceiling, and then curve your head all the way back, stretching outward through the chin. Take your head backward as the inevitable, natural expression of a total spinal stretch. Keep your neck soft. This feels fabulous. Experience yourself as a strong arc of curving energy.

**9** Take inventory. Merge whatever is on the floor into the floor. Continue pulling the abdominals inward, continue pressing the sacrum and tailbone foward, and continue squeezing inward with your legs. The thighs are now vertical. Aim the thrust of the pose upward through the chest, and stretch enthusiastically outward and backward through the chin. All these movements work together beautifully. From inside the shape of the pose, press outward in all directions like air in an expanding balloon. Fill out the shape you now are.

**10** Endeavor to be strain-free. Do what you have to do, but also be as relaxed as possible as you expand toward greater roundness. Breathe. Fill the pose with air and space. Expand. Watch it happen. Be here half a minute. When you sense that it's nearly time to come out of the pose, accelerate your energy for a few seconds, then release the pose.

**11** To come out of the pose, firmly press the top of your feet down, release your feet, and return to the kneeling position. Sit down between your feet in Virasana, Hero Pose, or rest in Child's Pose.

# Benefits: Camel Pose *or Ustrasana*

Tremendous chest and shoulder opener. Stretches front of body, increases circulation throughout. Stretches knees, thighs, groins, brings mobility to the spine, releases tension in upper back. Strengthens legs, buttocks, back, neck. Stimulates kidneys, adrenals. Breathing improves because of opening in rib cage and chest. Opens heart center, heightens perceptions. Exhilarating.

# 28 Upward Facing Bow Pose *or Urdhva Dhanurasana*

This is one of the very special poses in yoga. It's very energizing. There is nothing quite like a fantastic backbend. Be sure to work the Upward Bow in stages, though, and proceed slowly. If you have difficulty with this pose, spend more time with the other backbends, as well as with preparatory poses such as Dog Pose and its variations to increase your shoulder flexibility. Never press into the Upward Bow quickly. Move slowly and give your body time to acclimatize to each new edge. It takes more strength to go slowly; therefore, *by moving slowly you will build your strength.* You will also safeguard yourself against injury and, actually, end up deeper in the pose. The openings will be deeper, more long-lasting. I am giving the pose in five stages. Always move into the pose sequentially through stages, whether you do them all or not, and come out of the pose in reverse order.

## STAGE ONE

**1  Lie on your back with your legs bent, feet flat, and heels in close to the buttocks.** Have your feet hip-width apart with the inner edge of each foot pointing straight ahead, parallel with one another, and your toes spread. Place your palms flat on the floor beside your ears with the fingertips just touching the shoulders (photo 144). Keep the chin tucked down. Pause here for a moment before starting. Snuggle your hands and feet into the floor, become grounded, and establish a smooth flowing breath as you wait for the inner cue to begin. When you are ready, breathe in deeply.

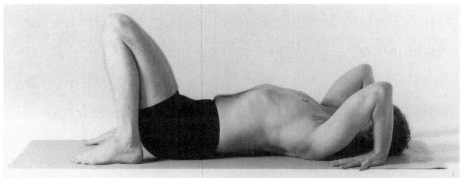

**144**

**2  As you exhale, lift your hips away from the floor until your body forms a straight line from shoulders to knees.** Pause here. Do not rush through this stage.

**3**  Check the alignment of your center: Pull the abdominals down, rotating the pelvis backward (cat tilt), and press the sacrum and tailbone upward as you stretch into your knees. This is the same action as in Camel Pose. Endeavor to make the pubic bone higher than the two frontal hip bones; if it isn't, then the pelvis has not rotated sufficiently.

**4**  The idea here is similar to Dog Pose, where it was important to be able to make a straight line through your arms and spine (Stage Two) before attempting to bow your spine toward the floor (Stage Three). Here, you must be able to make a straight line through your torso and thighs (in order to insure there is sufficient opening in the front of the thighs and groin) before pressing deeper into the pose. If you are unable to make a straight line here, and the two frontal hipbones are therefore higher than the pubic bone, it means there is insufficient pelvic rotation and that you will therefore overbend in the lumbar. If this is the case for you, spend time opening this area before proceeding.

**5** Keep the thighs parallel with one another. If your knees splay out, you will experience more weight on the outer edges of your feet and pressure in your lumbar spine. If this happens, move your knees closer together (without moving your feet) and bring more weight toward the inner edge of each foot. Press the whole sole of each foot firmly into the floor, aiming the line of energy toward the inner edge of each foot to prevent your knees from splaying out.

**6** Have your hands shoulder-width apart with your fingers fully spread. Hug inward with your elbows until the upper arms are parallel with one another.

**7** You should be sensing a stretch in the thighs and groins already, as well as an indication of how much strength is required to hold this position. Acclimatize to the stretch, try to be relaxed without losing the action of the pose, and breathe smoothly. Be here about half a minute. If you need to come down and rest for a moment before proceeding, by all means do so. When you are ready to proceed, breathe in deeply.

## STAGE TWO

**8** **As you inhale, lift your hips into Bridge Pose** (photo 145). Retain the feeling of stretch in your thighs as you press your feet evenly into the floor and elevate the hips. Keep the abdomen pulling downward toward the spine as you stretch the coccyx toward the knees and press upward through the groin.

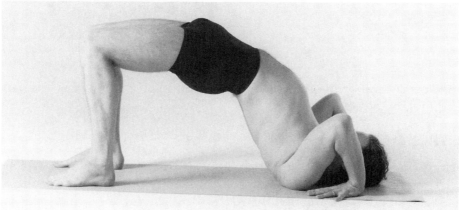

**145**

**9** Be here for several or many breaths, about half a minute. You're waiting for something to change and open before proceeding. Do not rush. Take your time. Open these early edges.

**10** **Come up on your toes.** This will enable you to take the pelvis higher, so do so. Keep the thighs parallel with one another, and prevent the ankles from falling outward by pressing downward through the inner edge of each foot. Go to your comfortable maximum, still being as relaxed as possible. Achieve maximum height here before proceeding.

## STAGE THREE

**11** **Come onto the crown of your head** by pressing downward with your hands (photo 146). You're still on your toes, still rotating the pelvis under, and still keeping the pubic bone higher than the two frontal hipbones. Press your feet downward, the buttocks upward, and open the groin toward the ceiling.

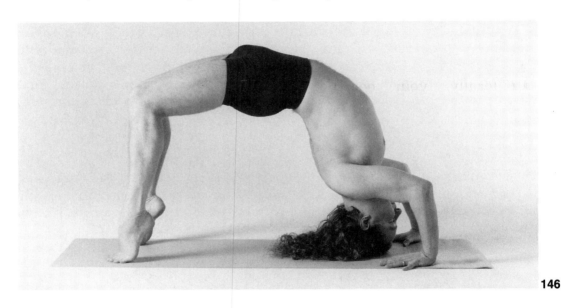

**146**

**12** Be here several or many breaths, again waiting for something to change as you acclimatize to the stretch.

## STAGE FOUR

**13** **Press your arms straight.** It may take several months before you have the strength and flexibility required to do this; therefore, think of moving the shoulder blades into your back and up toward the waist as you press your arms *toward* straight. Do not push suddenly or be aggressive; press a little, then wait, press, wait. Eventually, your arms will be straight. You're still on your toes.

**14** Walk your feet backward toward your hands if you can, but again, do not rush to your deepest extension. Be patient. Build strength by staying where you are, waiting for the musculature to release and open; then, at the right moment, take it deeper. Keep your weight on the ball of each second toe, ankles in, knees hip-width apart, thighs parallel with one another.

**15** Achieve maximum height with your pelvis. Press your hands and feet downward into the floor so the pelvis goes up, making your body round. The higher your hips, the easier it will be to straighten your arms.

**16 Lower your heels to the floor** (photo 147). Retain the height you achieved in your hips as you lower your heels. Snuggle your hands and feet into the floor and re-affirm your groundedness.

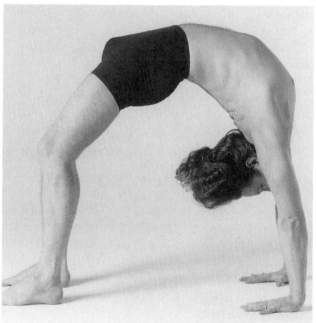

**147**

**17** Ideally, your body should form a round, bowlike shape with the highest point of the bow being just below the navel. The pubic bone, therefore, will no longer be higher than the two frontal hipbones. Now, the two frontal hipbones and the points of the lower ribs should be the same height. Try to align your armpits directly above the wrists so your arms are vertical, the knees over the heels so the shinbones are vertical, the pelvis high, body and torso round, and the hands and feet as close together as possible. The only way to get the hands and feet closer together and still keep both the arms and shinbones vertical is by moving your hips up. As the pelvis rises, you'll be able to walk your feet farther back, closer to your hands.

**18** Move your spine deeper into your back, the way you did in Camel Pose. Then, from your center, and with a deepening breath, press outward in all directions. Press your hands and feet down, your hips up, and attempt to bring your chest forward until the shoulders are directly above the wrists. It's the downward push through your hands and feet that gives height to the pelvis, rib cage, and chest, and this is what enables the chest and shoulders to come forward over the wrists. Spread your fingers fully, and press the whole palm of each hand evenly into the floor. Spread your toes, and press the whole sole of each foot into the earth. Become round. Experience yourself as one long curve of energy.

**19** Sometimes gaze at the floor between your hands, and sometimes lift your head and look for the navel. Most of the time, though, keep your head and neck straight, dangling loosely, ears in line with the upper arms, face vertical.

**20** Attempt to relax as you increase the intensity of the pose. Keep your breathing smooth.

**21** Savor this stretch. It's one of the best. Bring the pose to life with your breathing and create the degree of intensity that feels best to you now—sometimes more, sometimes less. Breathe with feeling. Merge with the pose. Feel what's happening. The inner feeling will guide you and tell you what to do as you go within and pay attention.

**22** Be in this position from half a minute to a minute. Come down and rest when you have had enough. It's difficult to stay in the pose for very long at first, and it is better to do several repetitions. Work toward staying in the pose for longer periods of time.

## STAGE FIVE—COMING DOWN

**23** **Come down in reverse order:** First, slowly lower yourself down onto the top of your head (Stage Three); pause here a moment. Then tuck your chin and lower yourself into Stage Two (Bridge Pose); pause here a moment. Then stretch the arms above your head, lift the heels, and slowly lower your hips, uncurling your spine in a smooth, rolling flow. When your sacrum finally rests on the floor, lower your heels to the floor, sweep your arms to your sides, and relax. Enjoy the way you feel.

# Benefits: Upward Facing Bow Pose *or Urdhva Dhanurasana*

Develops tremendous strength and flexibility of spine and whole body. Strengthens feet, legs, thighs, buttocks, upper back, shoulders, and arms. Stretches quadriceps, pelvic region, abdominals, full length of spine, chest, and shoulders. Exhilarating, energizing, calming, breaks up tension. Keeps body alert and supple, mind awake and clear.

## FORWARD BENDS

# 29 Seated Forward Fold *or* *Paschimottanasana*

Paschimottanasana is the basic seated forward fold. It has two lines of energy radiating from your center. One line travels outward through the legs, the other moves outward through the spine and arms. Your hips will be in dog tilt.

### STAGE ONE

**1 Sit on the floor with your legs extended straight** (photo 148). Have your feet hip-width apart so the legs are parallel with one another, wriggle the buttocks backward so you are on the tips of the sitting bones, and sit tall. Place your fingertips on the floor beside your hips, pointing forward.

**2** Roll your thighs inward toward one another until your kneecaps face the ceiling and the inner edges of your feet are vertical and parallel with one another. Be on the center of the back of each heel. Spread your toes.

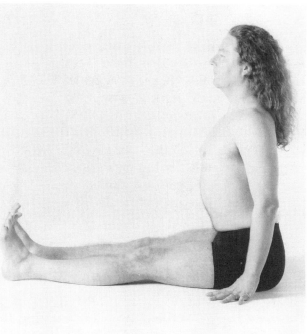

**148**

**3** Energize the leg lines by pressing the legs straight. Do this by firmly pressing the back of the thighs down and extending the heels away from you, lengthening the Achilles tendon. Then catch your heels on the floor, keep your toes spread, and press the ball of each foot away from you. Press through the inner edge of each foot so your legs spiral inward slightly, and direct the line of energy outward through your legs in the direction they are pointing. Do not strain as you do this. Create the perfect degree of intensity—not too much, not too little. Increase or decrease it as necessary.

**4** Align your torso and elongate your core by moving your shoulders backward and gently hugging inward with the elbows. Then press your fingertips down, lift and expand your chest, and bring your lower back in so your spine is erect, not rounded. Be alert not to lift your shoulders as you do this. Keep them down, away from the ears. Flatten the shoulder blades into your back, keep the abdominals in, and then elongate your core by moving the sitting bones straight down and the crown of your head straight up, away from one another.

**5** Breathe smoothly as you wait for the inner cue to proceed. Gaze straight ahead. Breathe in deeply when you are ready.

## STAGE TWO

**6 As you exhale, rotate your pelvis forward and clasp your feet** (photo 149). Clasp the outer edges of your feet, if you can; otherwise, hold your ankles or shinbones or use a belt to span the distance. I like to insert my thumbs between the little toe and ring toe and pull the outer edges of the feet backward with my fingers.

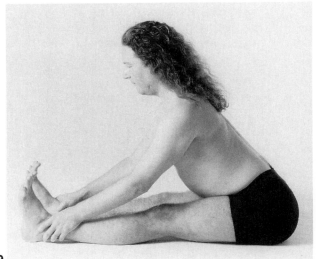

**149**

**7** Wriggle the buttocks backward, increasing dog tilt, and position yourself on the frontal edge of the sitting bones. Doing this will establish the alignment of your center and help propel your forward into the fold. Then strengthen the leg lines by pressing the back of your thighs down, spreading your toes, and pushing the ball of each foot away from you, as before.

**8 As you inhale, extend your spine up.** Press the back of your thighs down, concave your lower back—bringing it forward and in—and pull your spine up. Make the front of your body long.

**9** **As you exhale, fold forward** (photo 150). Bring your abdomen to your thighs, your chest to the knees, and snuggle your face into your shinbones—or as comfortably close to this as possible. Wriggle the buttocks backward to get as deep as possible, then clasp your hands around your feet, if you can. Do not be discouraged if you cannot fold this far yet. This is the goal. It takes most people several years to get this flat. Proceed slowly, intelligently, at your own pace, edge by edge. Do not rush to your deepest extension, and do not fold as deep as you can all at once. Eventually your torso will lie flat on your legs.

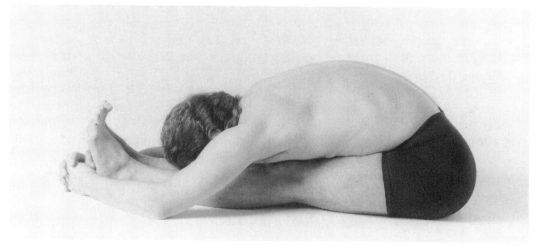

**150**

**10** Scan your awareness through your body. First, check your leg lines. Keep the legs strong, toes spread, ankles together. Then feel where your core is, from the tailbone to the crown of your head, and endeavor to elongate your core horizontally forward by moving the crown of your head closer to the toes. Slide the sternum forward, shrug the shoulders away from your ears, and pull gently with your hands. Bend your elbows outward, slide them forward, and then wriggle the buttocks backward again to make sure you're as deep as possible. Close your eyes and breathe smoothly.

**11** Counteract the tendency at this point for the shoulders to hunch upward toward the ears and for the neck to tense. Also avoid compressing the back of your neck by lifting your head and looking forward. Roll the back of your ears forward.

**12** Try to rest your chest flat on your thighs. Do not round your spine or gush your energy backward through the middle of your back. The way to get flat is by getting long, and the way to get long is by thinking forward.

**13** Monitor the intensity of stretch. Is it increasing, decreasing, or staying the same? Be willing to come up a bit if it is increasing. When the intensity decreases, it means the muscles have opened and are ready to go deeper, so do so.

**14** When you first attempt this pose, especially if your hamstring muscles are tight, do so with low current in your leg lines. Have your legs relaxed, even bent, but keep the inner edges of your feet parallel with one another and your toes spread. Later, when the hamstring muscles have lengthened and your legs are no longer inflexible, practice the pose with your legs straight. You'll notice that when your legs are straight and strong, your spine will extend outward more easily.

**15** Breathe smoothly, feeling your body gently ripple with the movement of breath. Endeavor to eliminate every trace of strain, both in your body and breathing.

**16** Immerse yourself in the sensations of stretch and the feeling-tone of the pose. Be the pose. Be one with what you're doing. That's the yoga, remember. This is more than just a physical activity. You are exercising your awareness and sensitivity as you exercise your body. Therefore, be interested in the quality of your participation. Be involved mentally. Be in the now. Practice moment-to-moment awareness by paying close attention to each new breath and every subtle change of sensation.

**17** Stay here anywhere from one to ten minutes. Increase your timings gradually. When you sense it's time to come up, take three more breaths. Never stay in the pose longer than seems right. Come up when you receive the inner cue to do so. Later, it will feel right to challenge your endurance edges by staying longer.

**18** **Come out of the pose.** Bring your hands alongside your hips, then slowly sit up. Bring your palms together in front of your chest, bow your head, and sit quietly for a few moments. Savor the aftereffects of the pose. Enjoy the way you feel.

# Benefits: Forward Bends

Forward Bends are soothing, calming, and very stretchy. They stretch and lengthen the entire backside of the body, thus releasing tension and improving circulation in the ankles and feet, legs, knees, hips, lower back, spine, torso, and neck. The spine, especially, is taught to lengthen, increasing the space and circulation between the vertebrae. This is important because the spine is the "freeway" to your brain, or the freeway from your brain to the entire body. The freer it is, the less congested, the better. Nerves throughout the body have their origin in the spinal cord. As they are freed and fed, nourished and healed, you will experience more vitality. As the spine and backside of the body is being stretched, the front side is firmed and toned. The abdominal organs receive a deep massage, thus stimulating the powers of digestion, elimination, and reproduction. Forward bends can be held for long periods of time, giving you more time to let go of tension and held energy. This is soothing to the nervous system and generates calmness, serenity, and a new outlook on life. Your kinesthetic sense, the feeling-tone of you, instead of being ragged or on edge will become smooth and even, more harmonious—and this feels good. Lengthening the backside of your body—legs, back, and neck—frees you from the past, so you're no longer bothered by events or circumstances that occurred earlier in your life, this life or past lives. This helps you experience your newness in the now. Done properly, forward bends simulate bowing and are humbling.

# Benefits: Seated Forward Fold *or Paschimottanasana*

Intense stretch to back of body—legs, back, neck. Lengthens and strengthens spine, thereby increasing vitality by improving energy flow. Massages and stimulates abdominal organs. Soothing, calming, rejuvenating. Refreshes mind and emotions. Promotes experience of peace.

# 30 Head to Knee Pose *or Janu Shirshasana*

Janu Shirshasana has two major lines of energy and a third minor line. The first major line travels up the spine and out the crown of your head. The second major line travels down the extended leg and outward through the foot. The third line presses into the heel from the bent knee, applying pressure to the tendon along the inner side of the extended leg's thigh. This is a minor line, but it helps insure your alignment by squaring the hips. It also helps propel you forward, enabling you to shift the weight of your body onto the straight leg. Your hips will be in dog tilt.

**1** **Sit on the floor with both legs extended straight in front of you.**

**2**  **Bend the right leg and place the sole of the right foot against the inner edge of the left thigh.** Bring the right heel near the pubic bone, then slide the right knee forward as far as it will go. Moving the knee forward will square your hips to the front and align your chest so it's facing straight ahead. Keep the inner edge of the left foot vertical and your toes spread.

**3**  Catch hold of the left foot with the right hand, placing your left hand on the floor adjacent to the left knee. If you cannot reach your foot, hold your ankle or shinbone, or use a strap to span the gap.

**4**  Wriggle the buttocks backward and position yourself on the frontal edge of each sitting bone. This establishes dog tilt. Then firmly press the back of your left thigh down into the floor, spread your toes, and push forward through the ball of your foot. Wait for the inner cue to proceed.

**5**  **As you inhale, elongate your spine upward** (photo 151). Use the inhalation to help you do this. Elongate your core, your invisible spine, by lifting the rib cage and chest upward, away from the waist. Relax the shoulders downward, away from the ears, keep the abdominals in, and pull gently with your right hand as you press downward with your left. Press downward with the back edge

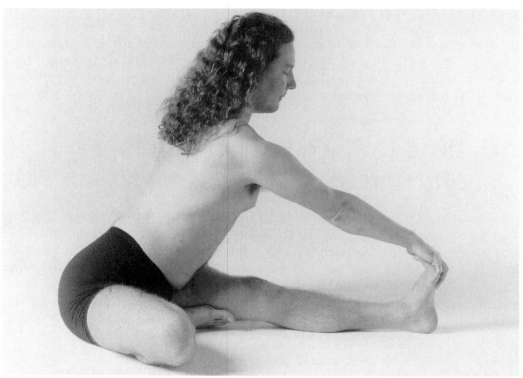

151

of your left leg and elongate upward through the fontanel, moving the tailbone and crown of your head away from one another. This will create a strong stretch in the hamstring muscles of the left leg. Be here several breaths, acclimatizing to the intensity of stretch, then breathe in deeply.

**6  As you exhale, fold forward.** Proceed slowly, edge by edge, always directing the energy flow forward and outward through the crown. Do not fold as deeply as you can all at once. Stop when you feel each new edge and wait for the sensations of stretch to diminish somewhat before folding deeper. Do this over and over until you cannot fold forward any farther. Eventually, the central line of your trunk and sternum will rest directly over the line of the left inner leg. Rest your abdomen on your thigh, your chest on your knee, and your face on the shinbone. Bring your nose down on the inside edge of the leg. Clasp the left foot with both hands, or clasp your wrist beyond the foot, then widen the elbows as you slide them forward and away from you (photo 152).

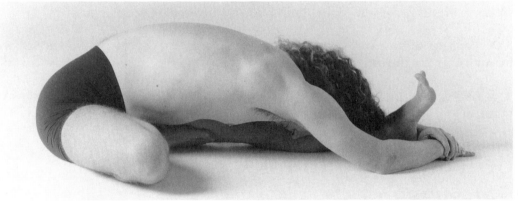

**152**

**7**  Energize the left leg. Press the back of the left thigh into the floor, tighten the quadriceps, and extend the left heel away from you, lengthening the Achilles tendon. Then, catching your heel on the floor and keeping your toes spread, press the ball of the foot away from you. Spiral your leg inward and direct the line of energy outward through the leg in the direction it is pointing. Simultaneously, flex the right heel and press inward from the right knee to square the hips.

**8**  Elongate your core horizontally forward. Maintain a subtle upward lift with the back of your neck so you are not resting heavily on your leg. Shrug the shoulders away from your ears, pull gently with your hands, and direct the stretch forward through the crown of your head toward your toes. Go forward toward the foot, not downward to the knee, and do not shorten the back of your neck by looking forward. Wriggle the buttocks backward so you're as deep as possible, close your eyes, and breathe smoothly.

**9** Monitor the intensity of stretch. Is it increasing, decreasing, or staying the same? Be willing to come up a bit if it is increasing. Increase or decrease the energy in your lines until the feeling-tone of the pose feels perfect. Orchestrate the whole event with your breathing.

**10** Bend your left leg if this stretch is too intense, but keep the inner edge of the left foot vertical and your toes spread. Acclimatize to the stretch in a relaxed manner. Be comfortable. Later, when your legs have lost most of their initial stiffness, you will desire more intensity. When this happens, generate more energy through the leg by pressing it straight.

**11** When you cannot fold forward any farther, stay where you are. Be still, breathe with awareness, and release all unnecessary effort and every trace of strain. Be here one minute. Enjoy the way this feels.

**12** **Come out of the pose.** Bring your hands alongside your hips, then slowly sit up. Sit quietly for a moment and savor the aftereffects of the pose.

**13** Repeat the pose on the other side. Straighten the right leg, fold the left leg in, and wait for the inner cue to proceed.

**14** When you are finished, sit quietly for a few moments and exult in the way you feel.

# Benefits: Head to Knee Pose *or Janu Shirshasana*

Tremendous leg stretch and strengthener. Relieves tension in lower back. Strengthens and elongates spine. Opens hips, knees, ankles. Stimulates and improves circulation through spine, torso, abdominal organs. Improves digestion, elimination. Quiets the mind.

# 31 Half Lotus Forward Fold *or Ardha Baddha Padma Paschimottanasana*

## STAGE ONE

**1** **Sit on the floor with both legs extended straight.**

**2** **Place the right foot in the crook of the left elbow and bring the right arm around the right knee, cradling the leg in your arms.** Flex the right heel, make the right shinbone horizontal, and gently pull the leg inward toward your chest as you elongate your spine upward. Sit tall. It requires hip and knee flexibility as well as tremendous spinal strength to pull the spine erect. Be here several breaths.

## STAGE TWO

**3** **Bring the right leg into Half Lotus.** Holding the right foot from underneath with both hands, bring the heel in toward the navel and then place the foot in the left groin, the crease formed by your left thigh and torso. Remove your hands, wriggle the buttocks backward, and sit tall.

**4** Bring the right arm around behind you and clasp hold of the right foot, then lean back on the left hand. Have your chest facing straight ahead, toward the left foot. If you cannot catch hold of the foot, then either use a belt to span the gap or simply lean backward on both hands.

**5** **Curve your head and chest upward** (photo 153). Do a backbend: First pull the abdominals backward toward the spine. Then move the shoulders backward and, as you inhale, lift the chest straight up. Expand the rib cage upward, away from the waist, then exhale as you press the shoulder blades forward into your back and arch backward. Roll the sternum upward and curve your head backward, bringing the whole chest and rib cage forward through the shoulders. Make your chest vertically round (from your pubis to your chin) and horizontally round (from shoulder to shoulder across the chest). Reach outward through the chin.

**6** If you are unable to clasp the right foot with your right hand, continue leaning backward on both hands as you do the back arch. This is similar to Stage One of the Fish Pose variations.

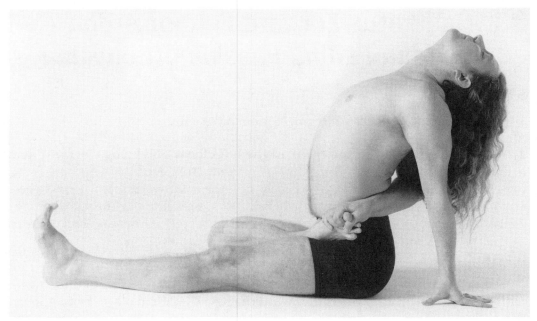

**153**

**7** Breathe. Use your breathing to expand the shape from inside.

**8** It is not uncommon at this point for the right knee to leave the floor, to float. Do not worry about this. The idea here is to lift and expand the chest. The more expansion and height you achieve in the chest, the easier it will be to squeeze the right knee gently downward toward the floor. Do that now. Gently squeeze the right knee down, but do it as a consequence of the chest expansion.

**9** Keep the left leg straight. Roll the left thigh inward until the kneecap faces the ceiling and the inner edge of the left foot is vertical. Spread your toes and press the ball of the foot away from you, spiraling the leg inward slightly. Press your left hand downward into the floor so your chest moves up, and pull gently with the right hand to increase the chest expansion. Breathe with feeling. Feel what's happening. This is a fabulous stretch. Be here several breaths, then bring your head to normal alignment.

## STAGE THREE

**10** **Fold forward into the pose** (photo 154). Do that by clasping your left foot with the left hand, resting your elbow on the floor, then widening the elbow as you slide it forward and away from you. This is the pose. Be here one minute. If and when your right arm gets tired, release it, bring it forward, and clasp the left foot.

**11 Return to a seated position.** Then undo Half Lotus, and perform the pose with your left leg in Half Lotus. Savor how you feel when you're finished.

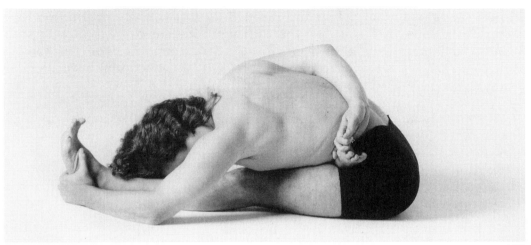

**154**

# Benefits: Half Lotus Forward Fold *or Ardha Baddha Padma Paschimottanasana*

Tremendous leg stretch. Increases elasticity of hips, knees, ankles, making full Lotus possible. Tones abdominal organs. Strengthens spine, opens chest, cures rounded shoulders. Calming, energizing.

# 32 Reclining Leg Stretch Series *or Supta Padangushtasana*

This Reclining Leg Stretch Series is a combination or cycle of five different poses done one after the other. You'll do the first four poses on the right side and then the left, and then you'll do the fifth pose. Of course, you can do each of these separately, but they flow together nicely like this.

## I KNEE TO CHEST

**1 Lie on your back with your legs bent, both feet flat on the floor. Bring the right knee toward you, clasp the knee with both hands, and gently pull it in toward your chest.** This is not strenuous. Be here several breaths.

**2** **Slide the left leg straight** (photo 155). Start on the center of the back of your left heel, then slide the heel away from you. Roll the left thigh inward until the kneecap faces the ceiling, spread your toes, and push outward through the ball of the foot, flowing energy outward through the leg. The leg line is now a long spiral. Press the sacrum down so there's a slight lumbar curve, pull with your hands, and flatten the shoulder blades into the floor, rounding your chest toward the ceiling. Keep your throat relaxed. Gaze into the sky, into infinity, and breathe smoothly. Be here several breaths.

**3** **Lift your head** (photo 156). Pull with your arms and try to touch your nose to your knee. Be relaxed as you do this. Keep the shoulders down, away from the ears. Be here several breaths.

**4** Uncurl your spine, rest your head on the floor, and slide the left foot back to starting position.

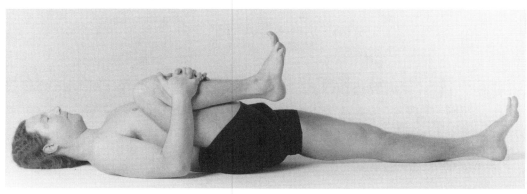

155

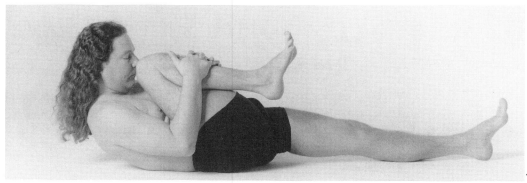

156

## II  LEG PULL

**1** **Straighten your right leg above your head and clasp the foot with both hands** (photo 157). I like to insert my left thumb between the big toe and second toe and my right thumb between the little toe and ring toe. This gives me a good grip and helps spread the toes. If you cannot reach your foot, use a belt to span the gap, or clasp your ankle, calf, or thigh.

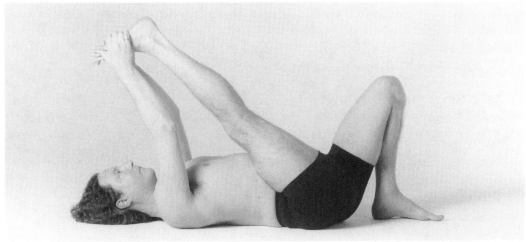

157

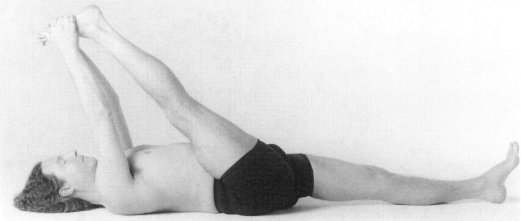

158

**2** Press the right leg fully straight, tighten the quadriceps, and extend the heel toward the ceiling. Then spread your toes and press the ball of the big toe away from you so the leg line spirals inward slightly and is directed outward in the direction the leg is pointing. As you do this, firmly press the sacrum down into the floor and gently pull the leg toward you, flattening the shoulder blades and rounding your chest. Breathe smoothly. Wait for the sensations of stretch to diminish before proceeding. Be here several breaths.

**3** **Slide the left leg straight on the floor** (photo 158). Start on the center of the back of the left heel, as before, and roll the left thigh inward until the kneecap faces the ceiling. Then spread your toes and push outward through the ball of the foot. Continue pressing the sacrum firmly down, keep moving your shoulders toward the floor so the shoulder blades flatten, and press both feet away from you as you gently pull the leg in tighter. Breathe smoothly and immerse yourself in the sensations of stretching. Be here anywhere from thirty seconds to two minutes.

## III   LEG TO THE SIDE

**1   Take the right leg to the right** (photo 159). Do this by letting go with your left hand, holding the right foot with the right hand only, and taking your leg to the right as you sweep your left arm to the left. Your arms will form a single straight line.

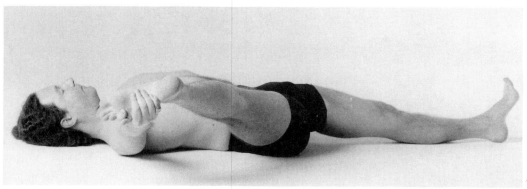

**159**

**2**   The tendency here is to tip to the right in the attempt to touch the right foot to the floor. Instead, keep the sacrum pressed flat into the floor and take the leg only as far as it will go without tipping. Do not allow the right foot to touch the floor unless you are also able to keep the sacrum flat. Prevent tipping by stretching more vigorously down the left leg, pressing the back of the left thigh down into the floor.

**3**   Lift your chest away from the waist, flatten the shoulder blades into the floor, rounding your chest, and press both feet away from you. Press the right foot into your right hand so the line of energy extends outward through the leg in the direction it's pointing, not backward through the knee.

**4**   Breathe smoothly, with feeling. Create the perfect degree of intensity, not too much, not too little. Bend your legs if this stretch is too intense. Flirt with it. Gaze into the sky. Be here anywhere from thirty seconds to two minutes.

## IV   SINGLE LEG RECLINING LUNGE

**1   Bend your right leg and clasp the right foot with both hands again** (photo 160). Move the knee to the side of your chest and make the shinbone vertical, positioning the right heel directly above the right knee. Then energize the left leg, sliding the heel away from you, and press the sacrum flat. This will make the left side of your body heavy and prevent tipping.

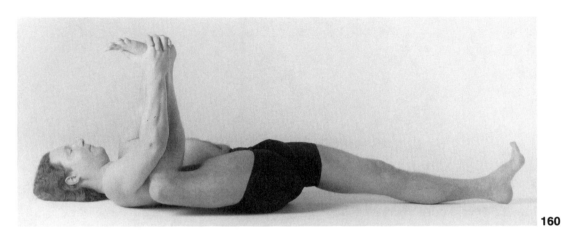

**160**

**2   Pull downward with your hands, attempting to touch the right knee to the floor.** Keep your sacrum flat and the left leg energized; do not tip sideways in your attempt to touch the floor. Move your shoulders toward the floor as you pull with your hands and round your chest. If this position is difficult for you, bend your left leg and slide the foot backward until it is flat. Breathe smoothly, emphasizing the pulling action as you exhale. Be here one minute.

**3   Slide the left foot backward, release the right foot, and return to starting position: both legs bent, feet flat.** Pause here a few moments. Absorb what just happened. Continue breathing smoothly.

Repeat Poses I–IV with the left leg. Then continue.

## V   TWO LEG RECLINING LUNGE

**1   Catch hold of both feet, legs bent** (photo 161). Hold the outer edge of the right foot with the right hand and the left foot with the left hand. Spread the knees sideways so they come off the chest, and make the shinbones vertical and parallel with one another. Allow your sacrum and lower back to curl off the floor; if necessary, cat tilt in order to lie backward, then rest your upper back and head comfortably on the floor.

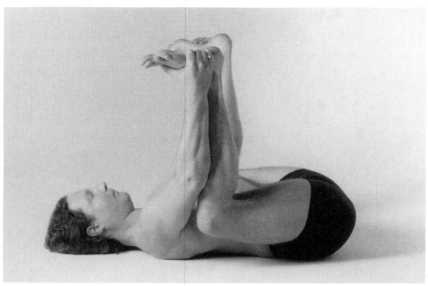

**161**

**2** **Press the sacrum firmly into the floor and pull straight down with your hands.** Move your shoulders toward the floor as you pull with your hands, flattening the shoulder blades and rounding the chest toward the ceiling. This stretch can be quite strong. Relax with the intensity. Breathe smoothly. Be here one minute.

**3** **Release the pose.** Come back to starting position: both legs bent, feet flat. Relax. Rest. Enjoy.

# Benefits: Reclining Leg Stretch Series

Tremendous leg stretch and strengthener. Opens hips, adductors, strengthens abdomen. Especially if your hamstrings are tight, these stretches are some of the best. The floor supports the back as the hamstrings stretch.

# 33 Upward Facing Spread Leg Forward Fold *or Urdhva Mukha Upavista Konasana*

## STAGE ONE

**1** **Lie on your back with your legs bent, feet flat. Bring the knees toward you, reach between your legs with your palms facing outward, and clasp hold of the shins. Then gently spread the knees apart, sideways** (photo 162). You will probably feel the stretch in the muscles along the inner thighs, the adductors.

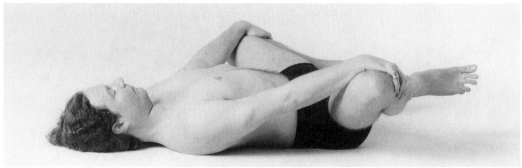

**162**

**2** Refine your alignment. Flatten the sacrum into the floor, move the shoulders toward the floor so your chest rounds, and wriggle the shoulder blades under until they are flat and comfortable. Some of the time, simply allow your arms and legs to relax and be passive so the stretch happens at its own pace, and some of the time pull gently outward with your hands and apply gentle downward pressure, delicately coaxing the knees toward the floor. Breathe smoothly as you do this. Relax with the intensity. Immerse yourself in the flow of breath and the various sensations of stretch. Savor this feeling.

**3** Be here one minute. Then pull your legs toward you as you bring them together and return to starting position: legs bent, feet flat.

## STAGE TWO

**4** **Stretch your legs toward the ceiling, then clasp hold of your inner thighs or calves with the palms facing outward.** Refine your alignment as before: Move your shoulders toward the floor, rounding your chest, and snuggle the shoulder blades and sacrum into the floor.

**5** **Spread your legs sideways** (photo 163). Energize the leg lines by spreading your toes and pressing the ball of each foot away from you. Stretch outward through your legs in the direction they are pointing. Try to straighten your legs fully. Some of the time simply allow your arms to relax and be passive, and some of the time apply downward pressure with your hands, gently squeezing your legs closer to the floor.

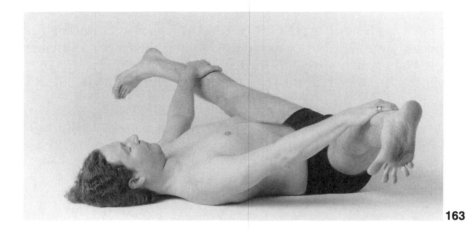

**163**

**6** Breathe smoothly and enjoy the way this wonderful stretch feels. Deliberately create the perfect degree of intensity, not too much, not too little.

**7** Be here one minute, then bring your legs to vertical again.

## STAGE THREE

**8** **Clasp your feet.** Hold the big toes or the outer edge of each foot, and then flatten the sacrum into the floor as you straighten and energize your legs.

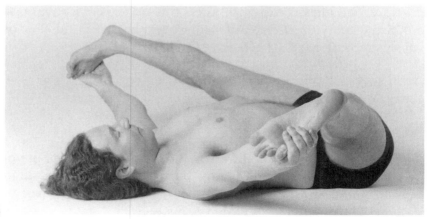

**164**

**9** **Spread the legs sideways** (photo 164). Press your feet into your hands as you press the sacrum down, and flatten the shoulder blades into the floor as you round your chest toward the ceiling.

**10** Breathe smoothly. Gaze into the sky. Be here one minute. Return to starting position: legs bent, feet flat.

# Benefits: Upward Facing Spread Leg Forward Fold *or Urdha Mukha Upavista Konasana*

Stretches hamstrings and adductors. Strengthens hands and back. Besides being an excellent pose in itself, the Upward Facing Spread Leg Forward Fold is perfect preparation for the next pose, the Spread Leg Forward Fold. Here, because your back is resting flat on the floor, the stretch can be directed very specifically into the legs.

# 34 Spread Leg Forward Fold *or Upavista Konasana*

**1** **Sit on the floor with your legs spread wide.** Place one hand on the floor in front of you, one hand on the floor behind you, then lift your hips and scoot forward to your comfortable maximum. Then use your hands to pull the buttock flesh backward so your sitting bones can merge with the floor.

**2** **Sit tall.** Establish the leg lines first. Turn the legs in or out until the kneecaps face the ceiling and the inner edges of your feet are vertical. Be on the center of the back of each heel. Press the back of each thigh firmly down into the floor, extending the heels away from you, then spread your toes and press outward through the ball of each foot.

**3** Align your torso and elongate your core. First, bring your lower back forward into your body so your spine is erect, not rounded. Then lift your chest upward away from the pelvis, move the shoulders backward, tugging gently downward with the shoulder blades, and then bring the navel backward toward the spine. Bring your palms together in namaste, prayer position, and then elongate your core by sinking the sitting bones straight down and floating the crown of your head straight up. Close your eyes, if you'd like, and become increasingly grounded, centered. Consciously establish your awareness in the now. Breathe smoothly. Let your face be soft. Be here until you are ready to proceed.

**4** **Lean forward and place your hands on the floor** (photo 165). Have your hands shoulder-width apart and your fingers spread. Snuggle your palms into the floor. Then wriggle the buttocks backward and position yourself on the frontal edge of the sitting bones, in dog tilt. This will help propel you forward into the pose.

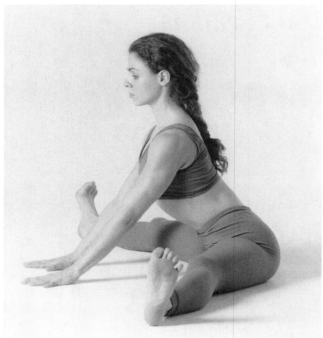

**165**

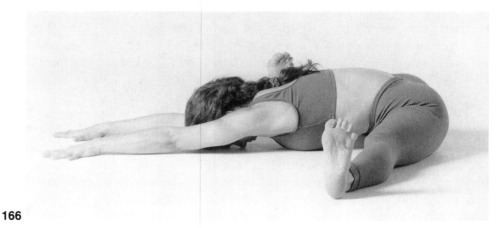

**166**

**5** **As you inhale, bring your lower back forward, press the backs of your thighs down, and stretch the front of your body up.** Elongate your arms; do not sag into the shoulders. Make the front of your body long.

**6** **As you exhale, fold into the pose by sliding your hands forward** (photo 166). Slide your hands forward until you sense a new edge, then stop. Do not let your legs roll in or out as you fold forward; the kneecaps should continue facing the ceiling. Wait for these new sensations of stretch to diminish somewhat, then fold deeper by sliding your hands farther forward. Maintain maximum extension from coccyx to fontanel to fingertips. Breathe smoothly.

**7** Proceed slowly, edge by edge; slide, stop, slide, stop. Do not fold as deeply as you can all at once. Stop when you feel each new intermediary edge, and wait for the stretch to ease up a little before folding deeper. Do this over and over until you cannot slide your hands or release your spine forward any farther. Eventually your torso—belly, chest, and forehead—will rest comfortably on the floor.

**8** Breathe smoothly, slowly. Feel the movement of breath ripple through your body. This is a lovely pose. Be here one to five minutes.

**9** **Come out of the pose.** Walk your hands backward and inhale as you return to a seated position. Bring your palms together in namaste, close your eyes, and experience the aftereffects of the pose.

# Benefits: Spread Leg Forward Fold *or Upavista Konasana*

Stretches hamstrings and adductors. Frees spine and hip joints, relieves sciatica, improves circulation in pelvic region. Tones abdominal organs. Calming, energizing.

# 35 Cobbler Pose *or Baddha Konasana*

### STAGE ONE

**1** **Sit on the floor with your legs bent and the soles of your feet together.** Wriggle the buttocks backward a few times, positioning yourself on the tips of the sitting bones, then pull the feet in as close as you can to the pubic bone.

**2** **Lean back on your hands, fingers pointing away from you.** Or be on the ball of your hands, if you prefer. Your first thought, as usual, is the alignment of your center, so pull the abdominals backward toward the spine.

**3** **Lift your chest upward and squeeze your knees downward.** Roll the shoulders backward, push down into your hands to lengthen the arms, and as you inhale, expand the chest away from the waist—up and up and up. As you exhale, stretch *outward* through the knees and squeeze them gently toward the floor, pressing the heels together. You'll probably feel a stretch in the adductor (inner thigh) muscles. Continue gazing forward. Be here several breaths.

**4** **Curve your head backward** (photo 167). Breathe in deeply to assist in lifting and expanding the chest, also push downward into both hands so the chest moves farther upward, then exhale as you thrust the chest forward through the shoulders and curve your head backward. Keep your neck soft. This is similar to Stage One of the Fish Pose variations.

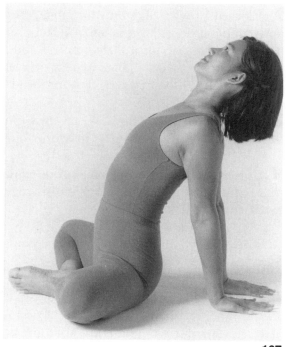

**167**

**5** Keep the abdomen pulled firmly backward toward the spine, open the sternum toward the ceiling, and from the base of your throat stretch outward through the chin. Get round, expanding from inside. Breathe deeply, filling the pose with air.

## STAGE TWO

**6** **Sit erect** (photo 168) **clasping hold of your feet.** Then firmly press the soles of your feet together, stretch the inner thighs toward the knees, and gently squeeze your knees toward the floor. Pressing the feet together helps move the knees *outward*, and because they are moving outward they will more easily move downward.

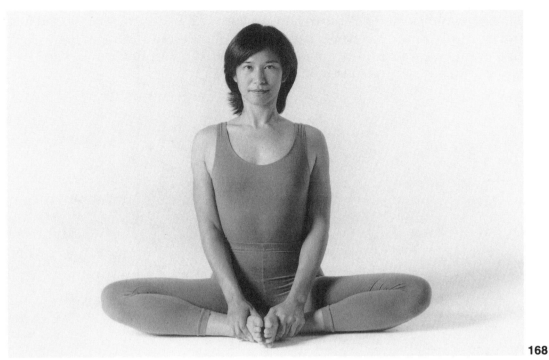

**168**

**7** Align your torso and elongate your core. Pull your spine erect. Press the sitting bones firmly down as you bring your lower back in and lift the chest. Pull with your hands, using your arm strength to help you do this. Move the shoulders backward, flattening the shoulder blades into your back, and then keep the abdominals in as you try to elongate your core. Go straight upward through the crown of your head and straight downward through the sitting bones.

**8** Breathe smoothly. Be here about a minute.

### STAGE THREE

**9** **Rotate the pelvis forward and place your hands on the floor in front of you.** Spread your fingers, snuggle your palms into the floor, and then wriggle the buttocks backward to position yourself on the frontal edge of the sitting bones.

**10** **As you inhale, bring your lower back forward, lengthen your arms, and stretch your spine up.** Make the front of your body long. Try to achieve maximum spinal extension. Move the coccyx and fontanel away from one another.

**11** **As you exhale, fold into the pose by sliding your hands forward** (photo 169). Slide your hands forward until you sense a new edge, then stop. Breathe smoothly as you wait for the stretch to diminish somewhat, then exhale and fold deeper. Keep sliding your hands away from you. Proceed slowly, edge by edge. Do this until you cannot slide your hands any farther. Eventually your chest will rest on your feet, your forehead on the floor.

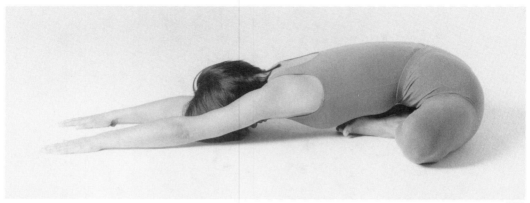

**169**

**12** The way to get flat is by getting long, and the way to get long is by sliding your hands farther away from you. Do not rush to your maximum extension. The slower you go, the deeper you'll get. Keep your palms flat, your arms straight and relaxed, and continue stretching outward through the knees, squeezing them down. Maintain maximum extension from coccyx to fontanel to fingertips.

**13** Direct your gaze toward the floor. Do not shorten the back of your neck by lifting your head and looking forward. Direct the energy flow outward through the crown of your head and arms.

**14** Breathe smoothly. Feel your body pulse with the gentle rhythm of breath. Be here one to five minutes.

# Benefits: Cobbler Pose *or* *Baddha Konasana*

Frees hip joints, stretches adductor muscles, strengthens back and spine. Improves circulation through hips, legs, and pelvic region. Good for meditation once comfortable.

# 36 Splits Pose *or Hanumanasana*

The Splits Pose is an advanced stretch, so please be careful with it. Approached intelligently, however, it is workable by just about anyone. It requires extreme flexibility in the quadriceps muscles of the rear leg and the hamstring muscles of the front leg. Be sure to stay well within your comfort zone at all times. Delicately nudge into your edges.

## STAGE ONE

**1  Start in lunge position with the right foot forward** (photo 170). Position the right heel directly below the knee, align the inner edge of the right foot so it's pointing straight ahead, and make sure the right shinbone is vertical. Spread your toes.

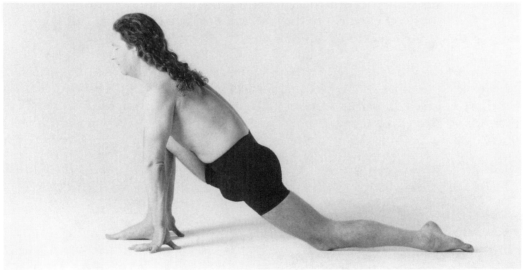

**170**

**2** Place your hands on the floor straddling the foot, fingers pointing forward. Be on the ball of each hand, if you prefer.

**3** Press your hands downward into the floor to lengthen the arms, lifting your torso upward so you are not sagging in the shoulders. Gaze at the floor and breathe smoothly. Establish your awareness in the rhythm of breath. Wait for the inner cue to proceed.

**4** Before moving on, though, be aware to keep the following two actions in mind as you do the pose. First, continue pressing downward into your hands and lifting upward, lengthening the arms for the duration of the pose. Stay up out of the shoulders as much as possible. This has been an important action in many of the poses. Second, stretch *outward* into the knees as you delicately pressurize your hips toward the floor. The knees should move away from one another, right knee forward, left knee backward. As this happens, there will be more space for your hips to sink downward into. The idea here is to create a straight line through your thighs from knee to knee. Sustain both of these actions for the duration of the pose, emphasizing the upward lifting action with each inhale and the hips-sinking-downward action with each exhale. When you are ready to proceed, breathe in deeply.

**5** **As you exhale, sink your hips downward toward the floor.** Do this gently. Your hips probably won't sink very far, at first; half an inch is a long way. Yet the intensity of stretch may increase dramatically. Let the weight of your body do the work for you. Release into it, rather than press into it. Stay where you now are as you inhale, lengthening the arms and lifting your chest, then release into it farther as you exhale. Continue stretching the knees away from one another. If this stretch is easy for you, be glad.

**6** Wait for the musculature to let you in. Be gentle and delicate, not aggressive. Do not create so much intensity that you also have to resist it. Be relaxed, strain-free. Lure yourself deeper into the stretch. Apply pressure as needed, increase the intensity of stretch when your body asks for it, yet also wait and be patient. Practice doing and not-doing at the same time. Allow the pose to deepen when your body is ready. Be here at least half a minute.

## STAGE TWO

**7** **Turn your left toes under, then straighten the left leg** (photo 171). Endeavor to keep your hips low, where they were in Stage One.

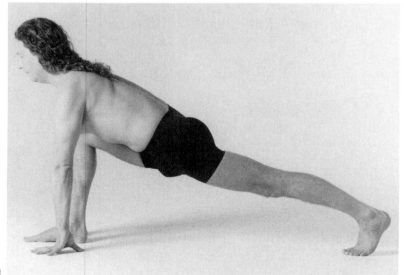

171

**8** This can be fairly strenuous at first. The trick is to keep the current in the back leg strong and steady so it feels relaxed. Continue sinking downward with your hips. Stay lifted out of the shoulders. Gaze toward the floor. Be here half a minute.

## STAGE THREE

**9** **Bend the left knee down to the floor again and point your left toes.** Your chest is probably pressed into your thigh right now. Keep your chest and thigh together as much as possible as you proceed with this stage.

**10** **Move your hips backward and straighten the right leg** (photo 172). Do this slowly, delicately. Lift your right toes off the floor, roll onto the center of the back of your right heel, and keep your chest pressed firmly into your thigh as you slowly straighten the leg. Bend your elbows toward the floor or straighten the arms and slide the hands away from you. Rest on your forehead. Your left thigh will now be vertical.

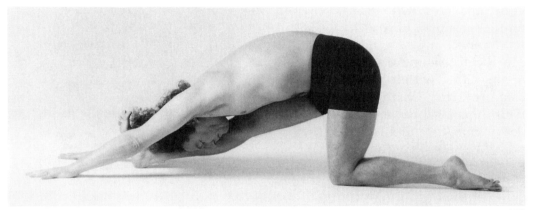

**172**

**11** As you straighten the leg, if the chest and thigh begin to separate, stop straightening the leg. This is your spot. It's where the stretch actually begins for you. Reaffirm the chest–thigh contact by pressing your chest firmly into the thigh again, even if you have to bend the leg a little; then, keeping your chest and thigh together, try to straighten the leg further. Only in the last few seconds or breaths of this stage should you allow them to separate, if at all. When you are able to straighten the leg fully without losing the intimate chest-thigh relationship, you will have a very tight forward fold.

**12** This is a strong stretch for most people. Do not forcibly press your way deeper into the pose. Do not be aggressive with yourself. Apply pressure, then wait for the musculature to release. Deepen the stretch edge by edge. Proceed slowly, carefully, with sensitivity. Stay within your comfort zone.

**13** Breathe smoothly. Be here half a minute or more.

### STAGE FOUR

**14** Slide your hands backward, straighten your arms, and lift your body away from the leg. Straighten the right leg and be on the back of the heel (photo 173). This is starting position for the slide into Splits.

**15 Slide into Splits** (photo 174): Using your hands for support, slide your right heel away from you. Slide a little, then stop; slide, stop, slide, stop. Do not be in a rush. Take your time, go slowly. Wait for the sensations of stretch to diminish at each new edge before sliding deeper. Again, stay within your comfort zone. Eventually, your hips will be on the floor; not the first day, probably, but eventually. Be patient and gently persistent.

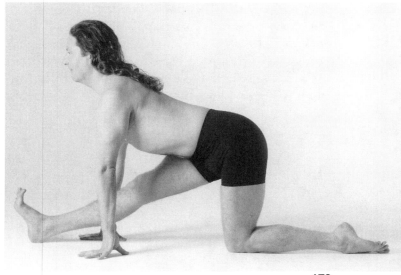

173

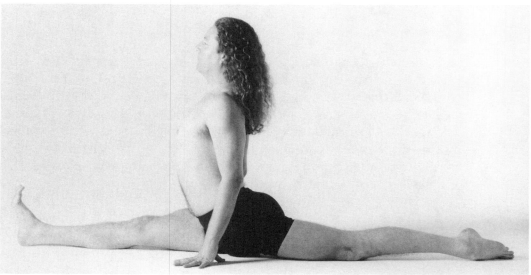
174

**16** Keep the right leg pressed fully straight as you slide into the pose, using your arm strength to prevent yourself from sliding too deep too fast. Hover lightly at your edges, letting the weight of your body sink you deeper into the pose. Pull the abdominals in and continue lifting your chest so your spine becomes increasingly vertical as your hips come down.

**17** When you can sit comfortably on the floor, take your arms up (photo 175). Press both legs straight, spread your toes, and roll both thighs inward. Pull the abdominals in, lift your chest away from the waist, and try to square your hips to the front so the abdominal plane faces straight ahead. Stretch vigorously upward through the arms and gaze into infinity through your fingertips. Be here several breaths. This feels fantastic.

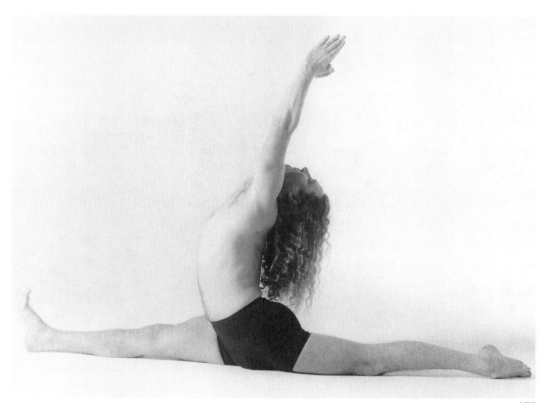

**175**

**18** Rest in Child's Pose (photo 176) when you are done. Then do the pose with your left leg.

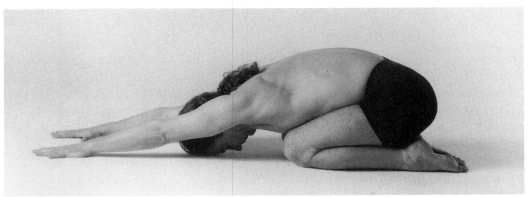

**176**

# Benefits: Splits Pose *or Hanumanasana*

One of the ultimate, classical poses. Requires tremendous leg and groin flexibility. Take your time with this one. Be gently persistent.

# INVERSIONS

# 37 Headstand *or Shirshasana*

The Headstand is a fabulous pose. It is also one of the easier postures once you've learned how to balance. For many people, though, it is an encounter with fear. This is because the perfect point of balance is where you feel nearly weightless, light, just before falling over backward. At first, this is a tenuous place to be, and you will not feel very secure in this lightness. As you become familiar with this spot, however, your balance will become steady, sure, confident. This is what you are looking for. There should be no strain anywhere.

It is important to do Shirshasana properly in order to keep it safe. Learn the fundamentals, stay aware to do the pose properly, and if you ever experience discomfort or pain in your neck or shoulders, come down immediately. You can always go back up. The foundation of this pose is the positioning of your arms, head, and shoulders. Learn the correct arm, head, and shoulder positioning before going up. If you are asymmetrical or crooked in your foundation, the entire pose will be distorted and under unnecessary strain.

## GETTING READY

## ARM PLACEMENT

**1** Correct arm placement is your first objective. Use a mat or folded blanket to pad your head and arms. Kneel on the floor, rest your forearms on the blanket or pad, and clasp hold of your elbows (photo 177). This will position your elbows so they are directly beneath your shoulders. Keep them shoulder-width apart, without moving, for the duration of the pose. This is step number one. Always do this. Every time you practice Headstand—for the rest of your life—start like this.

**2** Keeping your elbows exactly where they are, swivel your hands out, and interlace your fingers fully, even crossing the thumbs (photo 178). Conform your hands into the shape they'd be if you were holding a tennis ball. Tuck the bottom little finger inside the cup formed by your hands. Look at the overall shape of your forearms and hands and make sure they form a symmetrical, equilateral triangle. If your arms are not symmetrical, the base of your Headstand will be faulty and the pose will be crooked. Do not underestimate the importance of

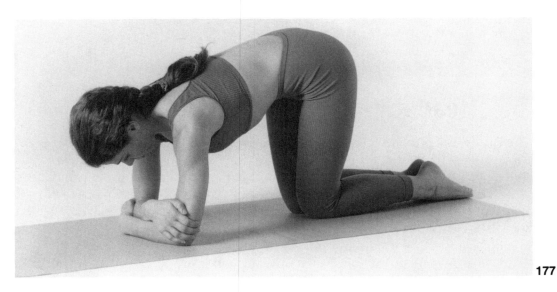

**177**

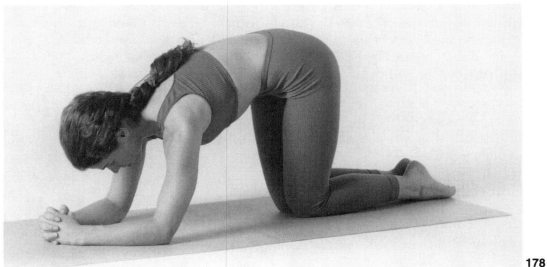

**178**

symmetry. Make sure this part of the pose is correct before placing your head on the floor.

## HEAD PLACEMENT

**3** Correct placement of your head is your second objective. If your arms are symmetrical, put the crown of your head on the floor with the back of your skull nestled up against the curve formed by your hands. Do not move your arms as you put your head in. Establish the arm positioning first, keep your arms stationary, and then put your head into your hands. Never place your head on the floor first (before establishing the correct arm positioning) because then you'll have no way of knowing whether your arms are symmetrical or not. Put your head into your hands, not the other way around.

**4** The center of the crown of your head should be on the floor, straight up from the ears. If you are too far forward toward the front of your head, the back of your neck will compress and be under strain. You will not be comfortable in the pose, nor will you feel weightless. If you are too far toward the back of your head, however, with the chin tucked excessively, the pose will again not be stable. Your neck will feel fragile, weakened, and be susceptible to injury. If the point of balance is off at all, your alignment will not be perfect. You will need excessive muscular effort to stay balanced and will probably experience some degree of strain in your neck. When the weight of your body comes straight down through the center of the crown of your head, however, the pose will feel weightless, there will be no strain in your neck, and your balance will be effortless. Gaze straight ahead at your knees.

## SHOULDER PLACEMENT

Your third objective involves learning to lift your shoulders away from your ears. This is an easy movement, and if you learn it on the ground before attempting Headstand, you should have no trouble doing it once you are up and balanced. Your shoulders must always be lifted. The strength of your shoulders, arms, and upper back will protect and take pressure off the neck. But you should also know what's right and what's wrong and be able to do both, so you can easily distinguish the difference once you're up. Lifting the shoulders is easy, it just takes a little remembering.

**5** With your head in your hands and your knees and feet still on the floor, practice lifting and dropping the shoulders. This involves shrugging your shoulders up, away from the ears, then letting them drop down. Do this ten times. Look closely at the photographs here, move from one position to the other slowly, and learn to distinguish between the two.

**Shoulders Down:** Let your shoulders collapse and fall inward toward your ears (photo 179). This is what they will look like once you're up in Headstand if you do not deliberately lift them up and away from the ears. This is not what you want, however. When your shoulders collapse inward toward your ears, your neck will feel thick and congested, and there will be too much weight on your head. Your forearms and elbows will feel ungrounded and loose because they are not firmly connected with the floor.

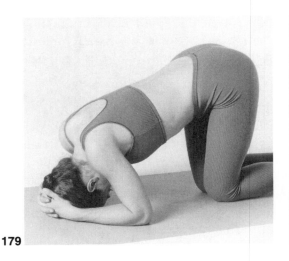

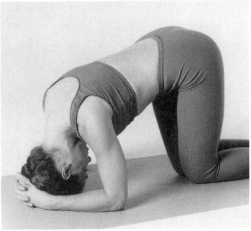

**179**　　　　　　　　　　　　　　　　　　　　　　　　　　**180**

**Shoulders Up:** To lift your shoulders, simply shrug them away from your ears as you press each forearm firmly into the floor (photo 180). Your neck will elongate, your chin will level, and the shoulder blades will spread sideways away from one another. You will experience a sense of relief on the top of your head and in your neck as you do this.

Make it a conscious habit always to go through these four steps before moving into Headstand: 1) Clasp the elbows, establishing correct arm placement, elbows shoulder-width apart. 2) Lace the fingers and insure arm symmetry. 3) Put the top of your head on the floor with the back of your skull nestled into the curve formed by your wrists and hands. 4) Lift and drop the shoulders several times, just to remind yourself, then lift them up and keep them up.

## GOING UP

**6** Lift your hips and walk inward toward your arms as far as you comfortably can (photo 181). Bend your knees and lightly touch them to your chest. Then, without yet lifting your feet from the floor, move your hips up and back—lifting them as high as you can—and straighten your legs. You are attempting to position your hips directly above your head so your spine is vertical, or nearly so. When your spine is vertical, your center will be directly over the base of support (the triangle formed by your arms). Be sure your shoulders are still up.

**7** Lift one foot, press your forearms and elbows into the floor, keep moving the raised foot up and back, and then gently push from the other foot to hop up into the pose. The higher you are able to lift your hips, and the more backward you are able to move the raised foot, the less you'll have to hop. Eventually, this will be a very smooth, fluid movement with no hopping. You'll find yourself lifting

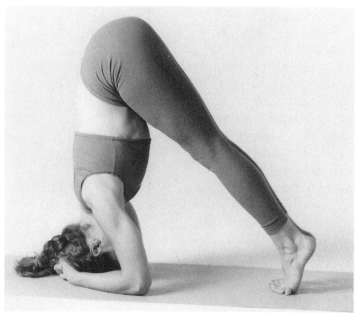

**181**

up effortlessly, as though you were floating. This may surprise you the first time it happens, so go slowly.

**8** You are now balancing (photo 182). Keep your legs bent, your feet and knees together, and pause here a moment. Do not be in a rush to take your legs up. The secret to the perfect balance is here. Acclimatize to the balance here while your center of gravity is still low. Check that your shoulders are up and that your elbows have not moved.

The trick to balance is awareness. Simply stay aware of the various sensations on your head, arms, and hands. You're already balanced, and there are certain definite sensations associated with this balance. All you have to do to maintain the balance is keep the sensations exactly as they

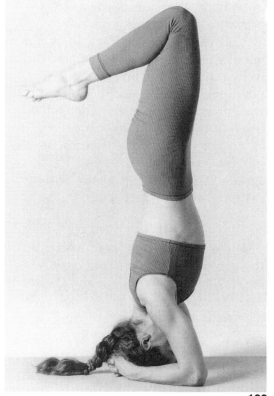

**182**

are now as you slowly take your legs up. If the sensations stay the same, it will be impossible for you to fall over. If the sensations begin to shift or change, it means your weight is shifting off-center and your balance is becoming uncertain. If you start tipping backward, for example, your elbows will begin to hover off the floor, your hands will experience more weight and pressure, your head and neck will become uncomfortable, and you'll lose the previous sensations associated with the balance. If your elbows get heavy and press into the floor excessively, it means you are leaning forward too much.

**9** Slowly take your legs all the way up (photo 183). Keep your feet together so your legs move as one. Stay aware of the sensations in your hands, forearms, and elbows, and the feeling of weight and pressure on your head. Keep the sensations steady. Maintain the shoulder lift. If the sensations shift or change at all as you're taking your legs up, stop moving. Get steady, reaffirm the shoulder lift, then go again, slowly taking your legs farther up. It's all a matter of awareness.

**10** Once you're up, stay aware of the sensations in your hands, forearms, elbows, head, neck, and shoulders. Try not to wriggle or shake. Be firm without being tense or rigid.

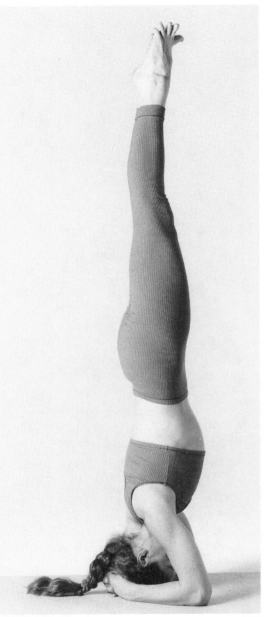

183

## HEADSTAND WITH THE WALL

Using the wall can be helpful if you are having trouble balancing or if you are fearful of falling over.

**1** Arrange your arms, head, and shoulders as before, going through the four steps. Your knuckles should be three inches from the wall.

**2** Walk your feet in, bend the knees in toward the chest, and keep the hips high. Lift one foot, press the elbows, and push from the other foot to come up. Bring your knees and feet together, keep the knees bent, and lightly touch the wall with the tips of your big toes. Do not rest your hips against the wall.

**3** The most important action to maintain at this stage is the shoulder lift. Press downward into your elbows, forearms, and wrists, and lift your shoulders away from the ears. Move your shoulder blades toward your waist. Always maintain this shoulder lift while upside down.

**4** Attempt to balance here with your knees bent and the tips of your big toes lightly touching the wall. To find your balance, simply flex your feet so your toes come off the wall. Balance. Be delicate. This is not difficult. It's easy to bring your feet off the wall without changing your position much. Just don't be in a rush to straighten your legs and don't push with your feet. Simply flex them. If you cannot balance here, you will not be able to balance with your legs extended. It's easier here because your center of gravity is lower. Keep your shoulders up and continue pressing the elbows, forearms, and wrists firmly down into the floor so they take root.

**5** Once you're able to balance with your legs bent, keep your feet together and slowly straighten your legs. If the sensations of balance change at all as you take your legs up, stop moving. If your shoulders begin to drop, stop moving. If anything changes, stop moving, Readjust, acclimatize, get steady, then continue straightening your legs. Remember, moment-to-moment awareness is the secret to perfect balance.

## ONCE YOU'RE UP

First, check that your shoulders are still strong and lifted, and that your elbows have not moved from their original position. Press your wrists into the floor as you lift the shoulder blades away from your ears. Make sure the foundation of the pose retains integrity and symmetry. Stay attentive for the duration of the pose to the sensations of weight and pressure on the top of your head and in your hands, forearms, and elbows. Then align your center and refine your balance. Move the thighbones backward as you press the tailbone forward. Draw the abdominals in, moving the back of your waist backward, and gently firm the buttocks in cat tilt. Bring your feet together, press the legs straight, and stretch straight upward through the inner core formed by the merger of your two legs. Spread your toes, opening the soles of your feet toward the ceiling, then from the root of your spine stretch upward through your inner legs and outward through your feet—so the line of energy flows freely upward. This will pull your torso and spine more erect. Remember, the pose should feel light, nearly effortless, and you will feel this way when you are vertical and straight through your neck, spine, and legs. Make subtle intuitive adjustments until you feel most weightless, most perfectly aligned. Correct and adjust the pose from inside, then ask a friend to check your alignment. From the side you should form a vertical line. Keep your eyes open and gaze straight ahead. Breathe smoothly. Stay in this position as long as you're able to maintain correct vertical alignment through the full length of your body and a strong shoulder lift—anywhere from a few seconds to five or ten minutes.

## UP AND DOWN WITH STRAIGHT LEGS

Eventually, you will want to move into and out of Shirshasana with both legs straight. This is actually easier, once you are able to do it, because there are fewer moving parts and less chance of error. It is easiest to learn the coming down phase of the straight-leg technique first, so let's start with that.

## COMING DOWN

**1** From Shirshasana, keep your legs together and straight and slowly lower your feet to the floor. Do this by tipping your hips backward (dog tilt) and firmly pressing your wrists, forearms, and elbows into the floor so the shoulders stay up. If you do this properly, your back will not round. Your upper back and spine will maintain an elongated upward integrity, your hips will be in a sharp dog tilt, and you'll simply hinge from your hips to lower your feet.

## GOING UP

The trick to going up with straight legs lies in learning to come down with straight legs. Spend a lot of time practicing the coming down part. When you are able to lower your feet all the way down without dropping the last few inches, you'll have no difficulty going up with straight legs.

**1** Lift your hips and walk your feet inward toward your head as far as they'll comfortably go. Do this without allowing your back to round; keep it as erect as possible. Push your toes into the floor, straighten your legs, and tip your hips backward. Then press your elbows firmly into the floor. Your feet will float up.

## WHEN YOU'RE FINISHED

Rest in Child's Pose with your head down and eyes closed.

# Benefits: Inversions

Inversions revitalize the whole system. They turn your body upside down, reversing the effects of gravity, and flood the brain with nourishment. Like twists, but more so, inversions are cleansing and nourishing at the deepest levels, and thereby engender tremendous systemic harmonization or health benefits. The entire physical system, under control of the brain, is energized and nourished as the brain is washed clean and flooded with rich new nutrients. The mind clears. Thinking improves. Understanding ensues. Headstand in particular activates the pineal and pituitary glands, the master glands of the endocrine system that controls the chemical balance of the body. Shoulderstand strengthens the nervous system and emotions by stimulating the thyroid and parathyroid glands, which regulate metabolism. Inversions in general, by elevating the legs, improve circulation, venous return, and lymph drainage, all of which nourish cells in the face, muscles, and skin, relieve strain and fatigue in the legs and feet, and stimulate intestinal sluggishness, improving digestion and elimination. They are a marvelous aid to sleep. Time spent upside down everyday is one of the best things you could possibly do for yourself. The ancient yogis were clever to have figured this out. Inversions turn you upside down and root you in the now. These poses are especially beneficial after a stressful day because they evoke calm, quiet an overstimulated brain, and soothe the nerves.

# Benefits: Headstand *or Shirshasana*

Irrigates the brain, stimulating pineal and pituitary glands. Strengthens neck, shoulders, arms. Relieves tired legs. Stimulates circulation, digestion, elimination. Centering, warming, develops concentration and focus. Energizing, calming, soothing to the whole body. Clears the mind. Heightens sensitivity. Conducive to meditation.

# 38 Shoulderstand *or Sarvangasana*

## SARVANGASANA PREPARATIONS

The three precursor poses to Sarvangasana are important. They increase mobility in the neck, spine, and shoulders and strengthen the neck, back, buttocks, and abdominals, all of which help make the Plow and Shoulderstand safe and easy. It is not necessary that you do all three precursor poses each time you practice Shoulderstand, but it's not a bad idea.

### TIP YOUR KNEES FROM SIDE TO SIDE

**1 Start on your back with your legs bent, feet hip-width apart, arms by your sides.** Pull your feet in tight toward the buttocks. Check that your feet are straight and parallel with one another, then snuggle them into the floor.

**2 As you inhale, sweep the arms up over your head to the floor.** Move smoothly, coordinating the breath and movement.

**3 As you exhale, tip your legs to the right.** Do this in order to shrug the *left* shoulder blade down your back, away from the ear, until it is flat on the floor (photo 184); then bring your legs back to center. It takes only a moment to do this. Then tip your legs to the left and slide the right shoulder blade down your back, then bring your legs back to center. The back of your neck, and the back of your arms and hands, should now feel more elongated than just moments ago, and both shoulder blades should be flat, stuck on the floor, actually pulled down your back by the floor. This is a subtle movement, but it dramatically improves alignment and energy flow.

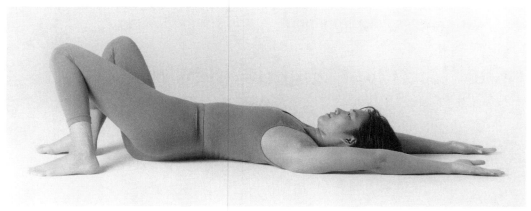

184

# BRIDGE POSE WITH ARMS OVERHEAD

**1** **Lift your hips away from the floor:** Breathe in deeply first, then exhale as you pull the abdominals down and rotate your pelvis backward in cat tilt; this will cause the coccyx and sacrum to lift an inch or two away from the floor.

**2** Gradually take your pelvis higher, breath by breath (photo 185). Lead with your tailbone as you very slowly lift your hips away from the floor. Let it feel as though an invisible hand were lifting you from underneath. Feel how your spine begins to arch and how the spine goes deeper into your back as the apex of the curve flows up your back. See how high you can get the curve. Keep your chin tucked down, your shoulders firmly grounded, and endeavor to bring the apex of the curve into your upper back, behind your heart, so that your pelvis moves upward toward the ceiling and your chest expands forward toward your face.

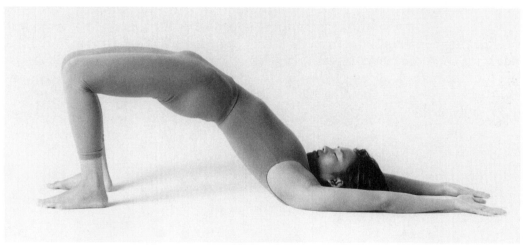

**185**

**3** Reaffirm the alignment of your center by pulling the abdominal muscles downward toward the spine and stretching the coccyx toward the knees. Open the frontal thighs and groins toward the ceiling and become increasingly grounded through your feet. Be solid, not stiff. Snuggle your feet into the floor. Because your feet are hip-width apart, your thighs will be parallel with one another. If your thighs splay out, however, you will compress the lumbar spine and experience more weight on the outer edges of each foot. If this happens, bring your knees toward one another without moving your feet until your thighs are again parallel, and press downward into the inner edge of each foot.

**4** When you cannot expand your chest or raise your pelvis any higher, stay where you are and hold this maximum position as effortlessly as possible. Try to release every hint of strain without losing the action of the pose. Be strain-free, yet strong. Be still, convinced. Breathe smoothly, expanding into the pose from the inside out. Keep the back of your neck elongating toward the skull. Be here one minute.

**5 Uncurl slowly.** This is an important movement. Pull the abdominals down, stretch the coccyx toward the knees in cat tilt, and slowly uncurl your spine to the floor. Keep the tailbone up as far as possible for as long as possible as your spine slowly makes sequential new contact with the floor—until finally your sacrum touches, rests, and relaxes into the floor. Be fluid, smooth, not in a rush. When your sacrum is flat, relax. Breathe smoothly. Enjoy how you feel.

## BRIDGE POSE WITH HANDS CLASPED UNDER HIPS

**1 Lift your hips into Bridge Pose again. Then sweep your arms up, take them down toward your feet, and interlace your hands beneath your hips** (photo 186). Straighten the arms, roll the upper arms out, and do "the wriggle." Wriggle the shoulders away from your ears, squeeze the upper arms inward, and slide your shoulder blades toward the back of your waist as you press the shoulders into the floor. Endeavor to be directly on top of the shoulders rather than on your back toward the shoulder blades. Breathe smoothly, deepening the pose as you're able. Be here one minute.

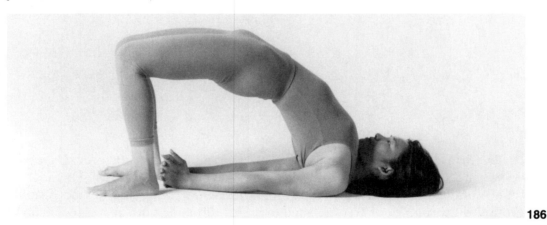

**186**

**2** When you are almost done, come up on your toes. This will enable you to raise the hips higher, so do so. Again, though, keep the knees inward, the thighs parallel with one another, and press downward through the inner edge of each foot. Then release your hands, sweep them up over your head again to the floor, and slowly uncurl your spine. When the sacrum reaches the floor, lower your heels and relax.

## HOW TO USE A BLANKET

Whether you choose to use blankets or not is up to you. It's a good idea to know how to use them for Shoulderstand, though, because they make the pose safer and considerably easier. Blankets elevate the shoulders. This takes the weight off your neck, which allows the neck muscles to stretch slowly and safely. Using blankets for Shoulderstand is not essential, by any means, but they do make the pose easier because less neck flexion is required in order to be straight. Practice the pose with blankets and without, and see which method you prefer.

**1** Place two or three folded blankets on the floor, then lie with your back and shoulders on the blankets and your head on the floor. Position your shoulders two to three inches from the edge so that when you roll into Plow and then raise your legs into Shoulderstand, the tops of your shoulders and the seventh cervical vertebrae (the protruding bone at the base of your neck) are on the blanket. Be sure the blankets are wider than your shoulders and as long as your back so that the shoulders, arms, and elbows are level and rest firmly on the blankets, and when you roll out of the pose after Shoulderstand you have a level surface for your entire back.

## BASIC SARVANGASANA SERIES

The Basic Sarvangasana Series has six stages to it. It may take you a while before you have the stamina required to do them all in a row without stopping, so be patient. Increase your strength, flexibility, and length of time you stay in the various stages gradually. Come down and rest whenever you need to. You can always go up again.

## EASY PLOW—HALASANA

**1** Lie on your back, legs bent, feet flat, arms over your head on the floor.

**2** Bring your knees in toward your chest, then straighten your legs toward the ceiling. Be here several breaths waiting for the inner cue to begin. When you are ready, breathe in deeply.

**3** As you exhale, bring your legs over your head into Halasana, Plow Pose (photo 187). Do this with as little momentum as possible. Be in an easy Plow with your toes turned under and your spine slightly curved. Relax in this position and acclimatize to the stretch. This feels exquisite. Breathe smoothly. If your neck and back are stiff, you may find it difficult to bring your feet all the way over to the floor. Take your time. Wait for the intensity to diminish before proceeding.

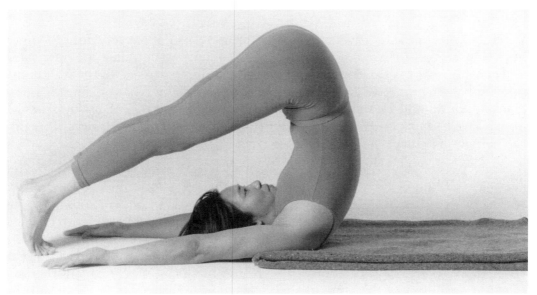

**187**

Do not use force. It's essential that this pose open up for you before attempting Shoulderstand.

**4** Be here one minute, though a few seconds may be enough for you at first; if so, come down. Do not stay in the pose if you are excessively uncomfortable. Repetition rather than duration is best at first. If this position is difficult for you, spend more time with standing poses, the three precursor poses, as well as the cat tilt portion of Cat Pose, in which you curl your head in and round your back to the extreme. Plow will make your spine strong, healthy, flexible, and free.

## KNEES TO EARS POSE—*KARNA PIDASANA*

**1** **From the Plow Pose, sweep your arms up, taking them to the floor behind your back. Interlace your hands, then roll the upper arms out, straighten the arms, and do "the wriggle."** Wriggle the shoulders away from your ears so you come on top of the shoulders, then extend a line of energy outward through the arms in the direction they are pointing.

**2** **Bend your knees down by your ears** (photo 188). Relax in this position and breathe smoothly. Acclimatize to the stretch, conform to this shape. Learn to be here with as little resistance or unwillingness as possible. This is the most important stage in terms of being able to achieve a vertical Shoulderstand because the cervical and upper thoracic areas of the spine are fully stretched. Wriggle deeper

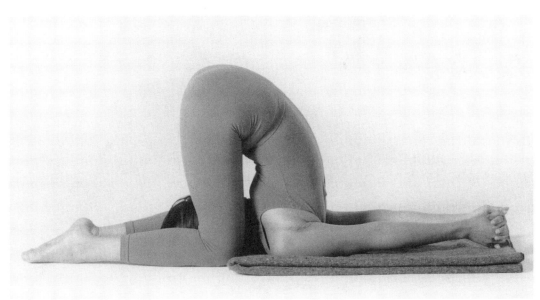

**188**

when you can and position yourself on top of the shoulders. Your toes can be pointed or turned under, whichever is more comfortable for you. Be here one minute.

**3** If this position is easy, bring your knees together on top of your head and slide them toward the floor, bringing your pelvis farther over your face. This is a fantastic stretch, usually requiring many months of practice. Be patient and gently persistent.

## DOG TILT PLOW—*HALASANA*

**1 Come into Plow Pose again, this time with your back straight and hips in dog tilt.** First, release your hand clasp, then bend your arms and place your hands on your back as close to the floor as possible. Press the ball of each index finger into your back and flatten the palms, pressing the rib cage forward. Then turn your toes under, straighten the legs, and straighten your back by turning your hips toward dog tilt.

**2** The idea is to elongate your spine vertically. Do this by pressing the shoulders and upper arms down as you stretch straight upward through the sitting bones. The neck will flex into a tight chin lock, and the upper back muscles will contract and draw inward toward the spine, causing the sternum to expand toward your face. As you push from your toes and rotate the pelvis strongly toward dog tilt, the spine will grow powerful as it lifts the hips and straightens, bringing the pelvis directly above the shoulders. This requires tremendous spinal strength and flexibility, but it also *develops* tremendous spinal strength and flexibility. Be here one minute.

**3** If you are unable to straighten your back, put your feet on a small stool, chair, or wall and do the correct action (photo 189). This will enable you to establish dog tilt and pull your spine straight. With practice, you will be able to do this with your feet on the floor, but it's more important at this stage to have your legs and back straight than it is to touch the floor.

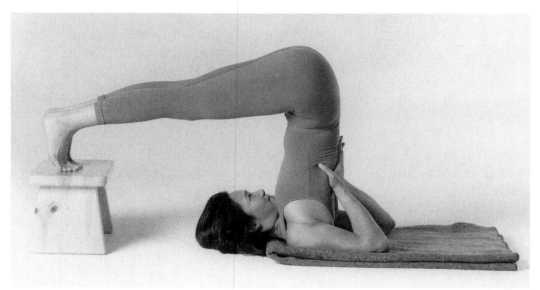

**189**

## HALF SHOULDERSTAND—*VIPARITA KARANI*

**1 Tip your hips backward and bring your legs up to a forty-five-degree angle** (photo 190). Push from your toes, tip your hips backward into a more pronounced dog tilt, and allow your feet to leave the floor, bringing them up until they point upward. Move your spine into your back, open and expand the chest, and make your back slightly concave. Align your legs by pressing them fully straight, rolling them inward until your kneecaps face forward, and keeping the ankles together. Spread your toes and gently press the inner edge of each foot away from you. Be here one minute. Breathe smoothly. This is an excellent back strengthener and preparation for Shoulderstand.

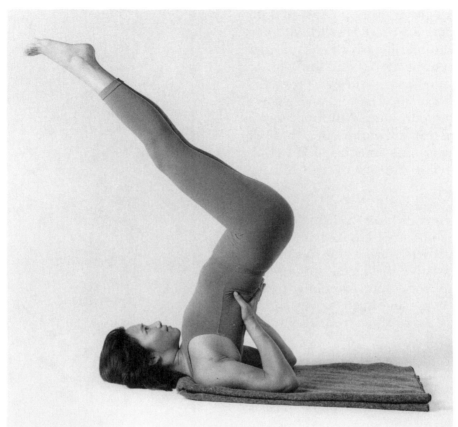

**190**

## SHOULDERSTAND—*SARVANGASANA*

**1** **Slowly raise your legs until they form a vertical line with your torso** (photo 191). Notice how your pelvis rotates toward cat tilt as your feet go up.

**2** Keep your legs together, your feet together, your kneecaps facing straight ahead, and your toes spread, then stretch straight upward through the inner core formed by the merger of your two legs. From the root of your spine, stretch upward through your legs and feet, so the line of energy flows freely upward. This will pull your torso and spine more erect, so that eventually, gradually, the core through your legs and the core through your trunk merge to become one long continuous core—an upward-moving, grounded flow. The tips of the sitting bones and the line through your legs will then point straight upward. Keep thinking upward through your feet—that's how you become straight.

**3** Wriggle your elbows inward until the upper arms are parallel with one another and slide your hands farther down your back (toward the floor) to brace yourself securely. Press the shoulders, upper arms, and elbows into the floor, squeeze the upper arms inward toward one another, contract the upper back muscles, and stretch your trunk upward away from the floor.

**4** Keep your head straight throughout the pose, not crooked, and never turn your face from side to side. Let the line down the middle of your face line up with your sternum, navel, pubic bone, and inner ankles so the ears are equidistant from the shoulders.

**5** Breathe smoothly, deeply, adjusting your arms and hands when necessary to insure that your spine is lifted, erect and supported. This is a wonderful pose. Do not strain. Enjoy the way you feel. Be here one to five minutes.

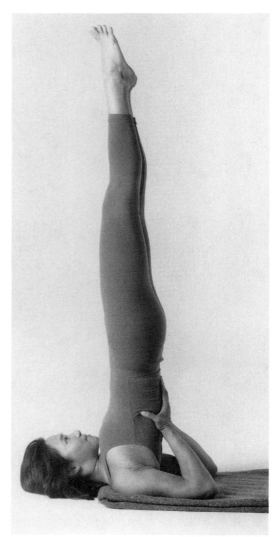

191

## TRANQUILLITY POSE—ANANDASANA

**1 From Shoulderstand, tip your hips backward (dog tilt) and lower your legs to a forty-five-degree angle.** Keep your back straight, even slightly concave.

**2 Reach up and place your hands on your thighs, just above your knees**

(photo 192). Keep your legs straight, thighs rolling in, toes spread, and then slowly press your arms straight. Balance. This is tricky at first, but once you find the balance it soon becomes very comfortable. Tranquillity Pose is like Half Shoulderstand, except for the different hand placement. Be here one minute.

**3** If you prefer, do Lotus Tranquillity. Cross your legs into Lotus, fold at your hips, reach up and place your hands on your knees, then straighten the arms. Here, also, you'll be in dog tilt. This pose is one of the best.

**4 To come out of Tranquillity Pose, bend your elbows and bring your feet to the floor.** You are now in the Easy Plow again. Stretch your arms toward your feet, straighten your legs, then slowly roll down your back keeping your legs close to your body. When your sacrum reaches the floor, bend your knees and place both feet flat. Sweep your arms to your sides and, without turning your head from side to side, rest quietly for a few moments. Enjoy the way you feel. This is a particularly good time to practice stillness.

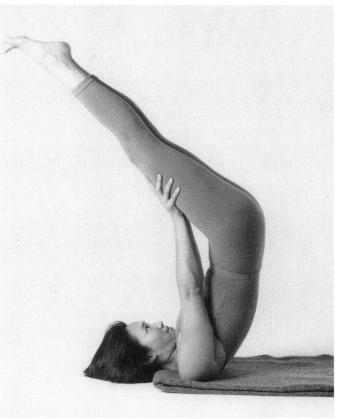

**192**

# Benefits: Shoulderstand Cycle *or* Sarvangasana

Irrigates brain, thyroid, parathyroid. Strengthens upper body. Opens chest. Stretches neck, shoulders, and upper back muscles. Stimulates circulation and energy flow through neck to brain and body. Improves digestion and elimination. Relieves fatigue. Relaxing. Aid to insomnia and exhaustion. Soothing, energizing. Calms and rejuvenates body. Nurturing effect.

## TWISTS

# 39 Easy Noose Pose *or Pashasana*

### STAGE ONE

**1** Sit on the floor with your legs bent, feet flat and together.

**2** **Wrap the left arm around the outside of both knees, catching hold of the right calf with your left hand** (photo 193). **Place your right hand on the floor directly behind you.** Put your awareness at the crown of your head and feel for any discernible sensations in that area, then move the crown of your head straight upward. Elongate your spine, press both sitting bones downward into the floor, and achieve maximum extension from your sitting bones and coccyx to the fontanel. Keep feeling that sensation at the top of your head.

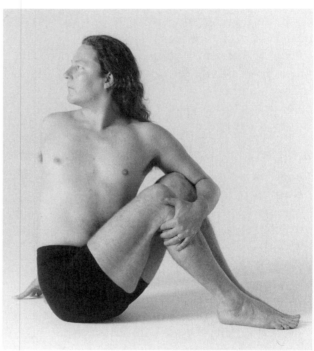

**193**

**3** **Twist:** As you inhale, lift your chest and pull your spine upward; as you exhale, rotate to the right. From there, inhale and elongate farther upward, then rotate deeper as you exhale. Press your right hand and sitting bones into the floor, pull with your left hand, and stretch upward through the crown of your head—then revolve your body and rib cage around your spine so you feel like a spiral of curving energy going up and around.

**4** Turn your head to the right some of the time, to the left some of the time, then in the direction your chest is facing. Breathe smoothly, with feeling.

## STAGE TWO

**5** **Bring the left arm to the outside of the right knee and place your left hand on the floor beside you. Walk the right hand farther around behind you** (photo 194).

**6** Elongate and rotate the spine, as before. This is more difficult now because of the position you're in. It's not as easy to pull the spine upward, and it requires more flexibility to revolve your body around your spine. Endeavor to do so as effortlessly as possible.

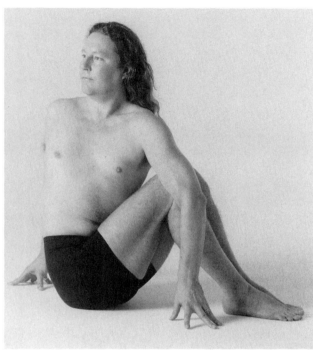

**194**

**7** Gently press your hands and sitting bones downward into the floor, lift the rib cage upward away from the waist, and move the fontanel straight upward. Then rotate your chest to the right, your head to the right, and roll both shoulders backward as you increase the spinal twist. Rotate as much as possible. Gaze straight backward. This feels exquisite. Gently wring yourself out. Breathe.

## STAGE THREE

**8** **Clasp hold of the right foot with your left hand** (photo 195). If you were able to rotate sufficiently in Stage Two, then it should not be too difficult to extend your left arm and clasp the right foot. Have your right hand on the floor directly behind you again, and then endeavor first to elongate and then rotate your spine in this new position. Stay immersed in the rhythm of your breathing. Focus on the sensations of stretch. Relax with the intensity and allow yourself to rotate deeper into the twist. Gaze into infinity. Allow the stretch to penetrate. Be here several or many breaths, anywhere from half a minute to a minute or two. Then do the other side.

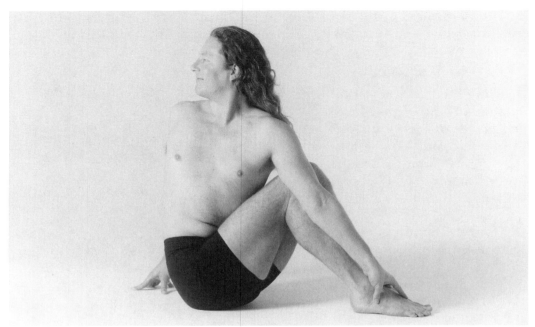

**195**

# Benefits: Twists

Twists wring out your body and thereby assist in releasing enormous amounts of tension. When you then release the twisting, wringing-out action, and the musculature relaxes again, that area becomes flooded with nutrients. This is both deeply cleansing and deeply nourishing. It feels good. Your body will like it. It feels better to be tension-free than it does to be tight and held in a contracted or semicontracted state. Wring yourself out with the various twisting postures, and then relax for a few moments after the pose to experience the benefit. Feel yourself being flooded with new nourishment, then do the other side.

Twists are especially good for the spine, strengthening the small muscles that link the vertebrae, and keeping the whole structure—from the base of the spine to the crown of your head—free and mobile. When compression or contraction sets in, microcirculation is diminished. And when circulation is impaired, then those areas become malnourished; in effect, they starve and dry up. With improved mobility, however, and the release of tension in the back muscles, spine, abdominal organs, shoulders, neck, and hips, there is improved circulation and energy flow. Those areas—the spine, especially—will then receive welcome nourishment. And since every nerve throughout the body stems from and originates in the spinal cord, every part of the body will rejuvenate, heal, and become vital. You, as an energy presence, will become both more comfortable and more powerful, more imbued with life force. A tense, dry sense of self will give way to a youthful, hydrated, strong, highly elastic, vital sense of self. As the trunk rotates, the kidneys and abdominal organs are activated and exercised. This improves digestion and removes sluggishness. Backaches, headaches, and stiffness in the neck and shoulders can all be eliminated or diminished. You'll also notice your perceptions becoming more acute. Hearing and eyesight can improve. A heightened sensitivity can help us be more in tune with ourselves, other people, the world and universe.

As you practice these poses, remember always to lengthen the spine first before twisting. Lengthening creates space between the vertebrae, which makes for safer, deeper twisting. There should be a spiraling, corkscrewlike feeling to the twist, going up and around, starting from the base and moving upward.

# Benefits: Easy Noose Pose *or Pashasana*

Teaches principle of extension during twisting movement. Strengthens and rotates spine fully, releasing tension, improving circulation and energy flow. Massages and stimulates abdominal organs, thereby improving digestion and elimination. Frees rib cage, expands chest, loosens shoulders and neck.

# 40 Sage Twist *or Marichyasana*

**1** **Sit on the floor with both legs straight. Bend the right leg, lift the right foot over the left leg, and place your right foot on the floor adjacent to the left knee.** Wriggle the buttocks backward so you are on the tips of the sitting bones, sit tall, and check that both sitting bones are pressed equally into the floor.

**2** There will be a tendency for the right buttock to lift from the floor as you deepen the twist and move through the following stages. Minimize this. Keep both sitting bones pressed down throughout the pose so the pelvis remains level. Only then can the spine be pulled up straight.

### STAGE ONE

**3** **Wrap the left arm around the right knee, positioning the knee in the crook of the left elbow. Clasp hold of your wrists or elbows** (photo 196). Gaze forward in the direction of your left foot.

**4** Roll the left leg inward until the kneecap faces the ceiling and the inner edge of the left foot is vertical, then spread your toes and press the ball of the foot away from you. Flow energy through your leg.

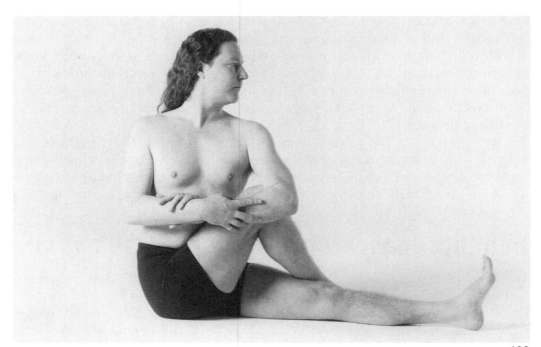

**196**

**5 Sit tall.** Align your torso and elongate your core. First, pull the abdominals in. Then press downward through both sitting bones, especially the right one, bring your lower back in and up, and elongate your core upward through the crown of your head. Lift the chest away from the waist and pull inward with your arms, squeezing the right leg toward your chest as you gently thrust your chest toward the leg. You'll probably feel the stretch in your right hip. Relax the shoulders down, and remind yourself that if you want one part of your body to rise upward, you press another part downward—whatever is on the floor. Here, press the right foot, left leg, and sitting bones downward in order to elongate your core upward. Tremendous spinal strength is required to do this, as well as flexibility in the right hip and buttock.

**6** Breathe smoothly. Let the stretch penetrate. Wait for the sensations of intensity to diminish before proceeding. As you are waiting, feel your way through the pose. Let your awareness roam around and through your body. Endeavor to release every hint of strain. Expand, relax where you can, yet maintain the action of the pose.

**7** Emphasize the upward spinal elongation during each inhalation, actually using the breath to coax the spine and rib cage upward; and gently squeeze inward with your arms during each exhalation. Inhale lift, exhale squeeze—back and forth with the breath. Feel the rhythm. Do not be in a rush. Immerse yourself in the flow. Be here until your body asks for more.

## STAGE TWO

**8** **Bring the back of the left upper arm to the outside of the right knee and place both hands on the floor** (photo 197). Be aware of the tendency for the right sitting bone to float away from the floor. Keep the right sitting bone grounded.

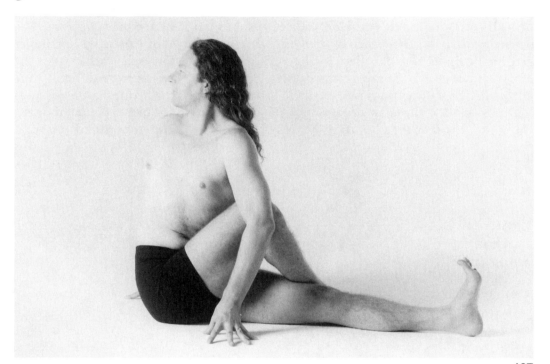

**197**

**9** **Twist:** Inhale as you press both hands downward into the floor and bring the lower back in and up to elongate the spine, thus achieving maximum spinal extension; exhale as you press the back of your left arm into the leg and rotate your rib cage to the right. First your belly turns, then your chest, then your head. Walk the right hand around behind you more, twist deeper, and gaze straight backward.

**10** The perineum and sitting bones go down, the hands press down, the fontanel goes up, and both shoulders pull backward as you lift and rotate the chest. This feels exquisite. Proceed slowly. Do not be in a rush to get to the deeper stages. You can twist your spine fully here. Savor the way this feels.

**11** Breathe smoothly, emphasizing the upward action as you inhale and deepening the twist as you exhale, even subtly. Gently spin your rib cage around your spine. Close your eyes and experience yourself as a strong curve of energy spiraling up and down and around. Feel the curve, become one with the curve, follow it deeper. Rotate. Be here until your body asks for a change.

## STAGE THREE

**12** **Clasp the left knee or right foot with your left hand** (photo 198). This will lock you into place. The ease with which you can clasp your knee or foot depends on how much you were able to rotate your rib cage in Stage Two. The deeper you twist, the easier this will be—because the right knee and left upper arm will contact one another closer to the shoulder and armpit, rather than the elbow. If the contact point is nearer the elbow, you'll have a more difficult time with this stage. Try, therefore, to have the contact point of your arm and leg as high toward the shoulder as possible. The closer it is to the armpit and shoulder, the easier it will be for you to catch hold of the left knee and, ultimately, the right foot.

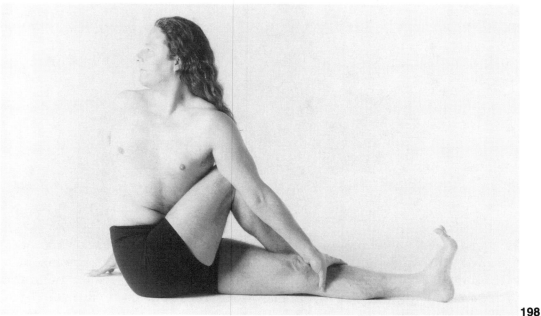

198

**13** Breathe smoothly, acclimatize to the stretch, then ease your way deeper. A fraction of an inch is a lot. Elongate your core as you inhale, rotate as you exhale. Have your right hand on the floor behind you for support, and use both the inhale and exhale to ease your way deeper into the pose. Relax as you deepen the twist, but do so without losing the action of the pose. Do and not-do at the same time.

**14** Check your alignment and take stock of where you are. The left arm is straight, with the hand holding either the left knee or right foot. The plane through your shoulders is on the same line as the left leg, and your chest is therefore facing sideways. The right hand is on the floor behind you, your gaze is straight backward, and because of this positioning, your spine and core will naturally spiral upward. Be here until you are ready for more.

## STAGE FOUR

**15** **Slip your left hand and arm through the triangular opening formed by your right knee. Clasp your hands behind you** (photo 199). The left hand does the clasping. Eventually, slide your right arm deeper and clasp hold of the right wrist. Pull the spine and chest upward and tighten the twist by rolling both shoulders backward.

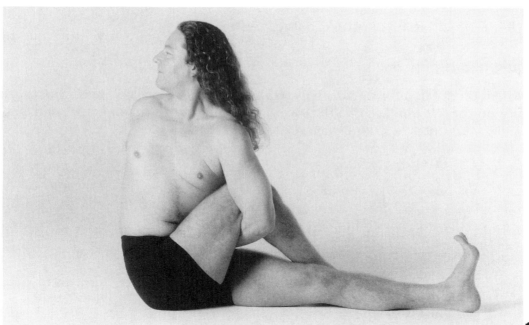

**199**

**16** Breathe smoothly, with feeling. Expand the shape from inside, using the breath. Gaze backward some of the time, forward some of the time. Be here half a minute to one minute.

**17** Remember, you can only fully enjoy something when you give your full attention to that thing; and the more you pay attention, the more you'll find to interest you. Therefore, now, immerse yourself in the rhythm of your breathing, the sensations of stretch, and the feeling-tone of the pose. Enjoy the way this feels. Learn to be guided from within.

**18** Reverse the legs and do the pose on the other side. Take your time. Give each stage its due.

# Benefits: Sage Twist *or Marichyasana*

Strengthens back, rotates spine fully, erases backache, stretches hip. Tones and massages the abdominal area, especially liver, spleen, intestines. Relieves lower back pain caused by muscular tension. Frees chest, makes shoulders elastic.

# 41 Rishi Twist I & II *or Bharadvajasana I, II*

Here are two variations of an exquisite twisting pose.

### RISHI TWIST I

**1** **Sit on the floor with your legs straight. Bend the legs and bring both feet beside the left hip.** Position the left shinbone in the arch of your right foot, and allow your knees to separate about a foot.

### STAGE ONE

**2** **Turn your chest so you are facing the right knee, then lean backward on both hands.** Pull the abdominals in and move the shoulders backward.

**3** **Curve into a backbend** (photo 200): As you inhale, lift and expand your chest upward, away from the waist; then exhale and press your chest forward and upward as you curve your head backward. Go up and over, like a fountain, letting your head come back last.

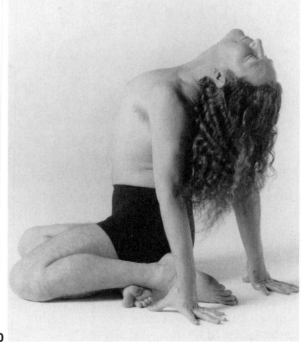

**200**

**4** Breathe deeply, with feeling. Use your breathing to expand the shape from inside. Close your eyes, go within, feel—then express the meaning of the pose without inhibition. Bloom your chest toward the ceiling. Get round. Be here half a minute.

**5** When you're nearly done, inhale deeply and, as you exhale, gently accelerate your energy through the pose. Then bring your head to normal alignment.

## STAGE TWO

**6** **Place the left hand on the right knee and the right hand on the floor behind you.** Bring your navel gently backward toward the spine.

**7** **Twist** (photo 201). As you inhale, expand the rib cage upward, away from the waist, and as you exhale, rotate your chest to the right. Do this over and over, breath by breath. Bring your chest up to the maximum, move the shoulders backward and down away from the ears, flatten the shoulder blades into your back, pull with your left arm to help you twist, and turn your head to the right as the natural consequence of your spiraling torso. Keep the navel firmly backward toward the spine, tighten the twist by turning your head fully, and gaze straight backward into infinity.

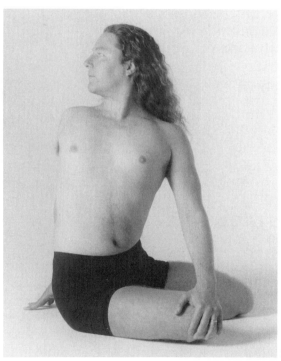

**201**

**8** Close your eyes, breathe smoothly, and immerse yourself in the feeling-tone of the pose. Experience yourself as a spiraling curve of energy. Go within and be guided by the inner feeling, intuitively making subtle internal adjustments until your alignment feels precise. Go where it feels best, where your energy flows best. Exercise your ability to sense this.

**9** When you are almost done, turn your head left. Inhale deeply, then exhale and rotate fully as you accelerate your energy for a few seconds—head left, torso right. Savor this part. Then release the stretch.

## RISHI TWIST II

**1** **Sit on the floor with the left leg in Hero and the right leg in Half Lotus Pose. Bring the right arm behind you and clasp the right foot** (photo 202). Use a belt to span the gap if you cannot catch hold. Separate the knees until your thighs are at right angles with one another, then turn your chest to face the right knee. The plane through your shoulders will now be on the same line as your left thigh. Rest your left hand on your left knee.

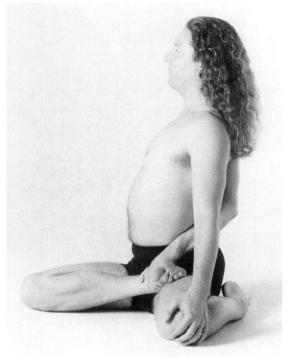

**202**

## STAGE ONE

**2** **Sit tall.** Merge downward into the earth through the perineum and sitting bones, become thoroughly grounded, then move your lower back in and extend your spine upward. Allow your chest to expand, softening the shoulders backward and bringing the navel backward toward the spine. Do not rock forward onto the frontal edge of the sitting bones in your attempt to be erect; that will create excessive dog tilt and cause you to become ungrounded. Instead, align your torso and elongate your core by moving the crown of the head and sitting bones away from one another, straight up and straight down.

**3** Allow the lotus knee to leave the floor, if necessary, in order to root both sitting bones and become grounded. Work toward keeping the knee on the floor—and staying grounded—as you pull upward through your spine and core. This will give you a deeper twist.

**4** Breathe smoothly. Acclimatize to this shape. Be here until your body asks for more, at least half a minute.

## STAGE TWO

**5** **Lean backward on your left hand** by pulling the abdominals in and moving the shoulders backward.

**6** **Curve into a backbend** (photo 203): As you inhale, lift and expand your chest upward, away from the waist, then exhale and press forward with your chest as you arch backward. Curve your head and chest upward, letting your head come back last.

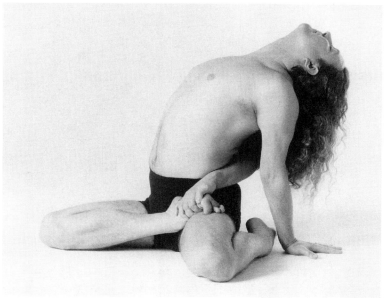

**203**

**7** Breathe deeply, with feeling, expanding the shape from inside. Close your eyes, go within, feel—then intuitively express the meaning of the pose. Bloom your chest toward the ceiling. Get round. Be here half a minute.

**8** When you're nearly done, inhale deeply and, as you exhale, accelerate your energy by pressing upward through your chest and outward through your chin. This feels exquisite. Enjoy what's happening. Then bring your head to normal alignment.

## STAGE THREE

**9** **Place the left hand on the right knee.** Check that you're still grounded, both sitting bones pressing equally into the floor.

**10** **Twist** (photo 204): As you inhale, lift and expand the rib cage upward away from the waist, and as you exhale, rotate to the right. Pull gently with both hands, move both shoulders backward, and squeeze the right elbow away from you. Continue lifting the chest, bringing it forward through the shoulders. Turn your head and gave over your right shoulder.

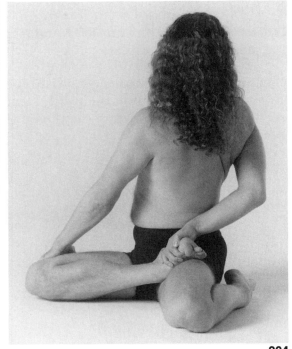

**204**

**11** Bring the pose to life with your breathing. Use your inhalations to lift and expand the chest—elongating your core and spine, even just a little. With your exhalations, rotate deeper into the twist, even a little—even just mentally. Immerse yourself in the rhythm and pulse of your breathing. When you cannot deepen the twist any farther, then be where you are and acclimatize to the stretch. Become more effortless without losing the action of the pose. Be here one minute.

**12** When you're nearly done, turn your head left. Inhale deeply, then exhale and rotate fully as you accelerate your energy for a few seconds—head left, torso right. Wring yourself out. Savor this part. Make it exhilarating. Then release the stretch and do it on the other side.

# Benefits: Rishi Twist I & II *or Bharadvajasana I, II*

Rotates spine fully, releases tension in back, neck, chest, and shoulders. Increases flexibility of ankles, knees, hips, chest, rib cage, shoulders, neck.

# 42 Extended Leg Half Lotus Twist *or* *Parivrrta Ardha Padmasana*

## STAGE ONE

**1** **Sit on the floor with the left leg straight and the right leg in Half Lotus, then take the right arm behind you and clasp the right foot.** Use a belt to span the gap if you cannot catch hold.

**2** Move the right knee away from the left knee until your thighs form a right angle, turn your body to the right so your chest is facing the right knee, and place your left hand on the left knee. The plane between your shoulders will now be on the same line as your left leg.

**3** **Sit tall.** Merge downward into the earth through the perineum and sitting bones and elongate upward through the fontanel. Lift and expand your chest, move the shoulders backward, shoulder blades down, and keep your navel gently backward toward the spine. Breathe smoothly. Wait for the inner cue to proceed.

## STAGE TWO

**4** **Slide your hand to the left ankle.** Look down your left arm and align the left elbow and shoulder directly above the left leg. Roll the upper arm out and shrug the left shoulder down, away from the ear. Pull the abdominals in and up. Exhale.

**5** **Twist** (photo 205): As you inhale, bring your lower back in and up, expanding the rib cage upward away from the waist; breathe upward into the sternum to elongate your spine and core. As you exhale, push into your left hand, twist into the pose by turning your belly, chest, and head to the right, and then pull gently with your right hand. Press the back of the left thigh firmly down into the floor, and as you rotate deeper into the pose, endeavor to move the right knee away from you. Retain the alignment of your left arm. Gaze straight backward.

**6** The tendency here will be to pull yourself toward the left leg with your left hand. Instead, *press* the left arm fully straight so you stay up, away from the leg. Push with the left hand and pull with the right, moving the right elbow backward. Expand your chest away from the waist, turn your chest and head to the right, roll both shoulders backward, and slide the shoulder blades down your back to help open the chest. Keep the navel backward toward the spine. Keep moving your chest forward through the shoulders.

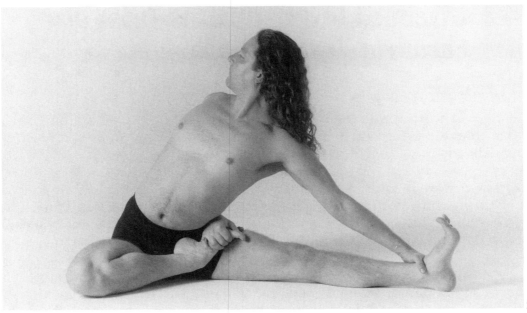

**205**

**7** Breathe smoothly, with feeling. Bring the pose to life. With your inhalations, expand the chest upward, moving the thoracic spine (behind the heart) in and up to open and support the chest. With your exhalations, gently rotate deeper into the twist.

**8** Gaze straight backward into infinity some of the time, and forward toward your left hand and foot some of the time.

**9** When you cannot rotate any farther, stay where you are, continue breathing smoothly, and acclimatize to the intense stretch. Fine-tune the alignment of your energy flow and try to be relaxed without losing the dynamic stillness of the pose. Go after the twist calmly. Be here one minute. When you sense that it is nearly time to come out of the pose, inhale deeply; then exhale and rotate fully, accelerating your energy for a few seconds. Enjoy the way this feels. Then release the pose and change sides.

# Benefits: Extended Leg Half Lotus Twist *or Parivrrta Ardha Padmasana*

Gives a tremendous stretch and rotation to chest and spine. Strengthens back, spine, core. Relieves tension in upper, middle, lower back. Frees rib cage, chest, and shoulders. Increases ankle, hip, knee flexibility for Lotus.

# 43 Reclining Twist I & II *or Supta Parivartanasana I, II*

### RECLINING TWIST I

**1** **Start on your back with your legs bent, feet flat and together.**

**2** **Bring the knees toward your chest.** Flatten your sacrum and lower back, and wriggle the shoulder blades under so your back is flat and comfortable. Flex your feet and spread your toes.

**3** **As you exhale, take your legs to the right.** Bring them upward toward your chest as you slowly lower them to the floor (photo 206). Slide the left shoulder blade down your back so the shoulder stays flat and the chest stays expanded. Turn your head and gaze toward your left hand.

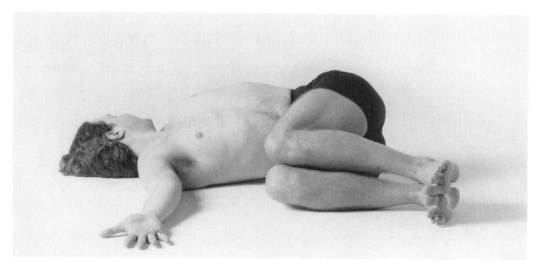

**206**

**4** Breathe smoothly. Let the stretch penetrate. Be here one minute.

**5** Repeat on the other side, then return to starting position.

## RECLINING TWIST II

**1** **Lie on your back with your legs bent, feet flat and together.**

**2** **Cross the left leg over the right leg.** Snuggle them together so there's no space between your thighs.

**3** **Shift your hips to the left a few inches, then exhale and tip your legs to the right** (photo 207). Endeavor to rest fully on the outside edge of your right hip and thigh. Your pelvis and shoulders will be at right angles to one another, giving the full length of your spine a superb twist. Weight the legs down with your right hand and reach outward to the left with your left. Lift your chest away from the waist, slide the left shoulder blade down your back so the shoulder, upper arm, and hand stay on the floor, and gaze toward the ceiling or in the direction of your left hand.

**4** Be here one minute, breathing smoothly. Let the stretch penetrate. Enjoy the way this feels.

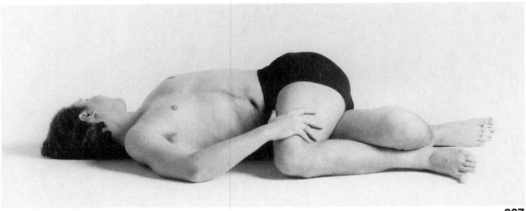

**207**

# Benefits: Reclining Twist I & II *or Supta Parivartanasana I, II*

Relieves tension in lower back and hips, tones abdominal area, frees chest and shoulders. Soothing to spine and neck. Improves digestion, elimination.

## FINISHING POSES

# 44 Relaxation Pose *or Shavasana*

**1  Sit on the floor with your legs bent, feet flat** (photo 208).

**2  Come down onto your elbows** (photo 209). Lift your pelvis away from the floor an inch or two, and turn your hips toward cat tilt, rotating the pelvis backward. Then, keeping your pelvis in cat tilt, place your lower back and sacrum on the floor again and allow them to relax into the floor.

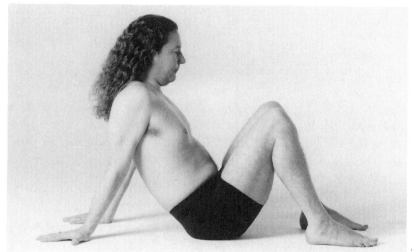

208

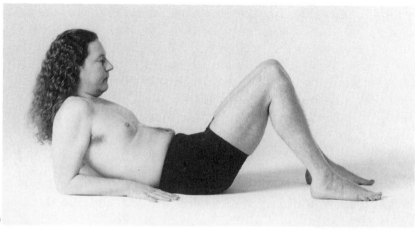

209

**3** **Lie flat** (photo 210). Move your elbows sideways and slowly bring your back down to rest on the floor. Extend your arms to your sides away from your body, palms up, then wriggle your back and shoulders, flatten the shoulder blades, and make yourself comfortable. Rest on the center point of the back of your skull.

**4** **Slide your legs straight, one at a time.** Have your feet about shoulder-width apart, and allow them to fall outward.

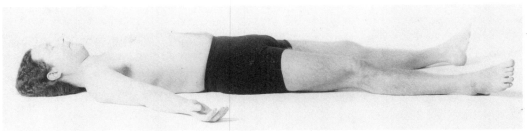

**210**

**5** Check that your legs are comfortably far apart, your arms are comfortably away from your body, and your head is straight. Do not have your arms or legs so close together that you feel cramped, held in, or claustrophobic, nor so far apart that your energy feels dispersed. Be symmetrical, comfortable. Find your perfect alignment, then give yourself permission to relax and do nothing for the next few minutes. Close your eyes.

**6** The technique is simple. Keep it simple. All you do is relax, everywhere—and then be aware of how you feel. Relax and feel. That's it, in brief. Relax every physical and mental tension, temporarily let go of everything you don't need, and then simply pay attention and see what happens. For these few minutes, willingly put aside your worries, fears, and concerns of the day, and release every discernible hint of tension in your body—and then be aware of how you feel. *Savor* the way you feel. Experience what's happening right there where you are.

**7** The tendency is to be unconsciously tense or anxious, both physically and mentally, and because it feels normal, we barely even notice it. The idea, there-fore, is to be increasingly conscious of tensions, of where your body is uncomfort-able or tight, even just a little, and then deliberately to release them and relax in order to experience what it feels like (what *you* feel like!) to be completely tension-free: not uptight anywhere, not contracted, not compacted or compressed, not deflated or depressed, not shielded, not in a posture of self-protection or self-defense, but voluntarily undefended and relaxed—and therefore expansive, spa-cious, clear, clean, wide open, and wide awake.

**8** This is more than just relaxing your body and muscles after an asana session, a way of getting relief. It's the essence of yoga made simple: going within and experiencing yourself. The feeling-tone of undefended, uncontracted, undistorted being is stillness, peace—and the peace of stillness feels good, not blah, not nothing, but good, positively blissful. Peace is a higher energy state than what we're used to. Peace is high-energy centeredness, dynamic calm. As you practice Relaxation Pose on a regular basis, then, and as the peace of Infinite Being becomes increasingly familiar to you as being the feeling-tone of your being, you will discover that it is *always* available to be experienced. The feeling of calm bliss is right there, here—always. It is not far away, hard to access. Nor is it something you create. It's something you let yourself relax into. It becomes a choice: Tension or relaxation? Contracted being or undefended being? Conflict, anxiety, physical discomfort . . . or peace? Deep, healing, soothing peace. If you want peace, relax. The choice becomes easy once you realize you have a choice.

**9** **Relax.** It feels like melting. Do this by scanning your awareness around and through your body—the space inside your body and the space around your body—alert to where there is unnecessary contraction, discomfort, tension, or excessive energy. Let go of every hint of holding on.

**10** Start at your hands. Rest your awareness in the area of your hands: the palms, thumbs, fingers, the space between your fingers, the fingertips, fingernails, the back of your hands, the wrists, the space inside your hands, and the space around your hands. Forget about what they look like, what you *remember* they look like, and instead immerse your awareness in the way they actually feel to you now. Go into your hands and *feel* them. Gradually, you may begin to sense heat or warmth, then a pleasant, tingling, electricity-like sensation. Feel the energy in your hands.

**11** As your hands relax, feel them expanding. Feel them becoming less dense, less thick, less contracted—more spacious inside, more comfortable. Feel this happening, and let them expand without limit. Notice how as they relax and expand, every tension evaporates, disappears. It may even begin to feel as though your hands aren't there, as though there's just wide open tingling space where your hands once were. Enjoy the way this feels.

**12** Allow this new sense of expanded and tingling openness to flow upward through your arms at its own leisurely pace, until your hands, arms, and shoulders feel tension-free, transparent, clear.

**13** Direct your attention to your feet. Go into your feet and *feel* them. Relax the sole of each foot, relax the arches, relax the toes, the space between the toes, the top of each foot, the ankles, the heels, the space inside your feet, and the space around your feet. Feel the energy in your feet. Again, forget about what they look like, what you remember they look like, and instead immerse your conscious awareness in the way they actually feel.

**14** When the tingling sensation in your feet becomes established in your awareness as with your arms, now allow it to flow slowly upward through your legs, torso, and head—until your whole body is experiencing this pleasurable tingling vibration.

**15** Savor the way your legs feel: the ankles, calves, shinbones, knees, thighs, inner thighs, back of thighs, all the way up into the hips, pelvis, genitals, and buttocks. Feel the energy in your legs and pelvis, feel the space around your legs, and allow your awareness to roam through this whole area at its own comfortable pace. Again, enjoy the way this feels, and allow yourself to be intrigued with your actual now-experience. Forget about what your legs look like, and instead experience yourself and body as you actually are. Experience your legs becoming transparent and clear.

**16** Relax your abdomen and belly, and let your breathing be normal, free, unrestricted. Feel your belly rise and fall with each breath, and experience how this gentle, continuous movement ripples through your whole body and can be felt everywhere. Ride the breath. Stay aware of your breathing. Savor the air on both the inhale and exhale.

**17** Keep bringing your awareness slowly upward through your torso, and let the movement of your breathing relax your lower back, diaphragm, ribs, chest, heart. Let this whole area relax, expand, and become tension-free. Release every hint of holding on. Let go completely.

**18** Relax your neck, throat, face, and head. Relax your mouth, the corners of your mouth, the lips, the jaw. Relax your nose, your cheeks, your ears, the back of your head, the scalp muscles, your forehead, your eyebrows, and especially your eyes. Relax the muscles around the eyes, the muscles deep in the eye sockets, the inner corner of each eye, the outer corner, the space between the eyes, the eyelids, eyelashes, the eyeballs themselves, the pupils. Be intimately aware of this whole area. Soften every tension you come upon, even little ones, even just a little. Relax areas that do not feel tense, too. Relax everywhere, letting your eyes fall backward away from the eyelids. Let go of all the usual tensions that feel like you. Feel the energy in your face. Glow.

**19** Feel the space inside your body and the space around your body. Notice that as you relax and expand, every tension evaporates, disappears. It may even begin to feel as though your body isn't there, as though there's just wide open tingling space. Be aware of what's happening. You're releasing tensions, melting, and therefore expanding—everywhere. You're deliberately letting go of all the lumps in your energy field, all the areas of compacted, held, blocked energy. You're clarifying, purifying, washing yourself clean with awareness. Your actual now-experience of yourself is becoming, more and more, that of being less dense, less blocked or held in, less physical, in a sense, and increasingly transparent or luminous, more consciously spiritlike. Notice how comfortable you are, how awake and at ease, unusual perhaps at first, but normal, familiar. It feels good to let yourself be this open. Enjoy the way you feel.

**20** Continue releasing tensions until there are none left, until you feel wide open like the sky. This spacious, conscious comfortableness is known as the "sky of Mind," or pure conscious awareness, and relaxing into yourself like this is how you can consciously experience your unity with infinity. Become thoroughly familiar with what it feels like to be this open, relaxed, fearless, and undefended. Feel the peace of stillness.

**21** As you relax you will expand. You will begin to feel big, huge, spacious. Pretty soon it will feel as though you—as awareness—are infinite; infinite in the sense of not finite, not limited, not what you thought you were, not "body" only, that you can't actually sense a limit or stopping point to where your consciousness is, to where you are—and that you are therefore not body only, nor body with mind, but the space, mind, or awareness *in which* everything you are aware of is happening. Your "real" body, therefore, is mental. The sound of that airplane or barking dog, for example, is happening within your awareness. The wind through the trees is happening within your awareness. Even your experience of "having" a body is happening within awareness. Everything you are aware of is happening within your awareness. And therefore, and this is the point, you are the Awareness in which everything is happening. You are Awareness being specifically aware. You are that big. You are infinite and specific, both at the same time. Relax inside, expand, forget about yourself as "body," and stay with your actual now-experience. Experience yourself as huge, spacious, without limit, infinite. Experience the peace of infinite Being.

**22** This is like a wave relaxing into itself and thereby experiencing its inherent ocean nature—that is, experiencing *itself* as the entire ocean (!) in both its infinite and specific aspects. There's a whole new sense of identity that comes about when this happens. It is not, in fact, a new identity. But it is a new *sense* of Identity—a less limited, more comfortable sense—because you cannot be comfortable if you entertain limited or false self-concepts. This is like trying to be comfortable in shoes that once fit but are now too small. It doesn't work. It can't work. But if you let go of all concepts, all ideas about who and what you are, all tensions, self-criticisms, and limited definitions—*and then be there for the experience*—you will experience yourself in a new and expanded way. You will experience the natural comfortableness or joy of being, which is the undistorted feeling-tone of your true nature. You will spontaneously come to new conclusions, new definitions about yourself and your Source, Mind. Therefore, be alert to what you find yourself Knowing when you are this open and relaxed.

**23** If any part of your body is tense or contracted as you lie in Relaxation Pose, then you are not as comfortable as you could be—even if it feels normal and you are not experiencing any obvious sensations of discomfort. You cannot be contracted or tense *and* comfortable. Tension is uncomfortable. Contraction is constriction, strangulation, blocked energy. But as you become increasingly sensitive to subtler sensations of tension and subtler degrees of holding on, and as you consciously release these tensions and experience yourself expanding, then the increasingly pleasurable experience of undistorted Being will emerge in your awareness as what you really are, and any areas of physical discomfort will disappear into wide open tingling space.

**24** Comfort is your natural state. Relax into it. Become one with it. Realize you are It, already. In other words, when you release every tension in your body and every sense of holding on or needing to protect yourself, it's not that *nothing* is then there. The tension will be gone. In its place will be the clear, undistorted experience of You: the experience of peace, bliss. Feel the bliss. It's right there, here. Slide into it. The more familiar you become with being this relaxed, the easier it will be to stay this way—and the more obvious it will be to you when you unconsciously contract and again become self-protective and defended.

**25** Relax into yourself and experience what's happening right there where you are. Ease into the idea that you are Consciousness being specifically conscious, and that your body, what you have until now identified with as "you," is actually an experience *within* the Consciousness that you are. You are not awareness within a three-dimensional body only, subject to birth and death. You are Mind, Awareness, Consciousness, being specifically aware, specifically conscious, and visibly tangible. This is not difficult to access or experience, because this is what you already are and have always been. It's simply a matter of letting go of everything you think you know about who you are and then staying with your actual now-experience—the experience of being conscious, that is, your being Consciousness.

**26** The technique, remember, is essentially simple. All you do is 1) relax your body; 2) feel the energy (Mind) you are made of, feel the bliss; and 3) be aware of what you find yourself Knowing when you are being this way. Keep it simple: Relax, feel, and pay attention to see what happens.

**27** Simply abide in this experience and pay attention to what's actually happening now. Enjoy the way you feel as you do this, and allow yourself to become thoroughly familiar with what it feels like to be thoroughly relaxed. Let it soak in deeply. Allow the profoundly soothing experience of deep inner peace to saturate your conscious awareness. Be aware of what's happening. You're not just relaxing your muscles. You're experiencing God! Melt into your actual now-experience. Let yourself be here where you are. Surrender, merge—totally. Let it feel as though you are relaxing the universe—or better, you are the universe relaxing. Let your whole body feel happy. This is what love feels like. Relax in Relaxation Pose for five to twenty minutes.

**28** When you've had enough, you'll know. At that point, ready yourself and open your eyes. Just before opening your eyes, though, be aware of how relaxed you are, how at ease, how peaceful, and then open your eyes without disturbing your peace—without shrinking and without tightening up. Stay relaxed, spacious, undefended, and wide open, and be like a child who is seeing the world for the very first time. Look at things without being quite so sure what everything means. Enjoy this awareness. Then roll to your side, linger there a few moments, and come to a seated meditation posture.

# Benefits: Relaxation Pose

Relaxing, refreshing, rejuvenating. Brings body, mind, and spirit into balance. Trains you to be tension-free, undefended, and wide awake at the same time. Gives you time to absorb and integrate benefits of other poses. Improves circulation, regulates blood pressure, reduces fatigue, induces calmness of mind. One of the best ways of learning to meditate. Introverts mind, develops faculty of self-awareness. Helps you feel the energy you are made of. Tremendous physical-psycho-spiritual repercussions. Gives experience of peace.

# 45 End Session Sitting Quietly

**1 Come to a seated meditation posture.** Sit erect, close your eyes, and allow the crown of your head to float straight upward, so your spine and core elongate. Simultaneously, become increasingly grounded. Go up and down at the same time.

**2 Relax.** For the next two or three minutes practice not moving and not thinking. Practice sitting absolutely still without holding yourself still, be thoroughly relaxed without losing your erect alignment, and instead of thinking, *feel*. Feel what's happening right there where you are. Be aware of your body breathing gently all by itself, ride the breath into the feeling-tone of you, and feel the energy you are made of. Become increasingly willing to be fully present. As you do this, mentally listen inwardly. Be aware of what you find yourself Knowing when you are not thinking of other things. Look for the feeling of peace.

**3** When you are experiencing the peace of your individual centered being, it is an indication that you are in perfect alignment with the Oneness. You will then spontaneously slip right through the center of you into the conscious experience of It/You/We. You will experience your oneness with the Oneness, the Self, the one and only I Am Presence. This is profoundly meaningful, transformative, healing. Therefore, willingly give your undivided attention to the clear, undistorted experience of You, the Self. For these few minutes, be consciously present in the now without concern for any other moment. Let your one concern be that of being fully present, here, in this now. It's wild!

**4** As you sit quietly, let your posture become more and more technically correct. Become more grounded through each sitting bone and the center of your core and, simultaneously, allow your core to elongate so the crown of your head opens and floats toward the sky. Be cosmic and grounded, both at the same time—without going anywhere except straight into the Now, Here.

**5** Let your whole body fill out and reconfigure to this new sense of expanding energy. Allow yourself to make subtle intuitive alignment changes until everything about you feels comfortable, spacious—so your hands are happy, your arms are happy, your shoulders are comfortable, your head delicately balanced on top of your spine without any tension or collapse in your throat or neck, your body grounded, and strong, relaxed, alive spinal energy coming up through your core. Sit like a king, a Buddha. Gently express the meaning of the moment. Bloom. Consciously experience yourself as part of God's infinite Self-Expression. Experience your inner beauty, your intrinsic worth—not because of anything you've done to earn or make yourself worthy of this uninhibited self-approval, but because of that which birthed you. *God* is great, in other words, and therefore so are you. You are That, This, in specific expression. And God is Love—and therefore so are you. Feel it now. Let this become your new normal state.

# Benefits: End Session Sitting Quietly

Grounding. Keeps you from being too spacy after Relaxation Pose. You're now ready to sit still. This is the most important part of the practice: experiencing yourself in stillness, like a wave relaxing into the ocean. Brings expandedness into daily life.

# PART

## FOUR

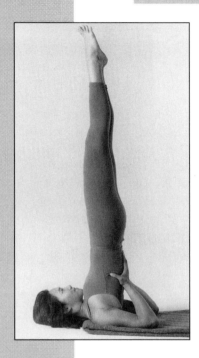

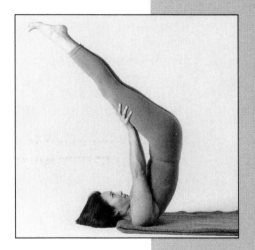

# 10

## MEDITATION

In the early days, thousands of years ago, when yoga was first being developed, the primary practice was meditation, or centering. The poses had not yet been invented. This was a highly cherished, esteemed practice because the ancients had found that by centering they were able to access a new way of knowing and being and thereby become more intuitive. They found that by consciously relaxing into themselves and experiencing their own consciousness with clarity, and by mentally listening inwardly and being as unthinkingly present in the now-moment as possible, they were able to experience the deeper nature of Consciousness.

Meditation, they discovered, was the most direct way of experiencing first-hand the meaning of God and Self. By the way, this was a nonintellectual practice. It was experiential. By *experiencing* the truth of who they were, they would **know** the truth of who they were. It wasn't a matter of thinking about it first and coming to intellectual conclusions. The conclusions or truths that arose did so out of personal experience and intuitive revelation.

The all-important revelation was that God and Self are one, that the individual wave is the specific expression of the entire ocean, that you and I are God-identified, God-specific. When one realizes this—when this becomes *real* for anyone—one acquires an entirely new understanding of himself or herself and the world. When this happens, it's as though you've come out of a haze or mental fog, or have just awakened from a dream and at last see things clearly. It will feel as though you now live in a new and different world because you're seeing all things anew, as though for the first time, with a different understanding. You'll feel different about yourself . . . more genuine, more authentic, more like the real you—happy. And you'll feel absolutely normal, finally. You'll feel, simply, wide-awake.

It was out of that centered meditative awareness that the poses evolved—or were, shall I say, channeled. They arose spontaneously out of the centered meditative mind. They were inspired, uncalculated actions. The ancients were simply moved to do them as a result of their meditative practice. Then they practiced and taught these to others as a way of finding or returning to that centered meditative state. The asanas were not only valued because they were physically beneficial, but because they were an especially effective way of both facilitating and sustaining the meditative state. The primary practice, however, was and *is* meditation—experiencing oneself in stillness.

Now, let's be very clear here. Meditation means listening, and the meditative mind is the "listening-to-Infinite-Mind" mind. The practice of yoga is a way of learning to be in this meditative listening state all the time. It's not only about how flexible your body is, or how many advanced and intricate postures you can do, though all of this is wonderful. It's about you and your specific mind listening to, being guided by, and communing with Infinite Mind, God.

The word yoga means yoke, and yoke means *union* and *joining*. Through the practice of yoga, you "join" your specific mind with the Infinite Mind through the act of listening for guidance, and thereby experience your already-existing oneness with the Infinite. In this way there is only one Mind in your awareness—not your mind *and* Infinite Mind, but Infinite-Mind-only expressing Itself as you.

The practice of meditation is about consciously establishing a line of communication between your mind and Infinite Mind—a line of communion. The result is ongoing nonverbal communion-communication with the Infinite in the form of spontaneous, intuitive revelation, specific and appropriate to the moment, wherever you find yourself. Through the regular practice of meditation you can learn to communicate with the ocean part of you, the as yet unclaimed part of you, the greater aspect of you that has always been you but that you have not yet recognized as yourself. And because of the undeniable effortless communion you'll experience, you will gradually realize that you are That in specific expression. It's inevitable.

In your attempt to express this verbally, both to yourself and others, you'll probably say something to the effect that "God" is in everything you're seeing, including yourself, and that God is all there is. An inherent oneness becomes obvious.

You'll realize that God is all there is of you and that your identity and existence are God-sourced. You'll especially realize that you did not create yourself. You exist because you were created. And therefore you are the specific Self-Expression of the Infinite Self Presence. You are That, This. You are God, Infinite Mind, Infinite Person, or Consciousness being specifically Itself as you. You are Consciousness being specifically conscious, an angle of awareness within the infinite arena of Awareness. You'll also realize that whatever it is you are, so also is everything else. *Everything* will begin to seem as though it's made of the same energy, the same cloth.

It's understandable, however, that this may seem preposterous, or at least unreasonable or wrong. Therefore, especially at first, be careful not to just accept or reject this idea. Live with it, test it out, see if it's true; and test it out in meditation. What you'll find is that because it **is** true, there will always be a part of you that knows it's true. Part of you will never quite give in to the ego sense of self, no matter how much you're brainwashed or conditioned into believing what's not true. Which means you will never be able to believe fully in the limited ego sense of who you are. Part of you *knows* that the most accurate, humble truth about yourself is that you are the direct expression of Infinite Conscious Being. Nothing less and nothing other than this.

Therefore, a very deep and knowing part of you will always be urging you to let go of your conditioning and limited beliefs in order to experience yourself as you actually are—in order to be congruent with life as it is. This part of you is always at peace, even when you are busy denying your own reality. It understands that there is absolutely no logical rationale for believing what's not true, and therefore it doesn't believe the suggestion that you are anything other than Consciousness or Divine Mind being specifically conscious. It knows you are the direct expression of the creative Life Principle.

And *if* this is true, and indeed it is, then that changes everything. It means that things—yourself included—are not what we thought they were and that life doesn't actually work the way we thought it did. We were close, perhaps—just as Newtonian physics was close when it presented a more comprehensive approximation of truth than the theories that preceded it—but close is not enough. And if life works differently from the way we thought, and if life is more incredible than we were previously aware, and if you and I are not who we think we are, then what's really going on? What is Consciousness, really? Who am I, really?

Be curious. Want to know. It's to your advantage to be intelligent and aware, not ignorant, and to know who you are and how life works—since everything is predicated on this. There is no reason to be hesitant, no sense in not investigating the truth of this claim. And don't be so sure you've already got it figured out, one way or the other. This may or may not be true, you may or may not be Consciousness being specifically conscious, but find out. Don't just accept it or reject it. See what it means. Look again. Experience yourself anew—directly. Consciously experience what it means to be conscious. We deserve to know the truth. We owe it to ourselves to prove it one way or the other, once and for all, and no longer to live out the suffering caused by inaccurate conceptions of who we are and how life works.

The only way you'll prove it to yourself is by ***experiencing*** yourself. This is the only way to discover what's true, the only way you'll become convinced. At the moment, though, we think it's egotistical to think we are fundamentally perfect expressions of a divine Life Principle. But, really, it's the ego (the limited sense of self, our conditioning) that is saying that it's ''bad'' to feel good inside about who we are—that it's selfish, arrogant, or egotistical, and that we've done so many cruel things in life that we don't deserve to experience the relief that comes from letting go of guilt, self-condemnation, and inner self-flagellation. Therefore, be willing temporarily to set aside the ego's admonition that this is a waste of time, that you *are* what you think yourself to be, and be open to a new experience.

Consider the possibility that you may be believing untruths about yourself, convictions that are causing you and others to suffer needlessly, and then consciously go inward and **experience** yourself. Allow yourself to experience the truth of your reality—your inherent creative goodness, and acknowledge your right to know the truth about yourself. And if doing that makes you feel absolutely fabulous for no apparent reason, then so be it. You'll find yourself feeling good about who you are because of what you are.

It's important to know this, or at least to suspect or consider it. The only reason we feel bad about who we are is because we engage in indiscriminate, inaccurate, inner self-criticism, and we therefore live in a fearful and defensive manner. We don't know any better. We believe what's not true and behave accordingly—not intentionally or maliciously, but ignorantly. We think self-appreciation is egotistical, but really it's just the reverse. It's egotistical not to feel good, not to be appreciative of the creative energy or Consciousness we are.

It is, in fact, exceedingly important to think well of yourself and to experience genuine Self-appreciation; and this happens spontaneously when you experience your undistorted truth. This is the source or well-spring of health, vitality, and aliveness, but you cannot force yourself to feel this way. You cannot make yourself feel good about yourself if you don't. You'll never quite believe it. But you can begin to loosen your grip on what you believe is true. You can introduce a little doubt and curiosity—*just in case* things are different from what you've thought. You can deliberately ease up on how convinced you are about yourself and everything else and temporarily suspend what you think you know in order to look again and experience yourself directly—and perhaps have a new experience. This will reveal the creative goodness in you *because* that is what's there.

It is not arrogant or egotistical to feel good inside. You had nothing to do with it. It's simply the honest response to clearly perceived Reality. It is arrogant, however, and egotistical (in fact, this is the definition of ego) to think that you are responsible for who you are and that you created yourself. To think this way is to think you can usurp the power of God. That's ego. On the other hand, it is the zenith of humility to recognize the Allness of God. When this becomes the obvious truth, your experience of yourself and the world will change radically.

The practice of meditation involves spending quality time alone every day with the discipline of centered sitting, and then to the very best of your ability carrying that meditative and centered listening mind with you all day long. And then doing it again the next day . . . and the next—so that a momentum is established. It's about 1) experiencing the truth of who you are, and 2) mentally listening inwardly for the wisdom and guidance of Infinite Mind, God—both in special times alone as well as all day long in the midst of daily life for as many moments as you can.

In this way you become the specific opening where the influx of wisdom and guidance from Infinite Mind can flow into human consciousness. By allowing and desiring yourself to be more open and being increasingly receptive and welcoming, and by consciously "joining with" the Infinite—from which you were never apart—you give permission for Life to flow through you unimpeded. You become less defended against letting it in or out, you become less blocked. And you thereby learn voluntarily to release your conditioned ego responses and instead become receptive to promptings from within. Your physical health will improve as you let the flow *flow*. You'll experience more vitality. Your mental outlook, as well, will become naturally optimistic, and a powerful, soothing calm will gently enfold you because you're beginning to see all things as they really are—infinite and divine. Life won't look so scary anymore.

When you first start experiencing the meditative mind, it may feel as though there is a you and a something else, as though you are experiencing something other and infinitely larger than yourself—like a wave experiencing the ocean, or a particle of air experiencing vast space. Many have referred to this as experiencing the "otherness." This is understandable. You're moving out of a limited or small sense of self. As you do this it will seem as though you—the wave—are joining with something other than you—the ocean; and yet, at the same time, it will also feel as though it is absolutely all you—that you are experiencing absolutely nothing external to you. The wave, for example, is not actually experiencing anything other than itself when it experiences the ocean, nor is the particle when it experiences vast space, and yet it *is* experiencing something infinitely larger than how it has thought about itself until now. Your small and limited sense of self will give way to a new and expanded Self-sense.

It is essential, however, that you somehow manage to let go or suspend what you now believe to be true about yourself, for at least a few moments, in order to have a new experience. You must clean the mirror a little in order to get a clearer picture of yourself. It's not necessary that you actually become different or change yourself in any fundamental way. You simply need to stop believing what you've always thought was true so that you're in a position to understand things in a new way.

Do this with meditation. The way to clean the mirror, achieve certainty, and access guidance from this seemingly "bigger-than-you" Consciousness, Mind, or Presence, God, is by centering and mental inner listening. Therefore, establish a daily twenty-minute meditation practice. Twice a day is even better. And as the days, weeks, and months go by, notice what's happening. You will not actually experience or hear anything other than yourself when you practice, but you will awaken to a whole new enlarged sense of who you are and how to be—one that contains tremendous fulfillment.

# The Practice

Think of your meditation practice as having three phases. The first is centering, becoming still, going within. In this part you let go of your usual moment-to-moment concerns and instead clearly experience this particular moment of conscious awareness. You relax physically and mentally, centering your awareness in the now, and then pay attention to what you are experiencing. What does it feel like to be centered and still? What's happening in this now? Again, this is like a wave on the ocean relaxing into itself and thereby experiencing the peace of the ocean's depths as the truest, deepest thing about itself. It's you sinking into your deepest experience of yourself and discovering—for yourself—that you are nothing less and nothing other than the specific Self-Expression of the divine Life Principle, the Father-Mother-Self of all, the Infinite Mind, God.

Centering is a technique for diving into yourself in order to experience the truth of who you are. It's a way of discovering the love within you. Love, you'll find, is the actual substance of everything—yourself included. And when you experience Love deep within you, you will feel deeply loved. This, not surprisingly, is tremendously nourishing and soothing; don't underestimate the transformative power of this experience. The first part of your meditation practice, therefore, say the first ten minutes of a twenty-minute session, should be geared toward becoming centered, peaceful, and still in order to experience the "ocean" within you. Once you're in there, soak it up. Relax the way you would in a hot tub and consciously savor the way it feels. As you do this you will feel yourself becoming the place where Love shines through effortlessly, naturally. You'll find yourself not wanting to block or hold it in. You'll center into yourself and then radiate outward and glow.

Let the second part of your meditation practice, say the second ten minutes, be about listening and communing inwardly. Mentally listen inwardly as though you were waiting to hear a message. This is a simple practice, yet it does require practice and discipline. Gently call out to the universe, God, mentally—into the vastness of your own quiet mind—and then simply listen for a response. Listen as though you had called out a note into the Grand Canyon and were waiting for the echoing response as reply. Simply be effortlessly attentive.

If there is a situation in your life that is troubling you, that needs resolution, that you would like clarification about—even if it's not a big problem—bring it into the arena of your quiet mind, lay it down at the feet of the Infinite, and listen for guidance about what to do. Ask for help. Ask a question. Bring your predicament to the seashore, place it on the moist sand at the edge of the water, and be there with it as it dissolves into the ocean. You'll find yourself mysteriously gaining clarity about what to do. Simply be patient, relaxed, and effortlessly attentive.

If there's nothing specific you need clarification about, then simply listen inwardly, experience inwardly, and see what transpires. Be open to revelation and new insights, new understandings, new teachings from the inner teacher about the nature of God and Self or anything else. Be in a place of openness and willingness. Be the student and let yourself be taught. Commune nonverbally.

As the listening phase of your meditation proceeds, continue centering. Let parts one and two be facets of one activity; that is, immerse yourself in your feeling-tone *and* practice listening. Feel the Consciousness that you are as you listen inwardly, and allow your awareness to float back and forth between listening and feeling and desiring to hear. Let one inspire the other.

Part three is your transition back into the world after your meditation. It's about continuing to feel the energy you are made of and continuing to listen inwardly for guidance, as you get up and go about your business. It's about being increasingly desirous of always wanting to know what God would have you do and of having no agenda other than being the place where clarity comes through. Part three is about your ever-improving skill at listening inwardly for guidance all day long, so you're engaged in nonstop continuous inner communion and then gladly doing and being as you are prompted from within.

Remember your deepest impulses—those coming from the ocean's depths— are *your* impulses. Doing God's Will, therefore, will not feel foreign in any way because it is your will also. There is no difference. It will feel supremely natural and deeply authentic to do increasingly as the ocean within you is wanting to do. Doing or being anything other than what your deepest being is urging you to do or be just won't feel right. It won't feel as good as it used to feel. Going with the flow will be so superior, so fulfilling, even when it's difficult, that at some point you're bound to realize it. You'll then relinquish every remaining trace of ego resistance and jump in willingly, totally.

This, again, is an example of the self-corrective nature of this transformational discipline. You'll find yourself less tolerant of mind-wandering, less tolerant of old-mind ego fears and projections, and less tolerant of not listening—not impatient, just less tolerant. You simply won't tolerate the not-listening egoistic state you've been operating from for so long. You won't tolerate it because it no longer feels right. In fact, it feels wrong. And it doesn't work as well as it used to work. That's the added incentive. And therefore you'll begin to want to listen. Inner listening will become your new way of being. And you'll be glad.

# 1 Feel the Energy You Are Made Of

Sit still. Ride the breath into the feeling-tone of you and feel the energy you are made of. Stillness = peace = joy = love.

Go about it something like this. Select a room where you can sit quietly by yourself and choose a time when you will not be distracted or disturbed. Set aside twenty minutes with the intention of giving your undivided attention to practicing the art of meditation, centering, and mental inner listening. Then sit down in a comfortably erect position, either on the floor with or without a zafu (Zen pillow), if you are comfortable sitting on the floor, or in a chair. You may also do this lying down, but there will then be a greater likelihood of falling asleep. Take your pick.

Assuming you are sitting erect, your first concern is to make yourself comfortable by finding the right alignment of your body. If your alignment is off, if you are crooked or slouched, you will become uncomfortable sooner than you would otherwise. You will experience physical discomfort and uneasiness instead of the pleasures of motionless sitting and inner listening, and this will make it more difficult than it needs to be. The more comfortably upright and erect you are, however, the more comfortable you'll be, and this will make communion more likely. Take a few moments to make sure your body is correctly aligned, and then endeavor to sit as straight as you comfortably can, without being rigid, for the duration of the meditation.

Do this by leaning forward and wriggling the buttocks backward until your two sitting bones are in contact with the cushion. The alignment of your center is now in an exaggerated dog tilt with the pelvis tilting forward. Bring your body to vertical again and delicately draw your belly backward toward the spine in order ever-so-gently to turn your hips under toward cat tilt. It will feel as though you are "plugging" both sitting bones into the cushion or chair, like plugging a light into an electrical outlet. Pay attention to the alignment of your lower back and spine as you do this, and stop the backward hip-turning movement when you sense that your sacrum is vertical, balanced, most weightless. Fine-tune and adjust your alignment here. Make it perfect.

Your center is now in "neutral"—not too much dog tilt, nor too much cat tilt. Let it feel as though you are doing both at the same time, just the right amount of each, so there's a sense of elongation and ease throughout the length of your entire spine and head. The root or base of your spine—your belly, your center, your sacrum, the sitting bones, that whole area—is now perfectly aligned and angled, grounded, which makes it easy and natural for your spine to grow straight upward from its grounded source.

Now, become more and more grounded. Spend a few moments here. Feel where you are touching the floor or cushion, and consciously allow the weight of your body to sink downward more into the floor. Become rooted, gently planted. Do not strain. Be effortless. Do less and less. Feel yourself being supported by the floor. Especially feel yourself grounding through the center of your core, in the area of your perineum, between the anus and genitals. Mentally feel around for the predominant sensation in that area and then allow it to sink farther downward. It may take you a moment to find the feeling. Once you've located it, lock your attention onto it. Don't strain, however; just don't let your attention stray from that particular focus. If it does stray, gently bring it back, over and over. Rest your attention in that area of yourself and experience what it feels like. Become grounded through the center of your core.

Then, starting from the floor, allow your awareness slowly to float upward through your core and body all the way up to the crown of your head. Feel it coming up slowly, at a leisurely pace. As your awareness floats slowly upward, allow yourself to expand and assume a new shape. Allow your chest gently to expand and lift up away from the waist, relax your shoulders back and down, rest your hands where they are comfortable, and balance your head perfectly on top of your spine. Lift or lower the chin until your head feels the most weightless, perfectly balanced. Then close your eyes and sense whether your face is slanting upward or downward excessively—even if it's minimal—and make subtle internal adjustments until it feels perfect to you now.

Allow all of this to happen. Enjoy this part. Make subtle intuitive alignment changes until your posture feels perfect. The straighter you are, the more comfortable you will be. Be comfortable. Then put your awareness at the top of your head, the fontanel, and feel around for any kind of sensation.

Effortlessly move the crown of your head straight upward as far as it will go, and feel your spine and body reconfigure to this upward thought. You'll notice many subtle changes occurring spontaneously in the alignment of your body as you do this, changes you are not personally responsible for, but that you allow to happen. Every subtle change will contribute to your overall sitting comfort.

Now, somehow, open the top of your head from the center of the fontanel. Do this mentally, gently. Let it feel as though the top of your head is opening and merging with the sky above. Take the lid off. Then, starting from the openness at the crown of your head, allow your awareness to slowly filter downward through your body—through your head, through your neck, through the shoulders, all the way down. As your awareness floats down, relax inside. Let go of every sense of holding, every subtle tension, every tightness and contraction. Wash your body clean with your gentle awareness. Soften and relax and feel what's happening—everywhere. Take your time doing this. Enjoy yourself. Savor what you are doing. Let your awareness filter down slowly, without losing the height of the crown of your head, and delicately touch and relax every part of you with your mind.

Notice that your body expands as you relax. It's not that you become limp and unable to hold yourself erect. It's that the contracted parts of you expand as they soften and release, much like what happens when you release a clenched fist. And since you're probably a little tense almost everywhere, it will feel as though all of you is expanding. This new expansion is what now holds you up effortlessly. It will feel as though you are becoming less dense or compacted, less thick, less solid, and you will literally experience more space in your body, more air, more comfort, less physicalness. In fact, it will start to feel as though you are only space, only awareness or Mind. You'll feel wide open, like a conscious sky, and you'll begin to suspect that what you really are is unlimited Awareness or Spirit—that even your physical body is, really, only energy. Inaccurate self-concepts will drop away effortlessly, and the Light that you are will shine more brightly. This is why you'll start to glow.

This is a skill. It is something you can practice. The more you practice being effortless expanded Being, simply being who you are where you are without inhibition or defense, the better you'll get at it. Practice relaxing your body, then, by gently moving your awareness around and through it and by being very sensitive to where you hold muscular tensions. Notice where you are unnecessarily or habitually contracted, and practice letting go. Deliberately relax. Consciously relax. Willingly release every sense of muscular holding, every hint or evidence of being uptight.

The tendency is unconsciously to hold on, and what's needed is the willingness consciously to let go. The more proficient you get at this, and the more relaxed and expanded you become, the more obvious it will be to you where you are still holding, where there are still unconscious subtle tensions that have become so ingrained and so familiar you hardly even notice them anymore. As you become internally more sensitive, more aware, more conscious in areas where you were previously unconscious, the more you'll be able consciously to relax even deeper. You'll be able consciously to let go more—not become more limp, but less uptight, less dense, less thick, less congested, more expanded and spacious, more consciously spiritlike. Sensitivity and awareness beget a deeper relaxation, which begets a clearer and more sensitive awareness, which begets an even deeper and more thorough relaxation.

You are now as tall and straight as possible, without being rigid, and as relaxed and expanded as possible. Elongate vertically straight up and down, allowing the crown of your head and your perineum to move away from one another, and effortlessly expand outward in all directions.

Now practice being still. Be motionless. Don't move. And practice being still without holding yourself still. Simply be so relaxed that no movement occurs. Let there be no holding anywhere in your body and no physical movement. You're not going anywhere. You're deliberately being where you are. Be here. Be with yourself right here where you are. And be completely relaxed. Be still. And in the midst of this stillness, in the midst of this not-movingness, be aware of the natural movement of life happening within you. Feel your body breathing all by itself.

Put your awareness in your nostrils where you can feel the air coming in and going out, and for the next few minutes simply be aware of your breathing. Feel the breath flowing in and out through your nostrils. There will always be some sensation in the nostrils caused by the movement of air. Be aware of these sensations and notice how they are constantly changing. Sometimes they are stronger and more obvious, sometimes they are barely perceptible. Be aware of your breathing body, savor the "taste" or fragrance of the air, and experience the subtle sense of overall satisfaction that accompanies breathing—of air-hunger arising and being satiated, again and again, continuously. Also notice that the air may be flowing more freely in one nostril than the other. Feel if this is so.

As you do this, be aware of the unconscious tendency to control the breath as you watch it, and instead allow it to flow in and out without obstruction, without your control, unimpeded, strain-free, at its own natural pace. Part of what you're learning in this practice is not to be in control. This is an especially important point that should not be overlooked. You're learning to be where you are, participating fully in your now-experience, without your usual willful control. You're learning to let go of your normal attempts to control what's happening in your life and instead to yield, surrender, be receptive to universal guidance and sensitive to the flow of Life. You're simply practicing here where it's easy.

When you surrender and become receptive to guidance, when you really become conscious of the movement of Life within you, you'll begin to understand that there is already something greater than you in control. There is already an underlying spiritual orderliness to all things. Be alert not to control or manipulate the breath. Practice leaving it alone. Let it be the way it is without intervening. Some breaths will be deep, others shallow. Each breath will be different. Allow it to be however it is, and with conscious awareness simply "ride" your breath.

Ride the breath in and ride the breath out. Feel it loop around gently at the end of each inhalation and exhalation. Be there with it all the way in and all the way out, over and over. Immerse yourself so thoroughly in the natural flow of breath that you establish an uninterrupted mental continuity. The breath is one long continuous ribbon; and so, make your awareness one long continuous watching. Make your awareness as continuous as the breath by watching the breath continuously.

Then, keeping your nostrils as the primary focal point, allow your awareness to expand to include all of you. Feel your whole body ripple with effortless breathing—even your elbows. Feel the obvious movements, and look for the less obvious. There will always be a discernible wavelike ripple somewhere in your body. Feel everywhere. Immerse yourself in the ceaseless flow. The more you get in there, the more fun this is. Do this for several minutes. Rest your undivided attention in the flow. Flow.

Then allow your attention to make a very subtle shift. Shift from feeling the breathing to feeling the feeling. Feel your feeling-tone, what you feel like. Experience you. And immerse yourself so thoroughly in this experience that you're not thinking about anything else. Practice not thinking. Instead of thinking, feel deeply.

For the next few minutes, immerse yourself as fully as you're able in your now-experience of you. Feel the energy you are made of. Feel life vibrating in your body. Feel what it actually feels like to be you. Focus, concentrate, in a relaxed and gentle manner, on your feeling-presence. Simply relax, expand, breathe and feel. Shift from thinking mode to feeling mode. Be in the now. Be where you are and feel what's happening. Savor what's happening. Be as unthinkingly in the now as you can, and experience the energy or substance that constitutes your being.

Realize that you are made of something. You are made out of some kind of energy or substance. You do exist. And so, what does that energy or substance feel like? What does it feel like to be you? Experience the fact that you exist, that there is a sense of presence to your existence, and that this existing presence has a feeling to it.

Experience what you feel like physically, feel the space inside your body, but also feel the space around your body. Notice that concepts like ''inside'' and ''outside'' have no meaning right now, that either one could be the other. Notice that, actually, there is no inside and no outside. There's just the experience of vast, open, undivided, indivisible space. There's just Awareness or Mind. And that's what you are. That's your actual now experience. You are Awareness being specifically aware. You are the Observing Self, the eternal constant. Therefore, experience the Consciousness or Mind that you are. Feel the energy that constitutes your being.

Sense into the depths of your energy field, your psychosphere, and notice there are no discernible boundaries or limits to where you are or aren't. Instead, you're experiencing yourself as unlimited, infinite, endless—without a discernible boundary of any kind. This is what it can actually feel like! And, therefore, if you are not limited, then you are the space or Awareness in which everything is happening. You are the universe experiencing Itself through you, and you—the universe—are now gently pulsing with what seems to be the rhythm of breath.

As you sit there, then, instead of thinking, feel the energy that you are. Feel it in your relaxed body and savor it with your thought-free mind. Notice what it feels like to have no tension or fear anywhere in your energy field, and be aware of the quality of your consciousness as you do this. Experience what it means to be conscious, aware of what's happening in every way you can.

The idea here is to immerse yourself in the feeling-tone of you and consciously access thought-free wakefulness in order to experience yourself with clarity. The practice is to be so unthinkingly in the now, so present, so involved with feeling what's actually happening now, that you override your conditioning about who you are—giving rise to a new experience of you.

Breath awareness during motionless sitting is one of the very best techniques for this because it effectively puts your awareness exactly where it needs to be in order clearly to experience the feeling-tone of who you are. Watching the breath places you squarely in the now. Each breath you take is only happening in the now. If you are feeling the movement of breath in your body, then your conscious awareness is precisely where it needs to be in order for you to experience with clarity the energy that you are. Riding the breath is a way of immersing yourself in the feeling-tone of you, and that's what you want. You want to feel what you actually are. You want to experience yourself so clearly that there is no longer any confusion or doubt.

Stay with the breath as a way of keeping your conscious awareness anchored firmly in the now, and continue riding the breath into the clearer experience of your feeling-tone. And don't move. Be absolutely still. Don't resist the temptation to move, simply let go of it when it arises and become more still. For these few minutes, immerse yourself fully in what you're doing. Get more and more involved. Become thoroughly familiar with what it feels like to be still and relaxed with no holding anywhere.

As you ride the breath into your feeling-tone and feel the energy you are made of, however, you may suddenly become aware that you are no longer with the breath or feeling-tone, that you have gone off on a thought tangent about something or other and are thinking of other things. Your attention may wander. Your interest level may fluctuate. You'll have many, many thoughts. You may feel compelled to get up and do something else, something important, something you really should be doing right now—like washing the dishes or cleaning the house.

When you notice this happening, gently bring your attention back to the breath. Mentally stop doing whatever you were doing and ride the breath, again, into the energetic feeling-tone of you. Consciously come back to the task at hand: Relax, be still, and feel the energy you are made of. Do this as many times as necessary.

As you do this, feel the peace that's beginning to emerge, the peace of stillness, and feel the joy inherent in that peace. Do not fight the thoughts or become upset with yourself for thinking or for the fact that thoughts keep arising, just repeatedly bring your conscious awareness back to the primary point of focus. Be interested in experiencing the peace of centered stillness. Give your attention to that. Be more interested in that. Do this gently, voluntarily, trying not to concentrate too intently. Allow your attention to rest lightly on the breath and feeling-tone. The more you do this the better you'll get at it—which means you'll have fewer thoughts distracting you from your breath and feeling-tone and more moments of quiet clarity and peace.

This is similar to what you did with your body when you first sat down. You began the meditation by establishing an erect and comfortable posture and then relaxed yourself physically by sweeping your awareness upward and then downward through your body, letting go of muscular tension. You relaxed your body by letting go of it. You consciously let go of every sense of muscular holding. As a result, you expanded and became more spacious inside. It was not just your imagination.

Do the same thing now mentally. In exactly the same way as you let go of muscular holding, let go of thinking. Relax and expand your mind, become more spacious in your mind by consciously letting go of thought. Do this by being aware of when you are thinking and then deliberately letting it go. Suspend the thought—ignore it—and instead of thinking, *feel what's happening.* Get involved with what's present to be experienced when you are not busy thinking about other things. Become perfectly one-pointed in the now, fully engaged in experiencing this instant of consciousness, and pay attention to what's happening. Immerse yourself totally in the experience of your now, of you being you, of Consciousness being conscious.

The tendency is unconsciously to be involved with thinking, and what's necessary is the willingness consciously to let that process go for these few minutes. This is how to relax mentally. You willingly let go of your usual worries and concerns, your habitual mental activity, and pay attention instead to the silence between thoughts. You'll find youself more and more willing to do this when you discover what happens when you do. Consciously accessing thought-free wakefulness gives you peace of mind. It's how you experience the peace of Mind. You'll find it alluring, attractive. It's also what readies your mind for intuitive revelation. It's where you'll find answers to every perceived problem. The "empty" mind has room for something new—a new perspective. You will see things differently, understand things in a new way.

Be aware of when you are thinking, be aware that as psychosomatic tension is released, thoughts will bubble up into your conscious awareness, but especially be interested in experiencing your peace. Be aware that a thought is floating through your mind, and instead of getting involved with it, simply let it go. Let it bubble up, and let it float away. Be more interested in experiencing the feeling-tone of the arena in which all of this is happening. Orient yourself toward the feeling of peace. You can always go back to the thought later, if you wish. For now, simply notice you are thinking, and deliberately—gently—stop. Stop thinking. Relax mentally. And be aware of how you feel as you do this. Experience what thought-free consciousness feels like. Experience the "empty" mind. Experience the peace. Experience what's happening! Go into the Void. Feel the Presence of Awareness. It's not nothing.

Something is happening right where you are. Life is happening. God is happening. God is all there is of you. Immerse your awareness so thoroughly in your feeling-tone that you are not thinking about anything else, and be aware that the energy you are experiencing is not something other than you. It's not you *and* the energy. The vibrating energy that feels like love is what you are. That's you. You are That. You are the creative God Force Energy in specific expression. And you can feel it right there where you are—and it feels good. In fact, it's lovely.

Whenever you notice that you have again forgotten about feeling the feeling and are instead thinking, again practice letting go of each specific thought in order to reaccess the thought-free state. Get back to feeling the feeling. This is like holding a balloon by a string. If you simply release the string, the balloon will float away. You don't have to do anything especially difficult. Each thought form is like a balloon on a string, and all you need do is mentally let go of it—ignore it—in order instantly to be back in the thought-free conscious experience of now.

This is not difficult, eventually, but it does require a tremendous amount of practice. The better you get at it, though, the more you'll want to do it, because this state is where inspiration comes from and where insight occurs. It's where illumination and revelation unfold. The thought-free conscious experience of now gently erupts with clarity and understanding, and thereby eradicates confusion and suffering. It's where you touch infinity and eternity and the birthless-deathless state. And it's right there, right here; it is not far off or elusive. And though you cannot make revelation happen, you can make yourself available to it. All of this will become apparent to you with your very first glimpse of stillness. This will increase your trust, willingness, and desire to pursue the silent mind and lure you deeper and deeper into the thought-free conscious experience of each new moment.

Therefore, in the same way that being relaxed in your body doesn't mean that nothing is going on—your body doesn't cease to exist, for example—so when you practice "not thinking" or mental relaxation, don't assume in advance that nothing will be there. When you are not busy thinking, you will still be *experiencing*. You will still be conscious. Your mind will not become null and void or cease to exist simply because it is not busy thinking. Instead it will be more open, more available, more sensitive to the stimulation of insight and guidance. You'll feel more awake than usual, and if you were to open your eyes, the world around you would appear more luminous.

Insight will occur spontaneously when you are in the thought-free now. Clarification will take place. Resolutions to problems will float into your awareness. Wisdom will arise. This will be much more satisfying than being worried or concerned with whatever your previous worries or concerns were. Therefore, practice accessing thought-free wakefulness, and find yourself spontaneously gaining clarity about what to do in any circumstance.

Test this out. See whether it's true or not. Suspend what you usually think in this regard and see for yourself. Suspend everything you think you know about who you are and find out for yourself what's really true. Put forth the small effort required to relax physically and mentally, let go of your usual concerns and habitual thinking, and experience with clarity who and what you actually, divinely are. It's worth the small effort required.

When you experience the energy you are made of, you will feel the love that you are. You will feel deeply loved, deeply nourished, deeply safe—effortlessly. It's effortless because this is what you already are; it requires no energy to become this way. It will also no longer matter that as a child you were not loved as deeply as you needed or would have liked. The fact that you didn't get it then doesn't matter now. You're getting it now. You're being fed now. You're feeling it now. You can therefore let everyone in your past off the hook for not giving you the love you needed. And this feels good. This is forgiveness.

It will therefore be blatantly obvious that if you choose to divert your attention away from the love you are experiencing now—to your anger or regret at not having received it in the past, for example—then, in effect, you're cutting yourself off from it again. When you realize this is what you're doing, you will be in a position to choose voluntarily not to do that—and instead reimmerse yourself in the thought-free conscious experience of you in order to stay present with the truth. As a consequence, you will become more loving. This is what it's all about.

But understand! It's not you *and* the love you're experiencing. You *are* the love. That's how you will experience yourself when you let go of every other self-concept and immerse yourself in the thought-free now. You will feel the love that you are. This won't feel phony, either. You'll know it's authentic. You'll have no doubt about what you are experiencing, at least for these few minutes. And when the revelation or clear perception wears off—if it does—and you're back to "normal" consciousness, you will not be as conditioned as you were before the revelation.

This new experience will help you overcome your doubting mind. You'll now have a legitimate argument, a direct and firsthand experience, with which to counter your objections to accepting this new "theory." In other words, it's not just a theory anymore. It's becoming your experience. Therefore, you do not blindly have to accept any of this as true. You do not have to brainwash yourself into believing something you are not ready to believe. You simply have to experience yourself as you are. Be the wave relaxing into the ocean that thereby experiences the ocean within itself. Experience your real Identity. Deliberately let go of everything you think you know about who you are, suspend it all, relax into the thought-free conscious experience of now and experience what's really so with clarity. Then you'll know, one way or the other.

Each moment of clarity, no matter how fleeting, is transformational. Each glimmer of illumination lessens the darkness of your conditioning, making it less dense, solid, and convincing. Every glimpse of Truth will cause you to doubt your previous (false) convictions about the nature of Reality. You'll begin seriously to question your assumptions and conditioned beliefs about yourself and the world, and this will put you in the position of being able to experience clearly what's really so.

# 2 Mentally Listen Inwardly as Though You Were Waiting to Hear a Message

Thus far the technique has been to sit motionless, ride the unbroken flowing stream of breath into the feeling-tone of you, feel the energy you are made of, and abide unthinkingly in the conscious experience of you.

Now, once you are quiet and centered and fairly well established in the thought-free conscious experience of now, let go of the technique and begin listening inwardly. If there is a problem or situation in your life that is troubling you, disturbing your peace, or if you have a specific question or concern, voice it mentally. Silently ask for clarification and then silently listen for an answer. Desire to know whatever you need to know. If there is nothing specific that you want clarification about, then ask for revelation or insight about anything that might be relevant to you. Say, "Is there anything I need to know right now?" Then mentally listen inwardly.

Listen inwardly to the stillness of your quiet mind. Be in the void and listen as though you were waiting to hear a message. Listen as though you were hearing beautiful music. Listen with the intent to hear. Do exactly what you do when you're on the phone with your best friend: Say what you want to say and then stop talking and listen. Do this mentally. Listen with the expectation of hearing. *Want* to hear. Want to know beyond your current level of knowing. Desire to know more, and then listen. Pay attention inwardly. Inner listening is what sets you up for intuitive revelation. It's what readies your mind for the reception of spiritual insight. Listen inwardly with the intent to hear.

Ironically, this may at first feel very similar to what you've always done in the way of mentally talking to yourself. This is because, in the deepest sense, you are. You are talking with the rest of who you are, the ocean part, the God part, the part of yourself you had temporarily forgotten about. It will also feel very different, however, because it *is* very different. It will feel potent and profound, and you'll know you're on the trail of something you were not previously aware of, something magnificent.

When you become distracted for one reason or another and notice that your mind has drifted away from listening, gently bring yourself back to the task at hand. Come back to listening. You're only going to be here for a few minutes. It's not interminable. Therefore, for the few minutes that you're here, be as involved as you can. Discipline yourself a little. Gently bring your attention back each time it wanders, and involve yourself again with listening.

If you find this difficult, or if your mind is simply too active or restless to engage itself in listening, then go back to part one: Consciously reground yourself and feel supported by the floor; elongate your core by allowing the crown of your head to float straight upward; relax and expand; be still; breathe; and feel. Reimmerse yourself in the energetic feeling-tone of who you are. Practice feeling. Practice being. Practice being present with what you're actually experiencing right now. Resume the technique and become centered again in your now-experience. Or start up one of the other techniques we've done;—Counting Backward, for example.

Once you're in there again, let go of the technique and once more say, ''Is there anything You would have me know?'' Then, as much as you effortlessly can, listen deeply and abide unthinkingly in the experience of what you are experiencing. Allow what's there—Consciousness! God!—to reveal itself. Immerse yourself in stillness and pay attention. Allow yourself to be taught.

Mentally speak into your quiet mind and ask for clarification. Ask for help, for understanding, for wisdom. And then simply listen. Be open to revelation and receptive to the influx of spontaneous knowledge. Allow insights and ideas and thoughts to bubble into your mind in response to your need. And *let* them bubble into your conscious awareness. Don't make your mind so still that you do not allow any activity. In other words, revelation will be felt as activity in your mind. There will be something happening as you receive clarification. Therefore, let the words bubble up. Allow clarity to form in your mind. And yet, if you find that you are distracted, or lost, or enmeshed in some extraneous mental tangent, and that you're not really listening, come back to the technique of riding the breath and feeling the energy. Deliberately bring yourself back into the thought-free now and then, again, resume listening.

From this point on, the meditation itself will guide you in how to proceed. You'll be taught from within. But in order for this to happen, you must be in touch with the ''within.'' You must become inwardly quiet and pay attention. You must take the steps necessary to go within. You must practice stillness and be willing to let go of everything you think you know in order to have a clear enough mind to be taught anew.

Let this happen. Be courageous enough to go into the not-knowing place all by yourself, even if you're slightly fearful. It's difficult not to be afraid at this point. Therefore, as in asana practice, relax with the intensity. Relax your body and relax your mind. Relax more as you ease your way into the unknown. Don't contract or become defensive. Stay defenseless, undefended. Allow yourself to not-know so you can be taught. Value the not-knowing place.

In doing this you will come upon a whole new experience and, therefore, new understanding of what's always been. You are allowing clarity to emerge about issues you may have thought were beyond your comprehension, in areas you may have thought you already understood, as well as in the activities of your everyday life. But, again, in order for this to happen, your mind must be pliable, swift, unknowing, and receptive.

Therefore, as much as you are able, immerse yourself in your now–experience of being conscious. Be there in your silence not knowing what you are supposed to do, and simply be attentive to whatever transpires. Don't be so sure you know what's supposed to happen when you meditate. Instead, allow yourself to be taught. Be still and pay attention. Be receptive. Learn.

At first you may not hear anything, or you may not feel much, or it may not feel very good, or your body may begin to ache, or you'll find yourself becoming bored or sleeply . . . or one thing or another. This is largely because we are not used to being this relaxed, especially mentally, while awake. Normally we're only this relaxed when we're asleep. As you approach this similar level of relaxation in your meditation practice, the tendency is to become sleepy. This is a good sign at first because it means you are relaxing, but you'll know you are progressing when instead of becoming drowsy you become more alert.

Simply persist with the practice day after day. When you notice yourself nodding off or losing interest, gently bring yourself back; and when it gets too much, stop for the day and try again tomorrow. More and more you'll be able to sit erect and still and relaxed with no holding anywhere, mentally immersed in the soothing experience of stillness, experiencing the tranquility and deep sense of well-being within you—communing with the Infinite.

For these few minutes, suspend your usual concerns and focus instead on experiencing your peace and listening. Feel the energy you are made of and mentally listen inwardly. Make this your concern for these few minutes. You'll be better able to resolve your other concerns once you deal with this one, of that you can be certain.

Give yourself the daily luxury of suspending your usual anxieties and concerns in order to have a few uncluttered minutes. Give a few minutes of your time daily to this other more important concern—that of experiencing the truth of who you are, of becoming receptive to intuitive revelation and universal guidance, and of experiencing God, Guru, and Self—all—within yourself.

You will feel relieved, not only because you are experiencing the God within you and are therefore spontaneously feeling good about yourself, but because you'll realize that you are in a world of other God-sourced entities. You are not in an inherently alien or hostile environment. You are safe. You are with family. You are with others like you. Therefore, you can dare to relax even more. You can release every hint of aggressive defensiveness and instead relax, be unafraid, and enjoy the movement of life.

# 3 When You're Done

When you are done listening, mentally say "Thank you." Express thanks in whatever way feels appropriate. "Thank you, Father, for being with me. Thank you, Mother. Thank you my dear Father-Mother God." Then bring your awareness back to the breath, to the sensations in your nostrils, the taste of the air, and the feeling-tone of who you are—and take several deep breaths before opening your eyes and completing the meditation. Savor the air as you breathe in and out. Breathe with the awareness that you are bringing in something valuable, something that you need and therefore want. Breathe with appreciation, gratitude, enjoyment. Pull in life with each inhalation, and release every sense of strain and fear with each exhalation. Breathe with feeling. Relish the way you feel. Notice how relaxed you are, how peaceful, how at ease. And as your eyes open and you come back into the visible world, be mindful not to immediately tighten up, contract, or shrink and become small again. Stay relaxed, wide open like space.

The only thing you can ever really experience with clarity is yourself. You are the closest thing to you. And when you take the time to become centered and still in order to experience yourself with clarity, you'll experience what is true. You'll experience the fact that God is all there is of you and that God is Love. You'll know this is true because as you get in there and experience yourself in a thought-free unbiased manner, what you will experience won't be nothingness or chaos. Instead, you will experience unblemished lovingness.

This is something you'll get in glimpses. You'll have an intuitive awareness or a sudden clarity that this is true, and then you'll flip back into your old way of thinking about yourself and others. You'll flip back and forth many times, and this may be quite disconcerting at first. Don't let it bother you. Be glad that movement is occurring and that you're not as stuck in your old world view as you used to be. If you were, you would not be flipping back and forth. The fact that you're flipping is a good sign. It means that the strength of your conditioning is weakening.

Be aware also, from that first intuitive glimpse on, that there is a persistent feeling in the back of your mind that what you intuited is what's really true. The remembrance of that glimpse will keep beckoning you, encouraging you to continue meditating even when it's difficult and nothing seems to be happening.

Stick with it. Out of the blue you'll have another glimpse, more revelation, and then you'll flip back—and another glimpse, more revelation, and again you'll flip back. And eventually you'll flip no more. You'll cross over and be convinced. And you'll know what's so.

When you experience yourself in a thought-free manner, it's not that there will be nothing there to experience. It's that your mind, your perception mechanism, will finally be clear enough to experience your reality without distortion. You'll learn that almost everything you thought about yourself was not true. Almost everything you were taught is not true. What *is* true is that God is Love and God is all there is of you. Therefore, when you experience yourself with clarity, without bias, that is what you will feel. You will know this is true when you experience yourself in a thought-free manner, and not until then.

This is not something you decide in advance and then give your allegiance to. It's something you can only fully give your allegiance to once you've experienced it as true, once you've experienced Reality—right where you are—without distortion. Until you've experienced it, this can only be an intellectual concept. It's an enticing one, however—one that, hopefully, will encourage you more willingly to practice these techniques so as to experience for yourself whether the concept is true or not. Therefore, be curious. Want to know. "What is the truth about me?" The only way you will ever really know one way or the other is by experiencing yourself in a thought-free manner.

This state is not so difficult, really. It's not *easy* at first, by any means. It can be extremely frustrating and require intense mental discipline. In fact, meditation will probably be one of the most difficult things you've ever undertaken. Don't be mistaken about this. It's rigorous. It'll push you to the edge. It will challenge your sense of sanity. But though it isn't easy, still, it *is* ultimately simple. It's only difficult to the extent that we're still trying to *become* different than how we naturally are, and we're doing this out of habit and conditioning. It's ultimately simple—once you get the hang of it. But, at first, it's not easy. Be prepared to work. Be aware that you'll probably stumble many times, and that you'll almost undoubtedly become confused and disoriented. But be aware also that if you will simply persist, it *will* become easier. You'll become a better meditator every time you practice.

It's ultimately simple because we are already That. We don't have to change or become fundamentally different from how we already are. We need to release the misperception—not become different! To the extent that we're trying to become different from how we actually, naturally, divinely are, it means we think that how we are isn't the way we're supposed to be—that there's something wrong with us that we need to change. And we believe this to the degree that we haven't yet experienced who we are with clarity. If you haven't spent sufficient time "at home" with yourself, free of other people's expectations, you most likely won't have come to an inner peace about who you actually are—by *experiencing* what's really so. And if you're not in touch with what's true about you, then you can't know that, in fact, there's nothing wrong with you.

The wave will stop trying to become other than how it is when it realizes that it already is everything—the entire ocean—in specific expression, and we'll stop trying to change when we experience our truth. This doesn't mean we'll stop growing. It means we'll stop feeling frustrated with ourselves. The absence of frustration is the perfect soil for real growth, for the flowering of consciousness. We'll stop trying to become different from how we are when we experience the calm bliss that is our natural feeling-tone.

You may think, ''Well, I must not be a very good meditator, then, because I'm not experiencing all these wonderful feelings,'' and feel the accompanying guilt of being a ''poor meditator.'' But this is simply an ego ploy to keep you away from experiencing yourself directly. If that thought catches your attention as it floats through your awareness, if you grab onto it, and especially if you buy into it or agree with it, then you have been effectively deflected from going within. You started moving toward your center, toward the thought-free conscious experience of now, but you made a quick left when you became aware of that thought floating by. You went after it. You became involved with that thought instead of letting it float by and continuing to relax deeply into yourself. And if you never really sink deeply into yourself, if you keep getting sidetracked, then, of course, you're not going to experience the profound peace—which feels like joy, like love—that is the feeling-tone of Being. Not that it's not there to be experienced, but *you're* not there. You're involved with some other mental activity—which is fine, but it's not how you come upon a clearer and more accurate experience of you. You won't experience the deep, powerful, confident peace of the ocean if you're bobbing around on the surface. You must go deeply within.

I'm not saying we don't need to change. We desperately need to change. We're suffering horribly. We're killing ourselves out of ignorance. We're making ourselves sick. We're polluting our environment. We're not happy. We're secretly afraid of everything. We're unfulfilled and miserable, and our behavior toward one another needs to change radically. The way to ''change,'' ''grow,'' or ''become different,'' though, is by taking the time to experience yourself as you actually are, so you have an accurate starting point. You'll come up with a radically different concept of who you are, who others are, what life is, and what's going on. Everything will take on new meaning. Life will be more meaningful. And your behavior will change and you will be different. But not different from who you've always been! Different from what you *thought* you were. You'll be minus the illusion. You'll be the you that you really are. Your Light will shine undimmed.

It's simply a matter of relaxing, both physically and mentally—and this may not be easy at first. Being relaxed physically means letting go of muscular tensions, and being relaxed mentally means letting go of thinking,—mental tensions. The idea is to become physically and mentally at peace for these few minutes by not moving and not thinking, and then to be there for the experience. See what's left. Feel the energy you are made of and the Consciousness that you are. Meditation is the cleanest and most direct route for doing this.

For these few quiet minutes of centered sitting, ease your way into thought-free being, and experience the energy you are made of. Instead of thinking, immerse yourself in what it feels like to be you and practice listening inwardly. Commune. Don't bog yourself down thinking this is something you will have to do forever. Do it for these few minutes only, but do it as totally as you can. Immerse yourself fully. Ease your way in. Try it. Simply be present and savor the energy. Savor Consciousness. Commune. Meditate.

Then, during the day, do and be as the energy—*your* energy—is prompting you to do or be. Move with the flow. Or rather, you are the flow, and if you simply let yourself be in the now—not knowing how you are supposed to be—the flow will move through you unimpeded, without your preconceptions, and it will be very clear to you how you should be and how you should respond. The energy will move you. You will be inspired to action. It will feel like you are running on free energy.

# 11

## LISTENING FOR GUIDANCE

# The Practice of Spontaneous Wisdom

When you experience yourself in stillness, you will intuit a new way of using your mind. You will be taught—from within the stillness—how to receive moment-to-moment inner guidance during the day from the Infinite Mind, and you will be given individually pertinent spiritual teachings.

These are two valuable and practical themes because with inner guidance and spiritual insight, you can know with certainty the most appropriate thing to do at any given moment in your life. Inner guidance is the means of right action. It is how you can know what to do. It is your deepest knowing made conscious. And as you learn to trust and make use of this faculty, it can become your decision maker. The more experience you have with it and the better you get at utilizing the information available to you, the more convinced you'll be of just how wonderful an attribute of mind this actually is. Listening for guidance is the technique of spontaneous wisdom.

The spiritual teachings you'll receive from within your silent mind will be the source of new meaning in your life, revealing to you life's inherent meaning. Spiritual teachings are communications of truth about the way things are. They will answer your conscious and unconscious questions concerning the nature of who you are and how the world works. Inspiring and guiding you in your thought, speech, and behavior, they will come in the form of clarifying insights and sudden inspirations, creative ideas, intuitive knowings, life circumstances, people and situations, hunches, premonitions, desires, attractions, and spontaneous impulses. Spiritual principles will then no longer seem foreign or irrelevant, divorced from daily life, and they will no longer be gleaned from books and teachers only. The teachings, taught from within, will be pertinent to you and your life. They will make sense to you, meaningful sense.

As this happens, life takes on a growing significance. You begin to understand and appreciate in a totally new way the fact that your life is indeed absolutely worthy of your fullest attention. And as you give it the undivided attention it deserves, moment by moment by moment, your life will become increasingly interesting. Remember, it's difficult to be interested in something if you are not paying attention to that thing. You may be listening to the most beautiful sonata in the world, but you won't know until you give it your attention and listen, if you *join* with it, do yoga with it, become one with it. As you do this with your life you will feel young again, renewed, refreshed, regenerated, optimistic, confident, secure, at peace . . . and you will experience authentic happiness. That is, happiness without guilt.

Experience yourself in silence, then—sit motionless, quiet your mind, immerse yourself in the feeling-tone of your own unique being, and then simply be aware of what you are experiencing of the world around you and within. This profound practice will clarify who you are and what your life purpose is and also make available the means to fulfill that purpose intelligently.

Of course, you will continue to experience life's exotic mystery, the wonderful attribute that makes total comprehension impossible, but the confusion will be gone. And as you allow yourself to savor the feeling-tone of your own mysterious being, you will clearly understand that you are a creation or expression of the creative God Force and that you are therefore literally and eternally connected to this Force because you are one with it. And this being so, you are in the wonderful position of being able to receive universal guidance that benefits all and is in harmony with every living thing.

# The Aerial Perspective

Imagine you are in your car driving down the freeway. It's a clear day, and from where you are in your car, you can see the road up ahead for the next mile or two. You can't see any farther than that, but from where you are the road appears clear. The traffic flows smoothly without congestion. But, say up around the bend in the third mile beyond your range of vision, there may be a traffic jam. And because you can't see it, you unknowingly drive smack dab into the middle of it.

This is why traffic helicopters were invented. From where a helicopter is—high above the earth—it can see the total picture. From where you are—on the ground—your vision is limited. You can't see around the corner, much less what's happening three miles in the future. To the helicopter, however, it's obvious that in three miles you'll be stuck. It easily sees the road congestion up ahead and can also easily see other routes where traffic flows freely. It sees the same picture as you see, but from a different angle, and so its view includes things yours doesn't. From the ground you cannot have the full perspective of the traffic that the helicopter has from the air. It has the aerial view, the superior perspective.

If you have a radio in your car, however, you can tune in to the helicopter's traffic broadcast that will suggest a quicker traffic-free route, or advise you about more scenic roads, or how to get to the beach from where you are. Whatever information you need, it can supply. This is clearly to your advantage, especially if you live in an area where traffic tends to be congested. But if your radio isn't turned on or if you are listening to a different station, you won't hear the broadcast. Maybe you're not even aware that such a broadcast exists and so won't know to tune in, and therefore you won't hear it even though it is always there.

Your mind is like your car radio, and the ''cosmic broadcast'' is continuously happening inside you. In other words, there is a larger perspective available to you—the aerial perspective—about what happens in your life. When you are on the ground, so to speak, your outlook and perspective on your life are necessarily limited, no matter how educated you are or how large your repertoire of life experience. You can only see so far and therefore have only so much information. But just as you can tune in to the helicopter's traffic broadcast with the aid of your car radio for instant access to an aerial perspective, so you can have ready access to an expanded knowledge, a larger perspective, a more inclusive outlook on your entire life with a simple shift of attention.

You have the capability to transcend your necessarily limited ground-level awareness for the vaster perspective of the helicopter. You can use your mind to hear the cosmic broadcast coming from the infinite Mind of God. The wisdom and information from this larger-perspective broadcast will help you navigate your way through life and make your most important decisions.

This broadcast is not a new phenomenon; it has been happening since the beginning. What may be new, however, is the awareness that it is going on—now!—and that you can tune in your mind and hear. Once you understand how personally and collectively advantageous it is to be attentive to the cosmic broadcast, you will gladly listen inwardly for guidance. Why spend your time stuck in traffic jams? Why drive through life with limited vision when you have such easy access to an expanded perspective? Why suffer when you have the means with which to end all suffering?

This ''new'' way of using your mind will help confirm your evolving perspective of yourself as a spiritual being in a spiritual universe composed of Mind. It is a way of accessing information, obtaining guidance and direction, and intuitively knowing what to do. It involves making conscious, deliberate, and practical use of your newly discovered but ever-existing connection with the creative God Force or Mind of All. It is a skill that will help you be less fearful and more authentic. It is a faculty you will want to use and improve once you perceive its value and begin to suspect that it might actually work.

This new way is about yielding to—following—the traffic helicopter's guidance. It is the car on the road in conscious communication with the helicopter in the air. It is you, your mind, in conscious communion with Infinite Mind, God.

And it involves voluntarily giving up or moving beyond your limited and partial knowing in glad exchange for the wisdom of the whole.

# The Divine Technique

Learning to rely on inner guidance takes practice and the development of trust. The best place to practice is in the midst of daily life, especially those moments when you are required to make a decision. If you feel the need to decide something, it means you are not clear about that thing. If you were clear, there would be no need of a decision. What to do would be obvious to you. "I am marrying this person and not that one," for example. There is no question about it, you are not really making a decision. You are clear.

The fact that you do have a choice, therefore—and a decision to make—indicates a lack of clarity. This lack of clarity is not a statement about you, however. You are not "bad" or inadequate simply because you are not clear about some aspect of your life. You are still who you've always been: the direct expression of God's Mind. Being unclear, however, means that you do not have sufficient information at your disposal to make a clear choice. Recognizing this, then, do not make up your own mind. Know you are looking at things from ground level. Recognize that your perception of the situation is necessarily limited and that any decisions you might make would be based on partial and incomplete data, and then do not make any decisions by yourself. Instead, suspend your best judgment about what to do and ask inwardly for guidance. Ask mentally, almost as though you were simply talking to yourself. Direct your question into the vastness of your mind—your mind being your personal conduit into Infinite Mind—and expect an answer.

It makes more sense to do this than it does to decide "by yourself." Therefore, decide not to decide. Make up your mind no longer to make up your mind. Deliberately suspend your partial knowing and ask the greater overview for advice. Turn on your radio, ask for clarification, and listen. This is a most intelligent thing to do. Accessing guidance through inner listening is how you get clear.

Whenever you have a decision to make during the day, observe your perspective on the situation and recognize when it is limited. Realize also that the so-called traffic helicopter or Infinite Mind has a superior view. Then, knowing it is in your best interest to access the larger knowledge, ask for it. Silently say, "I want to do what You would have me do. What would You have me do?" Memorize these sentences, use them frequently throughout the day, and do as you are prompted to do. Observe how your life moves and flows when you operate in this way.

Practicing yoga during the day is a matter of keeping your eyes on the road and one ear turned toward the Infinite. It's about listening inwardly as often as you can for your deepest impulses about what to say, think, do, or be. When you are in the store buying apples, for example, instead of choosing the ones you usually buy, pause inwardly for a moment and silently ask, ''Should I buy red, green, or yellow apples today?'' Buy the ones you are prompted to buy. Dare to do what your deepest impulses encourage you to do. Do this as many moments of the day as you can. Do it whenever you have a decision to make.

The practice is this: Ask, listen, and do. Ask for guidance, listen inwardly for your deepest impulses, and dare to do what these prompt you to do. Dare to gather information from more than your five physical senses only and go beyond your own best reasoning. Practice leaning into your intuitive ability. Practice accessing your greater capacity to be aware. Get better and better at hearing inner guidance. And practice on easy things, like what to buy, or what to eat, or what to wear, so that when you are faced with a decision about something more important, you will be in the habit of seeking silent counsel from the universal wisdom available to you in the depths of your own consciousness.

The gist of the new way, therefore, is to dedicate yourself to doing this on a consistent basis—listening for God's Will for you. It is the meaning of ''Thy Will be done.'' It is the conscious choice to suspend your best judgment of a situation and ask the bigger knowing instead. It makes perfect sense to do this, especially when you realize how little you actually know, how limited and partial your vision really is, and how in need you are of a perspective greater than your own. You will then find yourself surprisingly willing to inquire and listen to the bigger picture.

When you realize the limitations of your understanding, at first you may become depressed or despondent, but gradually you will experience your mind becoming more pliable, receptive, and eager to know more, which will enable you to embrace a larger truth. And as your understanding enlarges, as you trust, go with the flow, and do and be as you are prompted from within, you'll realize that life is not random nor governed by chance. Things will start happening more smoothly. You'll become ''lucky.'' You'll understand that you need not be suspicious or fearful that this faculty will lead you into trouble that culminates in regret or future suffering. And so you trust even deeper. You let go further.

And then you'll get it! God's Will and your own are one and the same. There are not two wills. The ocean and the wave are not essentially different. It is safe to trust in God, and it is also safe to trust in yourself. In fact—and this is the point—to do one is to do the other. It works both ways because who you are is the specific identification of God. The Will of God and the desires of your own heart are one and the same. And by listening to your deepest impulses to action, you will be hearing God's Will for you. You will no longer fear the Will of God, nor distrust the urgings of your own spontaneous being, and it will become increasingly easy to deepen your trust and dedicate yourself to listening. To do this is in your best interest.

Let's look at the three essential steps that develop the willingness to ask, the ability to hear, and the courage to act in accordance with your deepest impulses.

# 1 Know You Do Not Know

Surely, this is not hard to admit. All of us confront problems and situations we are unable to resolve. And understandably so. From ground level we do not have the best perspective on what's happening in our lives and certainly can't always know the right thing to do. We make choices and decisions with insufficient data and suffer to one degree or another because of it.

We can entertain the idea, however, that just as the helicopter has an obviously superior perspective on the overall traffic condition and we can use its information to help ourselves navigate down the road, so might there be some sort of bigger mind—even an Infinite Mind—that possesses a better or more all-encompassing perspective of our lives. We can entertain the idea because, even though it may seem remote, it does seem plausible. It doesn't sound too fantastic. It could be true. But even though it's plausible, still its truth must be demonstrated. Proof is required before any of us believe totally.

It's not difficult to be sufficiently willing to give inner guidance a try, though, because most of us have on occasion spontaneously experienced accurate intuitive knowings. The phone will ring, for example, and we know who it is. Or we think of someone we haven't seen or heard from in a long time and then receive a card from her the next day or bump into her on the street. We know what someone is going to say, and then he says it. Many coincidences happen that we had intuitively foreseen. It therefore seems likely that this just might work. And so, let's test it out and see. There's no danger in giving it a try, and if it works, great. Therefore, let's suspend what we think we know and experiment. Let's look anew at what's possible. It's in our personal and collective best interest to suspend any conclusions or decisions based on ground-level data and be willing, instead, to listen to the inner broadcast from the "aerial" perspective. It makes ground-level sense to do this.

The new way is the route to the resolution of any problem or question you may encounter. It involves accessing the wisdom of the whole. It is your "finite" mind connecting up with Infinite Mind. The willingness to do this surfaces when you realize how little you actually know about how life works and what's in your best interest. The logical next step is gladly to let go of your obviously limited and partial knowing and to open your mind to a larger and more comprehensive outlook.

The trick to doing this—to letting go of your partial knowing and thereby opening your mind to the larger perspective—revolves around how clearly you realize the limits of your knowledge. When you are aware of this it will make sense to let go of what you thought was true in deference to a second opinion. It will be eminently reasonable to desire and ask for assistance and then attentively listen for the inner promptings of universal guidance. When you know you don't know, it makes sense to ask.

If you were to get lost while driving through an unfamiliar town, for example, you wouldn't hesitate to stop and either ask someone for directions or look at a map. It is the same here; however, instead of looking at an external map or asking someone else for directions, you ask inwardly, using your mind to commune with Infinite Mind. You ask the traffic helicopter. You talk to God. You ask inwardly to your Self—like a wave to the ocean, a cell to the brain, or a cloud to the sky. You ask the larger portion of you, the part that knows. You ask and listen, and lo and behold . . . you find yourself knowing.

The important point to appreciate, however, is how limited the ground-level perspective actually is. Understanding this—that is, *knowing you don't know*—will dramatically heighten your motivation to learn the new way. When it's obvious to you that you don't know, and when you suspect that there is the possibility of knowing simply by asking, there will be increased willingness on your part to pursue this possibility. It makes more sense to listen for guidance than to do anything else. But unless you are clear about the limitations of what you know, you will continue to think you can answer your own questions and solve your own problems. And in your efforts to solve them with insufficient data, you will effectively deafen your ears to the inner voice.

The initial stumbling block for many people is in not allowing the first little willingness even to experiment with this, even to playfully consider it. This is because it takes courage to let go of what we know, even though we know it's partial, and begin trusting something that we do not yet know is fully trustworthy. You may feel brave, daring, as though you were taking a great risk, and you will almost undoubtedly experience fear. Your motivation to persist in spite of this involves the realization that if you could answer your own questions and problems, you would. Therefore, insofar as you have been unable to answer some of them, why not admit it? Be honest. Acknowledge the truth. There is nothing wrong with not knowing. Acknowledge honestly to yourself the limitations of your knowledge.

And notice that this in itself is an advanced kind of knowing! It is an accurate evaluation of the mind by the mind. Knowing you do not know satisfies the part of your mind that wants to know and be certain. Do not deny this part. Honor it. Be certain, convinced. This is not as self-demeaning as it may at first appear. Not knowing is your passport to knowing. It is your clear and open approach to truth. Value the not-knowing place. It's how you begin to *really* know. The moment you know you do not know is the moment you open yourself to true knowing.

# 2 Ask Inwardly for Guidance and Listen for a Reply

It may feel strange or a bit uncomfortable at first to talk to yourself so intimately. But don't be afraid of this, or let this feeling dissuade you from listening. Whenever you learn something new there are awkward moments. Just close your eyes and speak mentally, as though you were talking to a close friend, and then listen. And if, after listening for a few moments, you do not hear anything in response, then quietly, patiently, ask again—and listen more closely, in a more relaxed fashion. Do not strain to hear, however. Relax, be patient, wait. Let it come to you. Sit quietly, as though you were sitting at a bus stop waiting for the bus, knowing it will be here in just a moment. The more you do this, the better you will get at it.

There is a whole other language involved in listening inwardly for communications from the universe in this way. It is not always dependent on words. Instead it involves feelings, impulses to action, and meanings that can be put into words by you in order to be consciously accepted or communicated to others. In other words, you may not actually hear a voice. You may instead simply experience Knowing. You will know what to do without having figured it out. You will be prompted to do one thing rather than another. There will be a sudden clarity within you. More than anything else, listen to the way it feels—that is, listen to the way you feel. Consciously experience your feeling-tone. The messages that come from beyond lie in the feelings and impulses that arise from within.

You may, for example, have three or four things to do today. List them in your mind and mentally say, "I want to do what You would have me do. What would You have me do? Which one of these four things should I do first?" Then relax, listen and feel. Listen for a feeling, an insight or idea, or some sort of impulse to action. One of them will light up somehow as being the most appropriate one to do first. Do that one. Then ask, "Which one now?" And do the one that lights up. The answer will not always come in words. It might be a voice. It might never be a voice. It will probably come in the form of a sudden intuitive knowing without the use of any rational thought process.

This is one reason why the yoga asanas are important and why it is so valuable to learn to sit quietly in centered meditation. When your nervous system has been purified, calmed, and sensitized through asana practice and meditation, and when you are thoroughly familiar with the feeling-tone of being centered, at peace, and in harmony with yourself, the impulses coming from the Infinite will reverberate through you with more clarity. You will decipher the messages with greater ease. You will know what is right for you and what isn't. And it will be easy. Right feels right and wrong feels wrong. And the distinction will not be difficult to make.

# 3 Dare to Do As You Are Prompted to Do

The thing to be aware of at this point is that some of the guidance you receive may not make sense to you. This is understandable. From ground level, your perspective on what's happening is severely limited. From ground level, it is not logical to get off at the next exit as your inner voice may be suggesting when the road ahead appears to be clear and open. "Why should I get off here and go the long way around?" It doesn't make ground-level sense, and so the tendency is to disregard the intuitive knowing and ignore the inner signal. Only later, stuck in the traffic jam, do you realize why that would have been the appropriate and most intelligent thing to do and why "going the long way around" would have been a short cut. The aerial perspective takes everything into account.

This is how we learn. The next time you hear that little voice, even though the guidance may not make sense to you because from where you are the road looks clear, you may be a little more willing to do what it suggests. More and more, you'll realize it makes ultimate sense to trust your intuition and deepest impulses. And as your trust deepens, and as you allow yourself to do as you are prompted from within to do, you will realize there is no risk involved, that your best interests seem to have been taken into consideration, as well as everyone else's, and that it's intelligent to ask, listen, and do—which makes relaxing into it and trusting deeper even easier the next time.

Allow yourself more and more to trust the answers that arise from within, and pursue the fulfillment of your happiness by faithfully following instructions. Do those things your deepest impulses urge you to do. Be genuine, authentic. Eventually, in not too long a time, this won't even seem such a daring thing to do. It will simply make sense to let go of your limited knowing and open yourself to the larger wisdom. This willingness can take years or moments. Be ready for both. Do and be as your deepest, most current impulses are urging you to be.

## In the Morning

In the morning when you wake, lie on your back and be perfectly still. Silently say to yourself, "Today I will make no decisions by my-self." Say this several times, until you feel that you have meant what you are saying. Then add, "I will make no decisions by myself because it is no longer intelligent to do so. Instead, I will make all my decisions in silent counsel with the Infinite."

## During the Day

During the day whenever you are called upon to make a decision, do not decide by yourself. Instead, pause inwardly for a moment—and it only takes a moment—and ask for help in your decision making. Mentally say, ''I want to do what You would have me do. What would You have me do?'' Then dare to do as you are prompted to do.

If you know you have, say, four or five things needing to be done today, take a moment to be still, list them in your mind, and ask, ''Which one should I do first?'' Do the one that lights up. Then ask, ''Which one now?'' and do that.

## Requesting Clarification

If something is bothering you, or if there is an issue in your life that needs resolution or clarification, silently desire to know the answer and then silently listen for clarification. Say, ''I want to do what You would have me do. What would You have me do in this situation?'' Then listen deeply inside yourself for inspiration and be attentive to the way circumstances unfold in your experience. What does your deepest being, the deepest part of you, want to do? Desire and silent listening are the keys. Make the practice one of listening, listening, listening.

# 12

# REMEMBER TO REMEMBER

In order to test the traffic-helicopter hypothesis accurately and thereby gain an honest assessment about whether or not inner guidance actually works, you must give it a fair trial. You must deliberately use your mind to listen for the broadcast, intentionally directing your attention toward the Infinite in order to discover whether you actually do access a viewpoint larger than your own. You need to remember to ask for guidance, and to do it frequently.

Instead of driving through life with ground-level vision only—maybe you will hear a little voice telling you what to do and maybe you won't—the new "practice" is to start listening inwardly on a regular basis.

This is where *remembering* comes in. You must remember frequently during the day to suspend your normal impulses to action and instead ask inwardly for guidance about what to think, say, do, or be. You are conducting a test—an important test.

So decide to give it a try. Decide to check in and ask for guidance every half hour for the rest of the day. When the half hour arrives, ask for guidance about whatever is confronting you at that moment, even if it's something inconsequential like whether you should turn on the TV or not. What you're likely to find is how difficult this is to do at first. You remember to ask, and then, of course, the next thing you know it's been hours since you last asked. The first obstacle to listening is simply forgetting to ask. Therefore, remember to remember. Ask for guidance frequently throughout the day in order to see if the asking brings a response.

A beeper watch is especially useful at this stage as a reminder. You can set it to go off every hour, every half hour, every ten minutes—whatever you want. Each time it beeps, momentarily stop what you are doing, check in with the feeling-tone of your body, relax, and ask inwardly for guidance about whatever you are doing at that moment. There is always something you are making a decision about. The beeper may beep, and in that moment, for example, you may have been wondering whether you should call so-and-so. Instead of mulling it over and making up your mind, use the beeper watch as a reminder to pause inwardly and ask for guidance. Say, "I want to do what You would have me do. Should I make this phone call now or later?" And see what happens. You will have a subtle impulse about what to do. You will not have to figure it out. Then dare to do as you are prompted to do. Eventually the beeper watch will become unnecessary, but at first it can be of tremendous assistance.

One of the most interesting things about using the beeper watch is that it makes you very aware of how easy it is to forget to check in. It will catch you by surprise. Every half hour will seem to come around very quickly. By the end of the day, especially if you have set the watch to go off every ten, twelve, or fifteen minutes, your mind or brain will actually feel tired from having checked in so consistently. At first it will feel like doing mental push-ups, and by the end of the day you will have done quite a few. At first this is tiring. But each time you remember makes it easier to remember again, until eventually you are able to stay in touch all day long without forgetting and without getting tired. In fact, you will be invigorated from having been so consistently in the flow of Being.

Remembering to ask for guidance is an acquired skill. It is something you learn to do. It is also an especially wonderful way of using your memory faculty. Usually when you remember something you are recalling an event that occurred in the past, going back in time. Here, however, you are remembering to be present. You are not using your mind to reactive a past event. You are enlivening your experience of the present by improving the quality of your "now" participation. You are not remembering **an** experience, you are remembering **to** experience. And what you are attempting to experience with as much clarity as possible are your deepest impulses to action.

The impulses you receive from Infinite Mind in response to your asking will bubble up from deep within you and be experienced by you as *your* deepest impulses and desires. The practice of inner listening, then, is actually relatively easy, and ultimately simple, because your deepest impulses to action are inside you. They are not somewhere else, in someone else, or at a great distance from you. They are in you to be felt by you. They are yours. You simply need to listen quietly for them by sensing deeply into yourself in a relaxed, attentive, and effortless fashion. Yet you need to remember to do it.

Establish the strong intention to remember frequently throughout the day. Be motivated. Be interested in discovering for yourself whether or not you can access guidance through inner listening. Doing this will feel increasingly sensible, more and more the most intelligent thing to do. It is a good thing to be clear about. And when you actually begin to sense the potential for being guided by a cosmic, universal intelligence you'll find yourself lured, drawn by the process. You will not want to forget. You will want to access it more often. You will *want* to remember. And as you check in for guidance more frequently, it will eventually become all the time—"all the time" meaning "now"—and now—and now.

Remember to ask for guidance every time you think of it and at the very moment you think of it. If when you remember to ask for guidance you think, "Yes, I want to ask for guidance. I'll do that in just a moment," then you are developing the habit of putting it off until later. Be attentive at this point. Do not put it off until later. It takes only an instant, less than a moment, long enough to pause mentally. Putting it off each time you think to ask will only strengthen that tendency within yourself; instead, strengthen your remembering. Ask for guidance immediately each time you think to do it.

Each time you remember to ask for guidance makes it easier the next time. Eventually it will become habitual. When this occurs, it means you have successfully shifted to a new level of awareness, a new way of being, and are now living your life from your conscious connection with the Infinite. Want this. Desire this deeply. Understand how advantageous it is to you and everyone else to function from this awareness of your inherent connection with the All. We are all part of an incredibly vast, majestic and interconnected energy complex. Understanding this—and appreciating this!—is the basis and foundation of yoga. It is the knowledge required for living the divine life.

The best way to improve your ability to remember is by wanting to remember—by seeing the logic, the reason, the sense it makes deliberately to shift from intellectual or conceptual knowing to intuitive knowing. The more you realize how wonderful this is, the more you will desire it—and the more you'll want to remember.

# Intuition and Multiple Voices

The first obstacle to the regular, habitual use of inner guidance is not remembering to ask. The second obstacle is hearing three or four voices in response to your asking. The problem then becomes which one is real, which one do you trust?

This can be quite disconcerting at first because instead of gaining clarity about what to do, you may end up being more confused. Now you've got more choices than ever. But, as before, the best thing to do in this confused state when you are faced with a difficult decision is mentally to stop, become quiet, centered, and still, and then silently ask again.

Ask for clarification. And then be patient as you listen for an answer. Try not to be impatient. If you are splashing around mentally, being impatient and demanding, the waters of your mind will be agitated and muddied; there will be no clarity. But if you are calm and attentive and are truly desirous of an answer to your dilemma, and are therefore listening with open ears, the mental waters will become clear and calm and the most appropriate thing to do will be obvious. The more infinitely patient and open you are, and the less willful and demanding, the easier it will be to hear the answer. The impulse to action or inaction will be obvious and unmistakable. Although this takes practice, it is worth practicing. And you will know this is true in the very first moment when you actually begin to hear an answer.

If you are still confused about what to do, then do the only thing you can. Do the one you trust. You will be drawn to doing one thing more than the other. One of your options will seem the most credible. Do that one. Dare to do the one you trust most, the option that draws you most strongly. And practice on easy things, not on things that make a big difference to you. Practice on things like what to eat, or what to wear, or whether or not you should turn on the TV so that you build up a body of experience that will encourage your growing willingness to follow your inner feeling, as well as improve your ability to hear with clarity. Practice on easy things so that when you are faced with a decision about something that really does matter to you, you'll be in the habit of asking the Infinite for guidance and will have the learned confidence necessary to go with the flow by trusting your deepest impulses.

Now let's say you are driving in your car and you feel like listening to the radio. But just before you reach down to turn it on, you think, "The traffic helicopter! Let me use this moment as an opportunity to say mentally the sentences and practice accessing inner guidance." And so you temporarily suspend your impulse to turn the radio on and instead ask for guidance, saying "I want to do what You would have me do. What would You have me do? Should I turn the radio on or not?" And you listen inwardly. You relax your body and pay attention to what you feel like doing now.

As you pay attention to new subtle promptings from within, you'll notice yourself beginning to sense either a "yes" or "no" answer, and your arm will either feel energized to reach over and turn on the radio or it won't. You'll notice that as you gently pay attention and listen without bias, you'll find yourself quite able to clearly discern the meaning of the inner feeling. Which means asking does evoke a response. This is a new clarity. But it may be suggesting, for example, "No. For the next few minutes do not listen to the radio. Exist without the radio turned on." and you are hearing it clearly. And yet you may still want to listen to the radio. You may be unwilling to suspend your impulse to turn it on even though your inner guidance is clearly suggesting otherwise.

Remembering to ask for guidance and beginning to hear answers with clarity is no longer the problem. Now you find yourself unwilling to do as your guidance is suggesting. This is the third common obstacle.

At this point you will either ignore the guidance and do what you originally wanted to do anyway, or you will let go of what you thought you wanted to do—you'll suspend your desire to turn on the radio—and instead do as the inner feeling is suggesting. For the moment you'll refrain from turning on the radio and instead be open to experiencing whatever experience arises without the radio on.

Not a big deal. Not a big decision. Your life will not be drastically altered by turning or not turning on the radio. You will survive in either case. In all probability you can handle not turning the radio on if that is what the guidance is suggesting. Yet notice how attached we are to doing what we want to do! We squirm a little even on easy things like this. We want things our way, and this is understandable.

The important point to keep in mind is that whenever you ask for guidance, it is always because you have to make a decision. You are confronted with a choice, and having a choice always means that you are not clear. Now it is not "bad" to be unclear, but it *is* unintelligent to make decisions based on limited data when you have such easy access to more. It is no longer intelligent to make decisions by yourself without first consulting the Infinite within, especially now that you know about the traffic helicopter, the aerial perspective, and Infinite Mind. And it takes less than a moment to do this.

What's really important is the increasing willingness on your part to release your need to do what *you* want to do and gladly to do what the inner feeling suggests. Not heeding the guidance, especially once you start hearing it clearly, is like continuing to go straight because the road looks clear even though the traffic broadcast is blaring loudly and clearly about a traffic jam three miles ahead.

So, observe yourself in easy situations such as wanting to listen to the radio. Notice when you are willing to do what the inner prompting suggests to you and notice when you aren't. Willingness has a different feeling-tone from resistance and unwillingness. Become familiar with both.

Notice when you are willing to follow the guidance, and notice when you ignore it to do what you want to do. And be aware of the different feeling-tone of each of these responses. Be aware of how you feel when you flow with guidance and of how you feel when you ignore it. How do you actually feel when you stay fluid compared to when you are willful and controlling? Don't think too much or argue about the differences in your mind. Simply *feel* the difference.

This simple awareness is guaranteed to make you more willing, fluid, and at ease, and more consistently desirous of wanting to do *only* what the inner feeling prompts you to do—whether "you" want this or not. This occurs because inner guidance is really the most intelligent way to go about navigating your life, and also because being fluid and "going with the flow" feels so much better than being stiff, contracted, controlling, and willful.

And what's both mysterious and wonderful about this is that you change and embrace the guidance because *you* want to! You're doing what "you" want to do still, but now you are wanting to do God's Will. In a sense, you have shifted allegiance from your will to God's Will, and yet, in another sense, your allegiance is still the same. You are still interested in your own well-being and preferences, as you should be, but you are now more intelligent about how to secure them. You have found a better way of making decisions and being happy in the deepest sense. You are less addicted to doing what you thought you wanted to do and are instead more interested in knowing what the aerial perspective suggests you do.

Your attitude now is, "Thy Will be done." You want to do what Infinite Mind, God, suggests you do. You've learned enough to know that God's Will is what you want for you and no longer to ignore the guidance. You therefore voluntarily release your own tiny, little will—the *sense* of you that you thought was you—and join your will with God's. This "joining" is the meaning of yoga. In one sense, however, no joining actually occurs—because the parts were never really separate.

At this point of "joining," miracles start to happen. Spontaneous evidences of an underlying harmony and order begin to manifest in your experience. Now that you are asking for guidance and are, in effect, allowing yourself to be filled with what God is, you will start experiencing more energy and more love. More love-energy will start flowing through you. This makes your relationships, your contacts with other people, the events of your day, and your thoughts more powerful, more potent, more transformational.

Yet we are strongly attached to doing what we habitually want to do. This is where detachment comes in. Detachment is the ability or willingness to suspend what you think you want and instead remain fluid enough to flow with inner guidance. This is truly the most intelligent way to act. You'll find yourself using guidance voluntarily with full conviction and enthusiasm once you understand that the helicopter does indeed have the superior perspective. Infinite Mind sees what's happening to you and your life better than you do. It is infinitely more intelligent. Therefore it is to your personal advantage to do only what it suggests. It is no longer intelligent or fulfilling to decide by yourself or to attempt to solve your problems and issues without consulting it.

When you pause and ask for guidance, stop moving physically. Relax your body, breathe gently, and be aware of the feeling-tone of your body. This will move your awareness to your actual now-experience. Then listen inwardly as though you were waiting to hear a message. The inner feeling will give you a subtle, internal prompting about what to do or not do. All you do is pay attention and listen.

If something is right for you, it will feel right; if something is not right for you, it will feel wrong. This is logical, sane, practical, reliable, and easy to detect. Simply go by that which feels right. Let go of everyhing you think you know and experience the inner directive with clarity.

It will quickly become apparent that your interests are best served by following your inner feeling. You will also learn that the universal guidance that you can access through inner listening implies an enlarged and expanded self-concept: You are bigger than you thought you were. You really are a part of the One, an individual expression of universal Consciousness. And by tuning in to your own unique feeling-tone, felt most distinctly in the area of your heart, you avail yourself of the wisdom and guidance of the whole. And you will feel the difference this self-image makes in your daily experience of life.

At first, however, the idea of being guided by a "cosmic, universal intelligence" may seem strange, unreliable, unrealistic—perhaps irresponsible. The thought of trusting what feels right may even be frightening because we do not know ourselves well and are generally accustomed to navigating our lives by intellectual bias. Transcending the intellect seems foolish. It is, however, extremely reasonable.

Remember that you don't have to follow the inner feeling, you can always do anything you please. But as you penetrate stillness and experience yourself with clarity, evaluating the guidance you receive, you will be amazed at the superiority of its intelligence and insight. And because you have been so pure in your approach, alert to the possibilities of self-deception and honest in your intent to know the truth, you will be more convinced than ever.

This approach passes all the tests. Accessing inner guidance truly is the superior approach. Your mind will understand this and will be answered, silenced. It will gradually cease to voice objections or persuade you to do things that do not feel right. Rather, it will assist and applaud your every willingness to hear and follow the inner directive. This is not the abandonment of reason or intellect, but the flowering of reason, the intellect at its best. It is, in fact, where reason will ultimately lead you. Your mind, after reviewing all the evidence, will gladly choose intuitive knowing.

Sense yourself deeply, pay attention to your own unique feeling-tone, and allow the inner feeling to guide, direct, and advise you about your actions, words, and thoughts. Pursue that which *feels* right, attracts you. Do the things you like to do. Honor your deepest feelings and live the life that fulfills you and makes you happy.

The more you do this, the more refined your attractions will become. They will self-correct and change, and what used to attract you may no longer do so. One thing is certain, however. Your individual attractions and desires will come into alignment with those of the whole. What is best for you is best for the universe, and vice versa—and what is best for you is what makes you happy.

Your happiness and the universe's happiness are one and the same. This is important. It's true because you and the universe are one. You are not a separate entity somehow disconnected from the All. Herein lies the key to the whole thing: The universe is already happy! God is already happy! Consciousness *is* Happiness!

If you are experiencing unhappiness, it is always because you are not in touch with your core or with what's really true. You are misunderstanding things. In those moments you have forgotten your unalterable connection with the whole. You have identified yourself with something else and are, therefore, defining yourself as a separate being. You can do this because you have free will, but the unhappiness you subsequently experience will be the painful and direct result of thinking and believing yourself to be separate and alone, which makes you afraid. But you are not separate, you can never be separate, and thinking you are does not make it true. It makes you fearful and unhappy. It cuts you off from your conscious connection with the oneness, your true identity, and deprives you of intuitive knowing. These are not the ingredients of happiness. Therefore, what to do? Realign yourself with the creative God Force. Rejoin. Remember.

This is so easy to do and so tremendously important. And as you remember to ask for guidance frequently throughout your day, and as you dare to do as you are prompted from within, you are literally living yoga—living your life from your new understanding of being yoked to the Infinite. You will become increasingly happy, increasingly in harmony with everything around you, and increasingly in receivership of a steady stream of guidance from a reservoir of wisdom infinitely larger than your limited personal data bank of knowledge. Living your life like this is what yoga is really all about. This is how the world will grow into a more obvious manifestation of goodness.

You learn to be guided by the inner feeling in the postures and meditations. As you learn it there, within the safe arena of your own home, you will naturally start doing it everywhere. What was a specific learning becomes a generalized knowing. Yoga is your constant way of life.

## Listening on the Run

When you are in the supermarket buying apples, mentally ask, "Should I buy red, green, or yellow apples?" Then buy the ones you are prompted to buy. When you are getting dressed, mentally ask, "Should I wear the red shirt or the blue shirt today?" Wear the one you are prompted to wear. When you reach down to turn on the radio, mentally ask, "Should I listen to the radio right now or not?" Do not just mechanically turn it on. When you are driving home and you have the choice of turning left or right at an intersection, mentally ask, "Should I turn left or right today?" Turn the direction you are prompted to turn. Who knows, there may be something down the alternate route that would be interesting or valuable for you to see. Do this all day long, as many moments of the day as possible. Ask for guidance on easy, inconsequential things such as these and practice doing what the inner feeling suggests. Remember to do this.

## Before Sleep

Lie on your back and be perfectly still. Thank Infinite Mind for Its guidance during the day and reaffirm your dedication to listening for and carrying out God's Will, your will—the Will of the All expressing Itself as you. If there is an issue in your life that needs resolution or clarification, ask for help while you sleep. Then breathe gently and *feel* the energy that you are, the Consciousness or Mind that you are, the Spirit that you are, the Love that you are. Relax inside and sleep.

# 13

## THE ROYAL PRACTICE

In the early days when yoga was first being developed, the primary practice was meditation, or centering. The poses came later as spontaneous expressions of that centered state. In combination these became the "royal practice" because the ancients had found that through the discipline of yoga and quiet sitting they were able to access a new way of knowing and being and thereby become more intuitive and effective in all they were guided to do. This, they discovered, was the most direct way of experiencing firsthand the meaning of God, Guru, and Self.

They also discovered that intuitive revelation happens when one's mind, instead of thinking about other things, is unthinkingly attentive in the Now. The essence of the royal practice was not one of advanced thinking and coming to intellectual conclusions. It was, and is, the practice of communion and listening.

Happily, one of the most rewarding side effects of yoga practice and meditation is the renewed zest of life you will experience. This happens spontaneously when you simply take the time to sit quietly, relax, and consciously immerse yourself in the feeling of peace. When you go within and expand beyond your usual sense of self—when you "move into stillness" and experience the infinite I AM Presence—you will come alive with the enthusiasm of life. You will sense the creative movement or flow of ceaseless Being and find yourself charged with new energy, new creativity. You will feel moved to move, to express. You will be inspired to action. Your yoga and meditation practices will become even more meaningful and potent, and you'll find yourself practicing with renewed conviction.

Your job will be that of yielding to the flow. Traditionally, this has been called "surrender." It is the active choice for "Thy Will be done." It is the most intelligent, fulfilling thing to do. You surrender your best sense of what to do or not do, and instead trust in the flow of Being. This is when yoga becomes more than practice and practices—and becomes your way of life. Then you realize there is no such thing as practice! Never was. There is only the real thing, ever—and always.

# Appendix

## YOGA ROUTINES

Ten progressive yoga routines are included in this section. They encompass all forty-five poses and are designed to lead a beginning student safely to a fairly advanced level of proficiency. The speed with which you progress through the various routines will depend largely on how much time and enthusiasm you invest in your practice. There is no need to rush, however. Proceed intelligently. Spend as much time as you need with the Beginners Balanced Daily Sequence before progressing to the three Three-Day Cycles. Become familiar with the basics and establish a daily practice. Three to six months of daily practice with the Three-Day Cycle for Beginners will prepare you for the Three-Day Intermediate Cycle, and three to six months with that will prepare you for the Three-Day Cycle for Experienced Students. Please practice the poses in the suggested order and continue with each specific routine until you are fairly comfortable with it.

Routines as such are not what it's all about, however. Routines can easily become gods in their own right, threatening the very goals for which they were set up. The idea is to be creative in your practice, inspired, guided from within. Yoga is not mechanical. But until such time as you have learned to be guided from within, the various routines will be of value in helping you achieve this ability. Your goal should be to come up with unique routines that work well for you.

As a beginner the most important poses to work on are the standing poses. They are poses with big, whole-body movements. They strengthen your body and make the finer, more contortionistic poses possible. As an intermediate student you'll concentrate more on forward bendings, the counterposes for backward bendings; and as a more advanced practitioner you'll work primarily on backward bendings. So, as a general outline for practice, once you've become familiar with the basics think of it this way: Day One do a balanced practice but work primarily on standing poses. Day Two do a balanced practice but focus primarily on forward-bending poses. Day Three also do a balanced practice but focus primarily on backward-bending poses. Day Four do standing poses again; Day Five, forward bends; Day Six, backbends; and on Day Seven, take a day off and let your body rest. A day of rest, no yoga, is important. Practice what you can of inversions almost every day, though take your time with these, progress slowly, and do twists daily. Always include Relaxation Pose and seated meditation. Wear loose, nonrestrictive clothing, be barefoot, and do not eat for several hours before practicing.

# Beginner's Balanced Daily Sequence

Do this practice daily until you are familiar with the basics:

| | |
|---|---|
| OPENING: | Sit Quietly, Mountain I & II, Cat Pose, Quarter Dog, Half Dog |
| STANDING POSES: | Standing Side Stretch, Tree, Standing Forward Fold, Dog Pose |
| SALUTATIONS: | Half Salutes |
| MORE STANDING POSES: | Triangle, Standing Spread Leg Forward Fold |
| SHOULDERS AND HIPS: | Lotus Preparations, Lotus, Shoulder Stretches (1) sitting in Hero Pose* |
| BACKBENDS: | Locust Pose |
| FORWARD BENDS: | Reclining Leg Streches (1, 2) |
| INVERSIONS: | Bridge Pose |
| TWISTS: | Reclining Twist I & II |
| FINISHING POSES: | Relaxation Pose, Meditation |

When the foregoing practice has become sufficiently easy, begin this three-day cycle.

# Three-Day Cycle for Beginners

## BEGINNERS STANDING POSE EMPHASIS

| | |
|---|---|
| OPENING: | Sit Quietly, Mountain Pose I & II, Cat Pose, Quarter Dog, Half Dog |
| STANDING POSES: | Standing Side Stretch, Tree Pose, Standing Forward Fold, Dog Pose |
| SALUTATIONS: | Half Salutes, Lunge Salutes* |
| MORE STANDING POSES: | Triangle Pose, Bent Knee Side Stretch*, Warrior Pose I*, Warrior Pose II*, Standing Spread Leg Forward Fold |

SHOULDERS AND HIPS:    Shoulder Stretches (1, 2\*, 3\*) sitting in Hero Pose, Lotus Preparation, Lotus Pose

BACKBENDS:    Locust Pose, Cobra Pose\*

FORWARD BENDS:    Head to Knee Pose\*, Reclining Leg Streches (1, 2, 3\*)

INVERSIONS:    Shoulderstand Preparations\*, Shoulderstand Series (1, 2, 4)\*, Fish Pose\*

TWISTS:    Easy Noose Pose\*, Sage Twist\*, Reclining Twist I & II

FINISHING POSES:    Relaxation Pose, Meditation

This may seem like a lot to do, at first, If so, increase the number of new poses per group gradually, one at a time. Do more as you're able. Be especially attentive, however, to add the new pose in each successive group that you find most attractive. Look at the photographs of the new poses in each group and sense inwardly for what your body wants to do. Do the ones that have the most lure, the ones you feel like doing. Do the ones you're hungry for. And do not assume in advance that this means you'll only do the easy poses. Not necessarily. Instead of forcing yourself to be "disciplined" in the sense of doing things you don't really want to do, discipline yourself to sense inwardly more frequently—into yourself, like a wave into the ocean—for God's Will/your will about what to do or not do. *This is the yoga*, not the achievement of elaborate postures or the dutiful practice of prescribed routines. Yoga is not mechanical.

The idea is to sense inwardly for your deepest feelings. That's how you listen for God's Will/your will. Mentally pause long enough to *feel* what's most appropriate—even here in this simple context of yoga postures. And then do God's Will/your will by *doing* those poses that your deepest feelings prompt you to do.

This is the most intelligent way to progress. Do not force yourself to do more than you are ready for—or more than you want to do. Trust that you have your best interests at heart. Add new poses if and when you feel drawn to them. This is not a test, nor a race. Proceed voluntarily. Most important, and please always keep this in mind, learn to enjoy your practice *while you're practicing*. Do not overlook this! The more you enjoy your practice, the more one-pointed you'll be. Stay with each specific program until you can do it comfortably.

Also, if you feel like doing additional standing poses during the standing pose section of a routine, or more salutations, or more backward bends, forward bends, or twists, by all means do so. That's the whole point. Listen inwardly for what you feel like doing, for what you are prompted to do, and then do as you are guided. This is how you exercise your ability to be guided from within. Pretty soon, your whole session will be done like this. You'll be inspired into action.

## BEGINNERS FORWARD BEND EMPHASIS

| | |
|---|---|
| OPENING: | Sit Quietly, Mountain Pose I & II, Cat Pose, Quarter Dog, Half Dog |
| STANDING POSES: | Standing Side Stretch, Tree Pose, Standing Forward Fold, Dog Pose |
| SALUTATIONS: | Half Salutes, Lunge Salutes* |
| MORE STANDING POSES: | Triangle Pose, Warrior Pose I*, Standing Spread Leg Forward Fold |
| SHOULDERS AND HIPS: | Shoulder Stretches (1, 2, 3)* Sitting in Hero Pose*, Lotus Preparations, Lotus Pose |
| BACKBENDS: | Locust Pose, Cobra Pose* |
| FORWARD BENDS: | Head to Knee Pose*, Half Lotus Forward Fold*, Reclining Leg Stretches (1, 2, 3*), Upward Facing Spread Leg Forward Fold* |
| INVERSIONS: | Shoulderstand Preparations*, Shoulderstand Series (1, 2, 4)*, Fish Pose* |
| TWISTS: | Easy Noose*, Sage Twist*, Reclining Twist I and II |
| FINISHING POSES: | Relaxation Pose, Meditation |

## BEGINNERS BACKWARD BEND EMPHASIS

| | |
|---|---|
| OPENING: | Sit Quietly, Mountain Pose I & II, Cat Pose, Quarter Dog, Half Dog |
| STANDING POSES: | Standing Side Stretch, Tree Pose, Standing Forward Fold, Dog Pose |
| SALUTATIONS: | Half Salutes, Lunge Salutes* |
| MORE STANDING POSES: | Triangle Pose, Warrior Pose I*, Standing Spread Leg Forward Fold |
| SHOULDERS AND HIPS: | Shoulder Stretches (1–8)* Sitting in Hero Pose*, Lotus Preparations, Lotus Pose |
| BACKBENDS: | Locust Pose, Cobra Pose*, Bow Pose* |
| FORWARD BENDS: | Head to Knee Pose*, Reclining Leg Stretches (1, 2, 3*) |

INVERSIONS:          Shoulderstand Preparations*, Shoulderstand Series (1, 2, 4)*, Fish Pose*

TWISTS:              Easy Noose Pose*, Sage Twist*, Reclining Twist I and II

FINISHING POSES:     Relaxation Pose, Meditation

# Three-Day Cycle for Intermediate Students

Sample **intermediate** routines:

## INTERMEDIATE STANDING POSE EMPHASIS

OPENING:             Sit Quietly, Mountain Pose I & II, Cat Pose, Quarter Dog, Half Dog

STANDING POSES:      Standing Side Stretch, Tree Pose, Standing Forward Fold, Dog Pose

SALUTATIONS:         Half Salutes, Jumping Back Salutes*

MORE STANDING POSES: a) All the standing poses:
                        Triangle Pose, Bent Knee Side Stretch, Warrior Pose I, Warrior Pose II, Half Moon Pose*, Pyramid Pose*, Revolved Triangle Pose*, Standing Spread Leg Forward Fold
                     b) Standing Pose Flow*

SHOULDERS AND HIPS:  Lotus Preparations, Lotus Pose, Shoulder Stretches Sitting in Hero Pose

BACKBENDS:           Reclining Hero Pose*, Locust Pose, Cobra Pose, Bow Pose

FORWARD BENDS:       Seated Forward Fold*, Head to Knee Pose, Half Lotus Forward Fold, Cobbler Pose*

INVERSIONS:          Shoulderstand Preparations, Shoulderstand Series, Fish Pose

TWISTS:              Easy Noose Pose, Sage Twist, Rishi Twist I* & II*, Reclining Twist I & II

FINISHING POSES:     Relaxation Pose, Meditation

## INTERMEDIATE FOWARD BEND EMPHASIS

| | |
|---|---|
| OPENING: | Sit Quietly, Mountain Pose I & II, Cat Pose, Quarter Dog, Half Dog |
| STANDING POSES: | Standing Side Stretch, Tree Pose, Standing Forward Fold, Dog Pose |
| SALUTATIONS: | Half Salutes, Jumping Back Salutes* |
| MORE STANDING POSES: | Triangle Pose, Bent Knee Side Stretch, Warrior Pose I, Half Moon Pose*, Pyramid Pose*, Standing Spread Leg Forward Fold |
| SHOULDERS AND HIPS: | Lotus Preparations, Lotus Pose |
| BACKBENDS: | Hero Pose, Reclining Hero Pose*, Locust Pose, Cobra Pose, Bow Pose |
| FORWARD BENDS: | Seated Forward Fold*, Head to Knee Pose, Half Lotus Forward Fold, Reclining Leg Stretch Series (1, 2, 3, 4*, 5*), Upward Facing Spread Leg Forward Fold, Spread Leg Forward Fold*, Cobbler Pose* |
| INVERSIONS: | Shoulderstand Preparations, Shoulderstand Series, Fish Pose |
| TWISTS: | Easy Noose Pose, Sage Twist, Rishi Twist I & II*, Reclining Twist I & II |
| FINISHING POSES: | Relaxation Pose, Meditation |

## INTERMEDIATE BACKWARD BEND EMPHASIS

| | |
|---|---|
| OPENING: | Sit Quietly, Mountain Pose I & II, Cat Pose, Quarter Dog, Half Dog |
| STANDING POSES: | Standing Side Stretch, Tree, Standing Forward Fold, Dog Pose |
| SALUTATIONS: | Half Salutes, Jumping Back Salutes* |
| MORE STANDING POSES: | Triangle Pose, Bent Knee Side Stretch, Warrior Pose I, Warrior Pose II, Revolved Triangle Pose*, Standing Spread Leg Forward Fold |
| SHOULDERS AND HIPS: | Lotus Preparations, Lotus Pose, Shoulder Stretches Sitting in Hero Pose |

| | |
|---|---|
| BACKBENDS: | Reclining Hero Pose*, Locust Pose, Cobra Pose, Bow Pose, Single Leg Pigeon Pose*, Camel Pose* |
| FORWARD BENDS: | Reclining Leg Stretch Series (1, 2, 3, 4*, 5*), Upward Facing Spread Leg Forward Fold*, Spread Leg Forward Fold*, Cobbler Pose* |
| INVERSIONS: | Shoulderstand Preparations, Shoulderstand Series, Fish Pose |
| TWISTS: | Easy Noose Pose, Sage Twist, Rishi Twist I & II*, Reclining Twist I & II |
| FINISHING POSES: | Relaxation Pose, Meditation |

# Three-Day Cycle for Experienced Students

Sample routines for **experienced**:

## EXPERIENCED STANDING POSE EMPHASIS

| | |
|---|---|
| OPENING: | Sit Quietly |
| STANDING POSES: | Mountain Pose I & II, Standing Forward Fold, Dog Pose |
| SALUTATIONS: | Half Salutes, Jumping Back Salutes, Lunge Salutes |
| MORE STANDING POSES: | a) All the standing poses: Triangle Pose, Bent Knee Side Stretch, Warrior Pose I, Warrior Pose II, Half Moon Pose, Pyramid Pose, Revolved Triangle Pose, Standing Spread Leg Forward Fold<br>b) Standing Pose Flow 2X |
| SHOULDERS AND HIPS: | Shoulder Stretches, Sitting in Lotus Pose |
| BACKBENDS: | Hero Pose, Reclining Hero Pose, Fish Pose (in Hero), Camel Pose, Upward Bow Pose 3X* |
| FORWARD BENDS: | Seated Forward Fold Pose, Head to Knee Pose, Half Lotus Forward Fold, Spread Leg Forward Fold, Cobbler Pose* |
| INVERSIONS: | Headstand*, Shoulderstand Series |

| | |
|---|---|
| TWISTS: | Easy Noose Pose, Sage Twist, Rishi Twist I & II, Extended Leg Half Lotus Twist*, Reclining Twist I & II |
| FINISHING POSES: | Relaxation Pose, Meditation |

## EXPERIENCED FOWARD BEND EMPHASIS

| | |
|---|---|
| OPENING: | Sit Quietly |
| STANDING POSES: | Mountain Pose I & II, Standing Forward Fold, Dog Pose |
| SALUTATIONS: | Half Salutes, Jumping Back Salutes, Lunge Salutes |
| MORE STANDING POSES: | Standing Pose Flow 2X |
| SHOULDERS AND HIPS: | Lotus Pose |
| BACKBENDS: | Hero Pose, Reclining Hero Pose, Fish Pose (in Hero), Camel Pose, Upward Bow Pose 3X* |
| FORWARD BENDS: | All the forward bends: Seated Forward Fold Pose, Head to Knee Pose, Half Lotus Forward Fold, Reclining Leg Stretch Series, Upward Facing Spread Leg Forward Fold, Spread Leg Forward Fold, Cobbler Pose, Splits Pose* |
| INVERSIONS: | Headstand*, Shoulderstand Series |
| TWISTS: | Easy Noose Pose, Sage Twist, Rishi Twist I & II, Extended Leg Half Lotus Twist*, Reclining Twist I & II |
| FINISHING POSES: | Relaxation Pose, Meditation |

## EXPERIENCED BACKWARD BEND EMPHASIS

| | |
|---|---|
| OPENING: | Sit Quietly |
| STANDING POSES: | Mountain Pose I & II, Standing Forward Fold, Dog Pose |
| SALUTATIONS: | Half Salutes, Jumping Back Salutes, Lunge Salutes |
| MORE STANDING POSES: | Standing Pose Flow 2X |
| SHOULDERS AND HIPS: | Shoulder Stretches Sitting in Lotus Pose |
| BACKBENDS: | All the backbends: Hero Pose, Reclining Hero Pose, Fish Pose (in Hero), Locust Pose, Cobra Pose, Bow Pose, Single Leg Pigeon Pose, Camel Pose, Upward Bow 6X* |

| | |
|---|---|
| FORWARD BENDS: | Reclining Leg Stretch Series, Upward Facing Spread Leg Forward Fold, Spread Leg Forward Fold, Cobbler Pose |
| INVERSIONS: | Headstand*, Shoulderstand Series |
| TWISTS: | Easy Noose Pose, Sage Twist, Rishi Twist I & II, Extended Leg Half Lotus Twist*, Reclining Twist I & II |
| FINISHING POSES: | Relaxation Pose, Meditation |

\*indicates newly added poses